T0317441

Spectrums of Amyotrophic Lateral Sclerosis

Spectrums of Amyotrophic Lateral Sclerosis

Heterogeneity, Pathogenesis and Therapeutic Directions

EDITED BY

Christopher A. Shaw and Jessica R. Morrice

University of British Columbia, Canada

WILEY Blackwell

This edition first published 2021

Registered Offices
John Wiley & Sons, Inc., 111 River Street, Hoboken, NJ 07030, USA
John Wiley & Sons Ltd, The Atrium, Southern Gate, Chichester, West Sussex, PO19 8SQ, UK

Editorial Office
9600 Garsington Road, Oxford, OX4 2DQ, UK

For details of our global editorial offices, customer services, and more information about Wiley products visit us at www.wiley.com.

Wiley also publishes its books in a variety of electronic formats and by print-on-demand. Some content that appears in standard print versions of this book may not be available in other formats.

Library of Congress Cataloging-in-Publication Data

Names: Shaw, Christopher A. (Christopher Ariel), editor. | Morrice, Jessica
   R., editor.
Title: Spectrums of amyotrophic lateral sclerosis : heterogeneity,
   Pathogenesis and therapeutic directions / edited by Christopher A. Shaw and Jessica R. Morrice.
Description: Hoboken, NJ : Wiley-Blackwell, 2021. | Includes
   bibliographical references and index.
Identifiers: LCCN 2021003406 (print) | LCCN 2021003407 (ebook) | ISBN
   9781119745495 (hardback) | ISBN 9781119745501 (adobe pdf) | ISBN
   9781119745518 (epub)
Subjects: MESH: Amyotrophic Lateral Sclerosis–genetics | Amyotrophic
   Lateral Sclerosis–drug therapy | Genetic Heterogeneity | Spectrum
   Analysis | Models, Genetic
Classification: LCC RC406.A24 (print) | LCC RC406.A24 (ebook) | NLM WE
   552 | DDC 616.8/39–dc23
LC record available at https://lccn.loc.gov/2021003406
LC ebook record available at https://lccn.loc.gov/2021003407

Cover Design: Wiley
Cover Image: © Emma McEachern

Set in 10.5/13pt StixTwoText by SPi Global, Pondicherry, India
Printed and bound by CPI Group (UK) Ltd, Croydon, CR0 4YY

C9781119745495_020421

This book is dedicated to people living with ALS, their families, and those who care for them.

Contents

Contributors

Christen G. Chisholm, Illawarra Health and Medical Research Institute, University of Wollongong, Wollongong, New South Wales, Australia; Molecular Horizons and School of Chemistry and Molecular Bioscience, University of Wollongong, Wollongong, New South Wales, Australia

Roger S. Chung, Motor Neuron Disease Research Centre, Faculty of Medicine and Health Sciences, Macquarie University, Sydney, New South Wales, Australia

Robert A. Déziel, CNS Contract Research Corp, Charlottetown, Prince Edward Island, Canada

Patrick A. Dion, Montreal Neurological Institute and Hospital, McGill University, Montréal, Québec, Canada; Department of Neurology and Neurosurgery, McGill University, Montréal, Québec, Canada

Angela Genge, Montreal Neurological Institute and Hospital, Montréal, Québec, Canada

Daphne A. Gill, CNS Contract Research Corp, Charlottetown, Prince Edward Island, Canada; Department of Biomedical Sciences, University of Prince Edward Island, Charlottetown, Prince Edward Island, Canada

Manuel Graeber, Brain Tumor Research Laboratories, Brain and Mind Centre, The University of Sydney, Sydney, New South Wales, Australia

Cheryl Y. Gregory-Evans, Experimental Medicine Program, University of British Columbia, Vancouver, British Columbia, Canada; Department of Ophthalmology and Visual Sciences, University of British Columbia, Vancouver, British Columbia, Canada; Program in Neuroscience, University of British Columbia, Vancouver, British Columbia, Canada

Denis G. Kay, Alpha Cognition Inc., Charlottetown, Prince Edward Island, Canada

Charles Krieger, Department of Biomedical Physiology and Kinesiology, Simon Fraser University, Burnaby, British Columbia, Canada; Department of Medicine, University of British Columbia, Vancouver, British Columbia, Canada; Division of Neurology, Vancouver Coastal Health, Vancouver, British Columbia, Canada

Michael Kuo, Department of Ophthalmology and Visual Sciences, University of British Columbia, Vancouver, British Columbia, Canada

Audrey Labarre, Department of Neuroscience, University of Montréal, Montréal, Québec, Canada; Centre de recherche du centre hospitalier de l'Université de Montréal (CRCHUM), Montréal, Québec, Canada

Serena Lattante, Unità Operativa Complessa di Genetica Medica, Dipartimento di Scienze di Laboratorio e Infettivologico, Fondazione Policlinico Universitario A. Gemelli IRCCS, Rome, Italy

Albert Lee, Motor Neuron Disease Research Centre, Faculty of Medicine and Health Sciences, Macquarie University, Sydney, New South Wales, Australia

Thomas E. Marler, College of Natural and Applied Sciences, University of Guam, Mangilao, Guam, USA

Amber L. Marriott, CNS Contract Research Corp, Charlottetown, Prince Edward Island, Canada

Luke McAlary, Illawarra Health and Medical Research Institute, University of Wollongong, Wollongong, New South Wales, Australia; Molecular Horizons and School of Chemistry and Molecular Bioscience, University of Wollongong, Wollongong, New South Wales, Australia

Jessica R. Morrice, Experimental Medicine Program, University of British Columbia, Vancouver, British Columbia, Canada

Marco Morsch, Motor Neuron Disease Research Centre, Faculty of Medicine and Health Sciences, Macquarie University, Sydney, New South Wales, Australia

Alex Parker, Department of Neuroscience, University of Montréal, Montréal, Québec, Canada; Centre de recherche du centre hospitalier de l'Université de Montréal (CRCHUM), Montréal, Québec, Canada

Rowan A.W. Radford, Motor Neuron Disease Research Centre, Faculty of Medicine and Health Sciences, Macquarie University, Sydney, New South Wales, Australia

Jay P. Ross, Department of Human Genetics, McGill University, Montréal, Québec, Canada; Montreal Neurological Institute and Hospital, McGill University, Montréal, Québec, Canada

Guy A. Rouleau, Department of Human Genetics, McGill University, Montréal, Québec, Canada; Montreal Neurological Institute and Hospital, McGill University, Montréal, Québec, Canada; Department of Neurology and Neurosurgery, McGill University, Montréal, Québec, Canada

Mario Sabatelli, Sezione di Medicina Genomica, Dipartimento Scienze della Vita e Sanità Pubblica, Facoltà di Medicina e Chirurgia, Università Cattolica del Sacro Cuore, Rome, Italy

Kristiana Salmon, Montreal Neurological Institute and Hospital, Montréal, Québec, Canada

Natalie M. Scherer, Motor Neuron Disease Research Centre, Faculty of Medicine and Health Sciences, Macquarie University, Sydney, New South Wales, Australia

Christopher A. Shaw, Experimental Medicine Program, University of British Columbia, Vancouver, British Columbia, Canada; Department of Ophthalmology and Visual Sciences, University of British Columbia, Vancouver, British Columbia, Canada; Department of Pathology, University of British Columbia, Vancouver, British Columbia, Canada; Program in Neuroscience, University of British Columbia, Vancouver, British Columbia, Canada

Ted Stehr, ALS Society of BC Director, and person living with ALS

Andres Vidal-Itriago, Motor Neuron Disease Research Centre, Faculty of Medicine and Health Sciences, Macquarie University, Sydney, New South Wales, Australia

Justin J. Yerbury, Illawarra Health and Medical Research Institute, University of Wollongong, Wollongong, New South Wales, Australia; Molecular Horizons and School of Chemistry and Molecular Bioscience, University of Wollongong, Wollongong, New South Wales, Australia

Foreword

Charles Krieger

Department of Biomedical Physiology and Kinesiology, Simon Fraser University, Burnaby, British Columbia, Canada
Department of Medicine, University of British Columbia, Vancouver, British Columbia, Canada
Division of Neurology, Vancouver Coastal Health, Vancouver, British Columbia, Canada

The past decade or so has seen a substantial increase in the extent of research directly or indirectly related to amyotrophic lateral sclerosis (*ALS*). Unfortunately, this research has had limited impact on the clinical course of patients with ALS, suggesting that in many fundamental ways we do not really understand this disease. Numerous observations still defy a clear explanation. For instance, how is it that mutations in various genes, seemingly without a clear interaction in a signaling cascade or pathophysiologic mechanism, all result in a disease with a superficially similar phenotype, a phenotype that is shared with patients where no known gene mutations are present? How is it that the rate of progression of ALS is so rapid and unresponsive to modulation in some patients, yet a lucky few will have the disease course slow substantially? Why are there specific patterns of nervous system involvement in ALS such as "classic" ALS (Charcot type), bulbar ALS (perhaps better described by the original name of "glosso-labio-pharyngeal paralysis"), progressive muscular atrophy, and primary lateral sclerosis? What is the relation between the loss of motoneurons and their axons and the progressive decline in corticospinal and other descending connections? What is the basis of fasciculations? How does ALS "spread" so rapidly in the nervous system? These and other questions remain unanswered.

It is also interesting to look back at how our view of ALS research has changed over time. A clinician or scientist of 25 or 50 years ago would not have seen much investigation into ALS. To those of us who were involved with ALS at that time, the disease appeared neglected. Potentially, to a researcher investigating ALS 50 years ago, it also might have seemed that a treatment for this disease would be relatively straightforward, compared to the treatment of other neurological diseases like Alzheimer's disease or Parkinson's disease. ALS was characterized by the loss of neuronal populations that were well studied, even decades ago, and affected cells might be amenable to the delivery of intrathecal or intramuscular treatment to augment the health of dying neurons and so prolong patient survival.

How times have changed! Instead of being a neglected disorder, there has been considerable scientific and public interest in ALS, due not only to events like the Ice

Bucket Challenge, but also to social media and increasing public awareness. Second, the initial hopes that the disease would turn out to be treatable and responsive to trophic molecules and other factors that would improve the "metabolism" of moto-neurons have not yet borne fruit. In retrospect, it seems clear that given the com-plexity of motoneuron physiology, the difficulty of successful treatment may not have been fully appreciated. Furthermore, the scientific community generally has woken up to the challenge that ALS poses, and many labs around the world are investigating aspects of the disease: the genetics of ALS, the relation between viruses and ALS, RNA-binding proteins, risk genes and environmental toxins, as well as other topics that are reviewed in the present volume.

We can only hope that this new volume will be a stimulus for continued research on ALS and result in insights into this enigmatic, frustrating, and tragic illness.

Preface

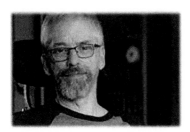

All humanity is on a train speeding through time. The name of the train is life. And like a train you might see in India, it's covered with people, inside and out. People inside are seated in different classes and are engaged in all manner of activities. The people on the roof would love to be inside. They are the sick. The wind buffets them, the rain drenches them, and the sun beats down on them. And each time the train jostles or turns, they have to quickly cling on to prevent them from sliding off and ending their journey.

The terminally ill cling precariously to the side of the train. They try to find perches on the thin window ledges or doorway openings. Some of them have ALS. They are exhausted from the relentless wind and weather, from standing, and from the strain of grasping whatever they can to keep from falling. Often the exhaustion is so great that they feel it might be easier to just let go. But something miraculous happens. People inside the train have given up their seats, walked over to the windows, and put arms around those desperate people. They say, "Don't worry, I have you. Relax for a while, and I'll hold on to you."

Who are these kind people? They are like those from the ALS Clinic or the ALS Society or its donors. By vocation, by volunteering, or by donating, they give help to people who urgently need it.

ALS patients like me need much more than the love and support of their care givers and healthcare providers. We need hoists and slings to move us; specialized wheelchairs to help us to get around; and hospital beds for support, care, and comfort. As our needs grow more complex, the list gets longer and more expensive. But this equipment often makes the unbearable bearable. Some of it literally keeps us alive.

Please donate to the ALS Society of British Columbia. When you do, you are saying, "Hang on, fellow traveler: I see that you need help. Grab my arm."

Typed on my eye gaze computer.
Ted Stehr

Acknowledgments

We thank Michael Kuo and Suresh Bairwa from our laboratory for their assistance. We also thank those at Wiley – Justin Jeffryes, Julia Squarr, Rosie Hayden, and Tom Marriott – for their guidance at all stages of the production of this book, and Tiffany Taylor for her hard work as the copy editor. Finally, we are grateful for contributor suggestions from David Taylor at ALS Canada.

CHAPTER 1

Clinical Heterogeneity of ALS – Implications for Models and Therapeutic Development

Serena Lattante[1,2] and Mario Sabatelli[3,4]

[1] Unità Operativa Complessa di Genetica Medica, Dipartimento di Scienze di Laboratorio e Infettivologico, Fondazione Policlinico Universitario A. Gemelli IRCCS, Rome, Italy

[2] Sezione di Medicina Genomica, Dipartimento Scienze della Vita e Sanità Pubblica, Facoltà di Medicina e Chirurgia, Università Cattolica del Sacro Cuore, Rome, Italy

[3] Centro Clinico NEMO adulti, U.O.C. Neurologia, Dipartimento di Scienze dell'Invecchiamento, Neurologiche, Ortopediche e della Testa-Collo Fondazione Policlinico Universitario A. Gemelli IRCCS, Rome, Italy

[4] Sezione di Neurologia, Dipartimento di Neuroscienze, Facoltà di Medicina e Chirurgia, Università Cattolica Sacro Cuore, Rome, Italy

INTRODUCTION

Amyotrophic lateral sclerosis (ALS) was first described in 1874 as a specific neurological disease by the French neurologist Jean-Martin Charcot, who chose this term to reflect both clinical observations and post-mortem pathological findings. *Amyotrophic* refers to clinical evidence of muscle atrophy as a consequence of the loss of lower motor neurons (LMNs). *Lateral sclerosis* refers to the pathological observation of hardness of the lateral columns of the spinal cord, following upper motor neuron (UMN) degeneration [1]. UMN degeneration is followed by the formation of a sort of scar. The disease leads to progressive paralysis, with death occurring due to respiratory failure within three to five years after symptom onset.

The classical form is characterized by the concomitant involvement of UMNs in the cerebral cortex and LMNs located in the brainstem and the spinal cord. Clinical manifestations of UMN damage are loss of dexterity of the hands and spastic gait

Spectrums of Amyotrophic Lateral Sclerosis: Heterogeneity, Pathogenesis and Therapeutic Directions,
First Edition. Edited by Christopher A. Shaw and Jessica R. Morrice.
© 2021 John Wiley & Sons Ltd. Published 2021 by John Wiley & Sons Ltd.

associated with overactive tendon reflexes. These signs are frequently associated with pathological reflexes, including Chaddock and Babinski signs (extension of the big toe after rubbing the lateral malleolus and the sole of the foot, respectively) and Hoffmann sign (flexion and adduction of index finger and thumb when flicking the nail of the middle finger downward). Corticobulbar involvement leads to slurred speech and difficulty swallowing, often with pathological crying and laughing. The consequence of LMN degeneration is weakness, which may involve any muscle of the body including those of the tongue, pharynx, or larynx (innervated by bulbar motor neurons); those of upper and lower limbs; and the respiratory muscles. Oculomotor and Onuf's motor neurons are usually spared. Muscular atrophy, reduced reflexes, and signs of hyperexcitability in motor neurons, such as fasciculation and cramps, are additional features of LMN degeneration.

The combination of the these symptoms and signs of UMN and LMN dysfunction results in a peculiar and stereotypical picture, which in most cases is easy for expert clinicians to identify. However, there is an evident clinical heterogeneity among ALS patients, which is determined by several independent elements. The age of onset and survival, two major phenotype features, show a marked variability among patients. Furthermore, the relative number of UMN and LMN signs may show substantial differences. An additional contributor to this heterogeneity is the evidence that the types of cells impaired in ALS may extend beyond UMNs and LMNs to include the frontal and temporal cortex, extrapyramidal system, peripheral nerves, and skeletal muscles, giving rise to variable and sometimes overlapping phenotypes.

Finally, genetic research has revealed that ALS is linked with several causative genes – a list that will probably increase in the coming years due to the rapid improvement of next-generation sequencing technologies. ALS-related genes are implicated in various cellular functions, including RNA metabolism, autophagy, and axonal transport, suggesting significant heterogeneity in disease mechanisms as well.

Thus, it appears that ALS is used as an umbrella term referring to a spectrum of disorders with diverse clinical manifestations, heterogeneous disease mechanisms, and (probably) different responses to therapies. On the other hand, all ALS patients, except carriers of superoxide dismutase 1 (*SOD1*) and fused in sarcoma (*FUS*) variants, appear to be unified by a single pathological signature: the presence of abnormal accumulation of the transactivation response DNA binding protein (TDP-43) in the cytoplasm of neuronal and glial cells [2].

CLINICAL HETEROGENEITY OF ALS

Familial and Sporadic ALS

The disease occurs sporadically in the majority of cases (sporadic amyotrophic lateral sclerosis [sALS]), and nearly 10% of patients have a positive family history (familial amyotrophic lateral sclerosis [fALS]) [3]. However, the dichotomy between fALS and sALS is less clear than previously assumed, since several clinical, pathological, and genetic observations support the view that they are linked with each other over a continuum. From a clinical point of view, patients with sALS are indistinguishable from those with fALS. Both conditions show similar pathological patterns – the presence of ubiquitinated TDP-43 positive inclusions in neuronal cells – with the only exception being patients with *SOD1* and *FUS* mutations in which the SOD1 and FUS proteins are detected, respectively [4]. Importantly, fewer than 50% of fALS patients show a clear Mendelian inheritance, usually autosomal-dominant (definite fALS). In the remaining fALS cases, the genetic architecture is less clear as familiarity is assumed by the presence of a single relative with ALS beyond the propositus. These cases are defined as probable fALS when the affected subject is a first- or second-degree relative and possible fALS when the subject is more distant than second-degree. Finally, the most consistent link between sALS and fALS is the observation that all genes involved in fALS are invariably found to be mutated in patients with apparently sporadic disease [3]. Genetic variants in major ALS genes have been detected in about 15% of sporadic forms [5, 6].

Age of Onset

ALS affects people of all ages, with a peak between ages 60 and 79. Recent population-based studies reported a prevalence of ALS between 4.1 and 8.4 per 100 000 [7]. Patients with onset in the first two decades are extremely rare; such cases are termed *juvenile ALS*. This appears to be a different condition than classic ALS as it is familial in most cases, generally has autosomal recessive inheritance, and shows a very pro-longed course. Patients with onset between 20 and 40 years are said to have *young-adult ALS*; this is otherwise classic ALS, although it has peculiar clinical features including predominant UMN signs, male prevalence, and more prolonged survival (usually greater than five years). It remains unclear whether distinctive clinical features of young-adult ALS are related to a different disease mechanism. Finally, very rare patients with onset before 20 years show an otherwise classic ALS with sporadic occurrence and an aggressive course. Most of the reported cases harbor a *de novo* mutation in the *FUS* gene.

Survival

The median survival of ALS is approximately three years from the onset, and about 70% of patients die within five years from onset. However, the duration of the disease differs widely in individual patients, ranging from a few months to over 10 years. Such remarkable variability is a major factor in favor of the hypothesis of ALS as a syndrome rather than a single disease. Median survival is worse in patients with bulbar onset ALS than with the spinal onset. Patients with disease onset before the age of 40 and patients with predominant UMN signs show a better prognosis. In most ALS patients, the cause of death is respiratory failure due to the degeneration of motor neurons controlling thoracic and diaphragmatic muscles. Of note, both the temporal and spatial patterns of the disease spread are important determinants of survival. Regarding the temporal pattern, the spreading rate of the degenerative process may vary among patients, with some patients showing a very rapid, aggressive course and others a slow progression. The spatial pattern is also important, since the sequence in which various body regions are involved is extremely variable and the survival changes if respiratory muscles are among the first or last to be affected.

Classic ALS, LMN Form, and UMN Form

By definition, ALS is characterized by a combination of LMN and UMN clinical and electrophysiological signs. However, the relative mix of UMN and LMN impairment is highly variable among patients, and clinical manifestations of ALS exist on a continuum whose extremes are represented by cases showing pure LMN dysfunction on one side and cases with pure UMN signs on the other side. Classic ALS (Charcot type) is the most frequent form, accounting for about 70–90% of cases, and is characterized by predominant LMN signs combined with slight to moderate pyramidal signs. Patients with pure LMN signs without any accompanying clinical or electrophysiological UMN signs are labeled as having progressive muscular atrophy (PMA) and represent about 5–10% of cases. However, the demonstration that UMN pathology is present at autopsy in 50% of PMA patients indicates that, in at least some cases, pyramidal signs are simply masked by LMN dysfunction on both clinical and electrophysiological grounds. For this reason, the presence of preserved but not hyperactive reflexes in atrophic limbs should be interpreted as UMN impairment. PMA and ALS are not distinct entities, as they show significant phenotypic and genetic overlap. About 2–5% of patients with motor neuron disease show a pure pyramidal form with predominant spino-bulbar spasticity, known as primary lateral sclerosis (PLS). The onset of PLS is generally after 40 years, and the disease duration is significantly longer than in classic ALS. A small proportion of PLS patients develop a clear ALS phenotype, usually within three to four years from the onset, while others show only minimal LMN impairment; most cases remain PLS for decades. ALS patients with predominant pyramidal signs consisting mainly of severe spino-bulbar spasticity are said to have upper motor neuron-dominant amyotrophic lateral sclerosis (UMN-D ALS). These signs are associated with slight LMN signs, usually in the hands. This phenotype is frequent in the young-adult group and males, and it has a better prognosis than classic ALS [8–10].

Site of Onset

ALS begins focally at a seemingly random location and progresses to involve other body regions through anatomically connected pathways and/or neighboring regions. Approximately one-fourth of patients show initial manifestations in the muscles innervated by motor neurons residing in the medulla (bulbar onset), one-third in the upper limb muscles, and one-third in the lower limb muscles whose motor neurons lie in the spinal cord (spinal onset). A small proportion of patients (2–5%) show respiratory symptoms at presentation. These cases are often difficult to diagnose because the absence of additional neurological signs can be misleading. The clinical phenotype at the onset, when temporal–spatial summation hasn't yet occurred, together with additional characteristics, may be important tools to delineate peculiar phenotypes, including spinal, bulbar, pseudopolyneuritic, emiparetic, and flail-arm forms. It remains to be clarified if these clinical pictures correspond to distinct noso-logical entities or are the simple consequence of stochastic phenomena.

Bulbar ALS usually presents with dysarthria and dysphagia due to a variable combination of impairment of LMNs located in the IX, X, and XII nuclei and of the corticobulbar fibers. Bulbar symptoms and signs may be the only manifestation for several months before limb symptoms occur and when only corticobulbar signs are present, the diagnosis of ALS is frequently overlooked. Bulbar onset is more frequent in females and has a worse prognosis than the spinal onset form. In pseudopolyneu-ritic ALS (Patrikios' disease), weakness and atrophy start in distal limb muscles with frequent absence of tendon reflexes, thus mimicking a neuropathy [11]. The flail-arm form (Vulpian-Bernhart syndrome) is characterized by symmetric, predominantly proximal, wasting and weakness of both arms with relative sparing of lower limbs in the initial phases. This ALS form is prevalent in males, starts after the age of 40, and shows a slightly slower disease progression than classic ALS [12, 13].

Diagnosis of ALS

To date, there are no reliable diagnostic tests for ALS, and clinicians rely on the clinical evidence of a combination of UMNs and LMNs in the same body region, electromyo-graphic confirmation of ongoing LMN degeneration, and the exclusion of mimicking conditions. Motor multifocal neuropathy, Kennedy disease, inclusion body myopathy, Sandoff disease, Morvan syndrome, paraneoplastic encephalomyelitis, inflammatory multineuropathies, and compressive myelopathies are conditions that may be con-fused with ALS and should be accurately evaluated. Criteria for the diagnosis of ALS have been established and are known as the El Escorial criteria, but they are more useful in the research field than in the clinical setting [14, 15].

ALS and Its Relationship with Frontotemporal Dementia and Myopathies

ALS has long been considered a paradigm of pure motor neuron disorder. However, genetic discoveries have shown that other cell types may be involved, linking ALS to other diseases. The most common and well-established condition connected with ALS is frontotemporal dementia (FTD). Frontotemporal lobar degeneration (FTLD) con-sists of the degeneration of the frontal and temporal lobes of the brain, leading to atrophy, and occurs with an incidence of 3.5–4.1/100 000 per year in individuals under 65 [16, 17]. Clinically, this is the second most common cause of early-onset dementia, referred to as FTD, and is familial in 20–30% of cases. Variants of FTLD have been described based on clinical signs. Behavioral variant frontotemporal dementia (bvFTD) is the most frequent form and is characterized by behavioral problems – apathy and disinhibition – and a decline in executive functions. Progressive nonfluent aphasia (PNFA) is characterized by language problems including nonfluent speech, dysarthria, poor articulation, and agrammatism with preserved comprehension. The third variant is semantic dementia (SD), also called progressive fluent aphasia (PFA), characterized by the loss of semantic and conceptual knowledge. All these FTLD variants have been described in patients with ALS.

Insoluble proteins aggregate in the neurons of patients with FTLD, leading to three different pathological variants: FTLD-Tau, characterized by the accumulation of the microtubule-associated protein and often by mutations in the gene encoding for the same protein (*MAPT*) (~30–40% of cases) [18]; FTLD-FUS, containing the FUS sarcoma protein (~10% of cases) [19]; and the most frequent, FTLD-TDP, with TDP-43 aggregates (~50–60% of cases) [18–21].

From a clinical point of view, FTD and ALS overlap since 15–18% of ALS patients have FTD and 15% of FTD patients show motor dysfunctions [22, 23]. ALS and FTD also share genetic and neuropathological features, thus leading to the definition of the ALS/FTD spectrum where ALS and FTD are the extremes of a continuum. From a genetic point of view, this idea has been consolidated by the identification of the gene *C9orf72* [24, 25], whose pathogenic expansion has been described in 30–50% of fALS, 25% of familial FTD, 5–7% of sALS, and 6% of sporadic FTD cases in different populations [26, 27]. Furthermore, other genes have been associated with the ALS/FTD spectrum: *TBK1, TARDBP, FUS,* and *SQSTM1* [28]. Finally, with regard to neuropathology, TDP-43 inclusions in neuronal cells are a hallmark of ALS as well as of a proportion of FTD.

Recent genetic evidence, along with clinical and pathological observations, indicate that ALS may be linked to primary muscle disorders as well. Mutations in valosin-containing protein (VCP), previously identified in a proportion of patients with hereditary inclusion-body myopathy (IBM), were later detected in a subset of sALS and fALS cases [29]. Additional genes, including *MATR3, hnRNPA1, hnRN-PA2B1,* and *SQSTM1,* have been identified, which are responsible for an ALS/myopathy spectrum with overlapping phenotypes [30–32]. Interestingly, most myopathies associated with ALS are distal myopathies with evidence of rimmed vacuoles at muscle biopsy. These structures represent the accumulation of autophagic vacuoles due to lysosomal dysfunction or protein accumulation.

Paget's disease of the bone, extrapyramidal syndromes, psychiatric disorders, and peripheral neuropathies are additional conditions that are mechanistically linked to ALS. The spectrum of clinical phenotypes associated with major ALS-associated genes is listed in Table 1.1 [24, 25, 29, 30, 32–66].

PLEIOTROPY OF ALS GENES

SOD1 is the only ALS-associated gene that has been associated exclusively with an isolated motor phenotype. A common phenomenon for all other ALS genes is pleiotropy, which means a genetic variant can be associated with multiple phenotypic traits. The same genetic variant can cause not only different ALS subtypes in families, in terms of age of onset and disease course, but also different diseases. Examples of

TABLE 1.1   Spectrum of clinical disease phenotypes associated with genetic variants.

	ALS	FTD	Myopathy	Parkinson's disease	Paget's disease	Others
SOD1	+[44]	–	–	–	–	–
C9orf72	+[24,25]	+[24,25]	–	+[45]	+/–[46]	Psychiatric disorders [33], Huntington disease [34]
TARDBP	+[47,48]	+[49]	–	+[50]	–	–
FUS	+[51,52]	+[53]	–	–	–	Hereditary essential tremor 4 [35]
NEK1	+[54]	–	–	–	–	Short-rib thoracic dysplasia [36]
TBK1	+[55]	+[56]	–	–	–	Herpes simplex encephalitis [37]
MATR3	+[32]	+[32]	+[57]	–	–	–
VCP	+[29]	+[58]	+[58]	–	+[58]	Charcot-Marie-Tooth type 2 [38]
SQSTM1	+[30]	+[59]	+[60]	–	+[61]	Childhood-onset neurodegeneration with ataxia, dystonia, and gaze palsy [39]
OPTN	+[62]	+[63]	–	+[64]	+[65]	Open angle glaucoma [40]
KIF5A	+[66]	–	–	–	–	Hereditary spastic paraplegia [41], Charcot-Marie-Tooth type 2 [42], neonatal intractable myoclonus [43]

Presence (+) or absence (–) of clinical signs in patients with variants in different genes is reported in the table.

pleiotropic genes are *C9orf72* and *VCP*. In the same family, *C9orf72* carriers can have only ALS, only FTD, or overlapping ALS/FTD phenotypes. Furthermore, the same pathogenic variant in *VCP* has been detected in patients with ALS, FTD, IBM, and Charcot-Marie-Tooth type 2 (CMT2) [67]. The opposite is also true: different pathogenic variants in the same ALS-associated gene can cause an identical phenotype.

High-throughput sequencing studies have shown that a consistent number of patients with the *C9orf72* expansion have additional variants in other ALS-associated genes, suggesting that pleiotropy can be explained by an oligogenic model [5, 27, 68–70].

With rare exceptions, it is not possible to establish a genotype–phenotype correlation in ALS. The variants p.D11Y, p.D90A, and p.G93D in *SOD1* are associated with a relatively benign form of motor neuron disease with distal limb distribution [71–74], while p.A4V and p.G85S are associated with a rapid course [75, 76]. Some mutations in *FUS,* including p.P525L and frameshift mutations, are frequently associated with juvenile-onset ALS with an aggressive course [77–79].

GENETIC MODELS TO STUDY ALS

In Vivo Models

ALS is currently untreatable. Riluzole and edaravone, the two drugs approved by the US Food and Drug Administration (FDA), increase survival by a few months, blocking excessive glutamatergic neurotransmission and preventing oxidative stress damage, respectively, but they are not able to halt or cure the disease [80]. Genetic models represent a very useful tool to identify the concrete target of new drugs. Of course, no model can fully reproduce the human condition, especially its clinical heterogeneity, but a combination of *in vitro* and *in vivo* models can help to investigate the mechanisms underlying the disease and explore epistatic interactions. Since the first genetic discoveries, molecular biology techniques have made it possible to insert gene mutations and express mutant proteins in a number of animal models (see details in Chapter 8). Small animals such as *Drosophila melanogaster* and *Danio rerio* (zebrafish), have been widely used due to the simplicity and rapidity of manipulations, especially for drug screening. The zebrafish has many advantages in this sense, mostly because it is a vertebrate and has high genetic homology with humans. The zebrafish can be used at the embryonic stage, taking advantage of egg transparency and its rapid development, which can be followed in real time; and also at the adult stage, using transgenic lines. Motor phenotypes can be easily detected and analyzed, and *in vivo* imaging can be promptly performed. Genetic interactions can be tested as well as mechanisms of action of pathogenesis. High-throughput drug screening can be done to test libraries containing thousands of chemical compounds at the same time. Since the zebrafish is not a mammal and does not have UMNs (the corticospinal and rubrospinal tracts are absent), it can be considered a very useful tool to study cellular dynamics *in vivo* and may be used prior to other models, such as rodents [81, 82].

A wide range of murine models has been created [83] but the most commonly used remains the first one developed: a transgenic strain carrying the SOD1^{G93A} pathogenic variant [84]. This model has been used to test most drugs in preclinical phases. It should be noted that these treatments are administrated at the pre-symptomatic stage, whereas ALS patients are treated after a disease onset that seems to be preceded by a long pre-symptomatic period. To better investigate the pre-symptomatic stage, a SOD1 pig model has recently been obtained [85]. Since pigs have a long lifespan, transgenic pigs, stably expressing the human pathological allele SOD1^{G93A}, have a pre-symptomatic phase of about 27 months. After this period, gait abnormality and concomitant dysphagia appear and progress rapidly with severe respiratory impairment. SOD1 animal models have been used in preclinical investigations of almost all drugs used in clinical trials. However, the principal limit of this model is that TDP-43 pathology, which is present in about 97% of all ALS subtypes, is not detected in *SOD1* mutated patients, suggesting different disease mechanisms. In addition, preclinical studies performed in mice have failed to be transferred to humans [86].

Considerable efforts have been undertaken to study the biological role of *C9orf72*, because its pathogenic expansion is the most frequent cause of ALS and FTD in populations of European descent. *Drosophila*, zebrafish, and rodents have been used to test various hypotheses of the C9orf72 mechanism, including loss of function, leading to haploinsufficiency of the gene, and gain of function, with the accumulation of RNA foci and dipeptide repeats (DPR) resulting from non-conventional repeat translation. TDP-43 inclusions are detectable in mice expressing the *C9orf72* expanded allele, suggesting that TDP-43 is downstream of C9orf72. Knockout mice show an inflammatory phenotype, thus implicating C9orf72 in immune regulation and the autophagic pathway [87]. Mice expressing the repeat expansion present with RNA foci and DPR, but they do not have a behavioral phenotype, suggesting that the gain of function is not sufficient to cause the disease [88, 89]. A combination of different mechanisms is probably required for disease development [90].

Different animal models, reproducing mutations in different genes, are needed to investigate ALS in its complexity along with the clinical overlap with other diseases of the spectrum. For example, a transgenic mouse has recently been described, carrying the *MATR3*^{S85C} variant. This model shows myopathic histological changes: TDP-43 aggregates in muscles, and respiratory problems occur due to myopathic changes in diaphragm muscles. Interestingly, the observed myotoxicity recapitulates the clinico-pathological features of distal myopathy and ALS [91]. Also, a *TBK1* mouse, recently developed, reproduces the main symptoms of ALS/FTD. Mice carrying the conditional neuronal deletion of *TBK1* show memory deficits and reduced locomotor activity. Interestingly, TBK1 overexpression extended the lifespan of symptomatic mice not only for TBK1 knockout strains but also for SOD1^{G93A} mice, thus suggesting that TBK1 and SOD1 are probably part of the same pathway and can be targeted by the same drugs [92].

By comparing phenotypes across ALS models carrying mutations in different genes, it is possible to study the disease as broadly as possible.

In Vitro Models

The combination of *in vivo* and *in vitro* models can be a good strategy to investigate disease mechanisms in depth. In recent years, a number of studies have been performed on commercial cells engineered to carry mutations in ALS-associated genes. In recent years, the innovative possibility of reprogramming somatic cells obtained from patients opened new avenues for ALS research. Hopefully it will lead to significant improvements in the future of regenerative medicine. Generating cells from patients has two significant advantages that are unique in this model:

1. It is possible to obtain human motor neurons, glial cells, and microglia, the cell types that are primarily affected by the disease and that have been studied in the past only as post-mortem samples.

2. Cells obtained from patients carry exactly the same genetic background as the patient. This means there is no need to insert the genetic mutation artificially: it is possible to study cells as they are in nature. In this context, it is possible to investigate the disease mechanism in all ALS subtypes, including those with known and unknown genetic defects. Moreover, a genetic mutation that arises spontaneously can be corrected using gene-editing techniques to revert the phenotype.

Two different strategies have been set up to reprogram cells from patients. The most commonly used is the generation of induced pluripotent stem cells (iPSCs) from skin fibroblasts [93] and their subsequent differentiation into motor neurons. The second strategy is the direct conversion of skin fibroblasts into motor neurons or glial cells [94].

Fibroblasts can be easily obtained through a skin biopsy, which is not invasive and is very well tolerated by patients. Specific transcription factors (Oct3/4, Sox2, Klf4, and c-Myc) can be introduced by retroviral transduction into somatic cells to convert them into iPSCs [93]. To avoid side effects caused by the use of retroviruses that integrate in the genome, various tools have been developed, such as non-integrating virus and mRNA transcription factors. The iPSCs have the ability to self-renew in culture and can differentiate into cell types of all three germ layers while maintaining the patient's genetic background. Direct conversion of neuronal cells from fibroblasts allows us to bypass the pluripotent stage and can be obtained by overexpressing a combination of transcription factors [94]. Thanks to this strategy, the maturity of the cell, as well as its epigenetic signatures, are preserved; and stem cells can be a better method to study late-onset diseases.

Once obtained, iPSCs can be differentiated into every kind of cell. The most recent innovative approach consists of generating three-dimensional cell cultures called *organoids*, with the aim of better reproducing intercellular interactions and physiological properties. Organoids are particularly useful for drug testing since they better mimic patient's response and tolerability.

CONCLUSION

Recent genetic discoveries and progress in neuropathology have completely changed the perspective on ALS. The current idea is that ALS cannot be considered a single entity (as it was until a few years ago) but rather is part of a clinical spectrum of disease. Various clinical manifestations can be described depending on familial history, age of onset, site of onset, disease duration, and overlap with other conditions as cognitive impairment or myopathies. Animal and cellular models have been established to better characterize the disease pathogenesis and to link the disease to different biological pathways. All these models have the same goal: looking for treatments that can stop or at least significantly slow the disease progression.

CONFLICT OF INTEREST

The authors declare no potential conflict of interest with respect to research, authorship, and/or publication of this manuscript.

COPYRIGHT AND PERMISSION STATEMENT

To the best of our knowledge, the materials included in this chapter do not violate copyright laws. All original sources have been appropriately acknowledged and/or referenced. Where relevant, appropriate permissions have been obtained from the original copyright holder.

REFERENCES

1. Rowland, L.P. and Shneider, N.A. (2001). Amyotrophic lateral sclerosis. *N Engl J Med* 344 (22): 1688–1700.
2. Neumann, M., Sampathu, D.M., Kwong, L.K. et al. (2006). Ubiquitinated TDP-43 in frontotemporal lobar degeneration and amyotrophic lateral sclerosis. *Science* 314 (5796): 130–133.
3. Byrne, S., Bede, P., Elamin, M. et al. (2011). Proposed criteria for familial amyotrophic lateral sclerosis. *Amyotroph Lateral Scler* 12 (3): 157–159.
4. Saberi, S., Stauffer, J.E., Schulte, D.J., and Ravits, J. (2015). Neuropathology of amyotrophic lateral sclerosis and its variants. *Neurol Clin* 33 (4): 855–876.
5. Lattante, S., Conte, A., Zollino, M. et al. (2012). Contribution of major amyotrophic lateral sclerosis genes to the etiology of sporadic disease. *Neurology* 79 (1): 66–72.
6. Renton, A.E., Chiò, A., and Traynor, B.J. (2014). State of play in amyotrophic lateral sclerosis genetics. *Nat Neurosci* 17 (1): 17–23.
7. Longinetti, E. and Fang, F. (2019). Epidemiology of amyotrophic lateral sclerosis: an update of recent literature. *Curr Opin Neurol* 32 (5): 771–776.
8. Sabatelli, M., Madia, F., Conte, A. et al. (2008). Natural history of young-adult amyotrophic lateral sclerosis. *Neurology* 71 (12): 876–881.
9. Sabatelli, M., Zollino, M., Luigetti, M. et al. (2011). Uncovering amyotrophic lateral sclerosis phenotypes: clinical features and long-term follow-up of upper motor neuron-dominant ALS. *Amyotroph Lateral Scler* 12 (4): 278–282.
10. Swinnen, B. and Robberecht, W. (2014). The phenotypic variability of amyotrophic lateral sclerosis. *Nat Rev Neurol* 10 (11): 661–670.
11. Cappellari, A., Ciammola, A., and Silani, V. (2008). The pseudopolyneuritic form of amyotrophic lateral sclerosis (Patrikios' disease). *Electromyogr Clin Neurophysiol* 48 (2): 75–81.
12. Hu, M.T., Ellis, C.M., Al-Chalabi, A. et al. (1998). Flail arm syndrome: a distinctive variant of amyotrophic lateral sclerosis. *J Neurol Neurosurg Psychiatry* 65 (6): 950–951.

13. Gamez, J., Cervera, C., and Codina, A. (1999). Flail arm syndrome of Vulpian-Bernhart's form of amyotrophic lateral sclerosis. *J Neurol Neurosurg Psychiatry* 67 (2): 258.

14. Ludolph, A., Drory, V., Hardiman, O. et al. (2015). A revision of the El Escorial criteria −2015. *Amyotroph Lateral Scler Frontotemporal Degener* 16 (5–6): 291–292.

15. Agosta, F., Al-Chalabi, A., Filippi, M. et al. (2015). The El Escorial criteria: strengths and weaknesses. *Amyotroph Lateral Scler Frontotemporal Degener* 16 (1–2): 1–7.

16. Ratnavalli, E., Brayne, C., Dawson, K., and Hodges, J.R. (2002). The prevalence of frontotemporal dementia. *Neurology* 58 (11): 1615–1621.

17. Harvey, R.J., Skelton-Robinson, M., and Rossor, M.N. (2003). The prevalence and causes of dementia in people under the age of 65 years. *J Neurol Neurosurg Psychiatry* 74 (9): 1206–1209.

18. Mackenzie, I.R., Neumann, M., Bigio, E.H. et al. (2010). Nomenclature and nosology for neuropathologic subtypes of frontotemporal lobar degeneration: an update. *Acta Neuropathol* 119 (1): 1–4.

19. Neumann, M., Roeber, S., Kretzschmar, H.A. et al. (2009). Abundant FUS-immunoreactive pathology in neuronal intermediate filament inclusion disease. *Acta Neuropathol* 118 (5): 605–616.

20. Mackenzie, I.R., Neumann, M., Baborie, A. et al. (2011). A harmonized classification system for FTLD-TDP pathology. *Acta Neuropathol* 122 (1): 111–113.

21. Mackenzie, I.R., Rademakers, R., and Neumann, M. (2010). TDP-43 and FUS in amyotrophic lateral sclerosis and frontotemporal dementia. *Lancet Neurol* 9 (10): 995–1007.

22. Burrell, J.R., Kiernan, M.C., Vucic, S., and Hodges, J.R. (2011). Motor neuron dysfunction in frontotemporal dementia. *Brain* 134 (Pt 9): 2582–2594.

23. Lomen-Hoerth, C., Anderson, T., and Miller, B. (2002). The overlap of amyotrophic lateral sclerosis and frontotemporal dementia. *Neurology* 59 (7): 1077–1079.

24. DeJesus-Hernandez, M., Mackenzie, I.R., Boeve, B.F. et al. (2011). Expanded GGGGCC hexanucleotide repeat in noncoding region of C9ORF72 causes chromosome 9p-linked FTD and ALS. *Neuron* 72 (2): 245–256.

25. Renton, A.E., Majounie, E., Waite, A. et al. (2011). A hexanucleotide repeat expansion in C9ORF72 is the cause of chromosome 9p21-linked ALS-FTD. *Neuron* 72 (2): 257–268.

26. Majounie, E., Renton, A.E., Mok, K. et al. (2012). Frequency of the C9orf72 hexanucleotide repeat expansion in patients with amyotrophic lateral sclerosis and frontotemporal dementia: a cross-sectional study. *Lancet Neurol* 11 (4): 323–330.

27. van der Zee, J., Gijselinck, I., Dillen, L. et al. (2013). A pan-European study of the C9orf72 repeat associated with FTLD: geographic prevalence, genomic instability, and intermediate repeats. *Hum Mutat* 34 (2): 363–373.

28. Nguyen, H.P., Van Broeckhoven, C., and van der Zee, J. (2018). ALS genes in the genomic era and their implications for FTD. *Trends Genet* 34 (6): 404–423.

29. Johnson, J.O., Mandrioli, J., Benatar, M. et al. (2010). Exome sequencing reveals VCP mutations as a cause of familial ALS. *Neuron* 68 (5): 857–864.

30. Fecto, F., Yan, J., Vemula, S.P. et al. (2011). SQSTM1 mutations in familial and sporadic amyotrophic lateral sclerosis. *Arch Neurol* 68 (11): 1440–1446.

31. Kim, H.J., Kim, N.C., Wang, Y.D. et al. (2013). Mutations in prion-like domains in hnRNPA2B1 and hnRNPA1 cause multisystem proteinopathy and ALS. *Nature* 495 (7442): 467–473.

32. Johnson, J.O., Pioro, E.P., Boehringer, A. et al. (2014). Mutations in the Matrin 3 gene cause familial amyotrophic lateral sclerosis. *Nat Neurosci* 17 (5): 664–666.

33. Arighi, A., Fumagalli, G.G., Jacini, F. et al. (2012). Early onset behavioral variant frontotemporal dementia due to the C9ORF72 hexanucleotide repeat expansion: psychiatric clinical presentations. *J Alzheimers Dis* 31 (2): 447–452.

34. Beck, J., Poulter, M., Hensman, D. et al. (2013). Large C9orf72 hexanucleotide repeat expansions are seen in multiple neurodegenerative syndromes and are more frequent than expected in the UK population. *Am J Hum Genet* 92 (3): 345–353.

35. Merner, N.D., Girard, S.L., Catoire, H. et al. (2012). Exome sequencing identifies FUS mutations as a cause of essential tremor. *Am J Hum Genet* 91 (2): 313–319.

36. Thiel, C., Kessler, K., Giessl, A. et al. (2011). NEK1 mutations cause short-rib polydactyly syndrome type majewski. *Am J Hum Genet* 88 (1): 106–114.

37. Herman, M., Ciancanelli, M., Ou, Y.H. et al. (2012). Heterozygous TBK1 mutations impair TLR3 immunity and underlie herpes simplex encephalitis of childhood. *J Exp Med* 209 (9): 1567–1582.

38. Gonzalez, M.A., Feely, S.M., Speziani, F. et al. (2014). A novel mutation in VCP causes charcot-marie-tooth type 2 disease. *Brain* 137 (Pt 11): 2897–2902.

39. Haack, T.B., Ignatius, E., Calvo-Garrido, J. et al. (2016). Absence of the autophagy adaptor SQSTM1/p62 causes childhood-onset neurodegeneration with ataxia, dystonia, and gaze palsy. *Am J Hum Genet* 99 (3): 735–743.

40. Rezaie, T., Child, A., Hitchings, R. et al. (2002). Adult-onset primary open-angle glaucoma caused by mutations in optineurin. *Science* 295 (5557): 1077–1079.

41. Reid, E., Kloos, M., Ashley-Koch, A. et al. (2002). A kinesin heavy chain (KIF5A) mutation in hereditary spastic paraplegia (SPG10). *Am J Hum Genet* 71 (5): 1189–1194.

42. Crimella, C., Baschirotto, C., Arnoldi, A. et al. (2012). Mutations in the motor and stalk domains of KIF5A in spastic paraplegia type 10 and in axonal charcot-marie-tooth type 2. *Clin Genet* 82 (2): 157–164.

43. Duis, J., Dean, S., Applegate, C. et al. (2016). KIF5A mutations cause an infantile onset phenotype including severe myoclonus with evidence of mitochondrial dysfunction. *Ann Neurol* 80 (4): 633–637.

44. Rosen, D.R., Siddique, T., Patterson, D. et al. (1993). Mutations in Cu/Zn superoxide dismutase gene are associated with familial amyotrophic lateral sclerosis. *Nature* 362 (6415): 59–62.

45. Xi, Z., Zinman, L., Grinberg, Y. et al. (2012). Investigation of c9orf72 in 4 neurodegenerative disorders. *Arch Neurol* 69 (12): 1583–1590.

46. Rubino, E., Di Stefano, M., Galimberti, D. et al. (2020). C9ORF72 hexanucleotide repeat expansion frequency in patients with Paget's disease of bone. *Neurobiol Aging* 85: 154.e1–154.e3.

47. Kabashi, E., Valdmanis, P.N., Dion, P. et al. (2008). TARDBP mutations in individuals with sporadic and familial amyotrophic lateral sclerosis. *Nat Genet* 40 (5): 572–574.

48. Sreedharan, J., Blair, I.P., Tripathi, V.B. et al. (2008). TDP-43 mutations in familial and sporadic amyotrophic lateral sclerosis. *Science* 319 (5870): 1668–1672.

49. Kovacs, G.G., Murrell, J.R., Horvath, S. et al. (2009). TARDBP variation associated with frontotemporal dementia, supranuclear gaze palsy, and chorea. *Mov Disord* 24 (12): 1843–1847. https://doi.org/10.1002/mds.22697.

50. Quadri, M., Cossu, G., Saddi, V. et al. (2011). Broadening the phenotype of TARDBP mutations: the TARDBP Ala382Thr mutation and Parkinson's disease in Sardinia. *Neurogenetics* 12 (3): 203–209.

51. Kwiatkowski, T.J. Jr., Bosco, D.A., Leclerc, A.L. et al. (2009). Mutations in the FUS/ TLS gene on chromosome 16 cause familial amyotrophic lateral sclerosis. *Science* 323 (5918): 1205–1208.

52. Vance, C., Rogelj, B., Hortobágyi, T. et al. (2009). Mutations in FUS, an RNA processing protein, cause familial amyotrophic lateral sclerosis type 6. *Science* 323 (5918): 1208–1211.

53. Yan, J., Deng, H.X., Siddique, N. et al. (2010). Frameshift and novel mutations in FUS in familial amyotrophic lateral sclerosis and ALS/dementia. *Neurology* 75 (9): 807–814.

54. Kenna, K.P., van Doormaal, P.T., Dekker, A.M. et al. (2016). NEK1 variants confer susceptibility to amyotrophic lateral sclerosis. *Nat Genet* 48 (9): 1037–1042.

55. Cirulli, E.T., Lasseigne, B.N., Petrovski, S. et al. (2015). Exome sequencing in amyotrophic lateral sclerosis identifies risk genes and pathways. *Science* 347 (6229): 1436–1441.

56. Freischmidt, A., Wieland, T., Richter, B. et al. (2015). Haploinsufficiency of TBK1 causes familial ALS and fronto-temporal dementia. *Nat Neurosci* 18 (5): 631–636.

57. Senderek, J., Garvey, S.M., Krieger, M. et al. (2009). Autosomal-dominant distal myopathy associated with a recurrent missense mutation in the gene encoding the nuclear matrix protein, matrin 3. *Am J Hum Genet* 84 (4): 511–518.

58. Watts, G.D., Wymer, J., Kovach, M.J. et al. (2004). Inclusion body myopathy associated with paget disease of bone and frontotemporal dementia is caused by mutant valosin-containing protein. *Nat Genet* 36 (4): 377–381.

59. Rubino, E., Rainero, I., Chiò, A. et al. (2012). SQSTM1 mutations in frontotemporal lobar degeneration and amyotrophic lateral sclerosis. *Neurology* 79 (15): 1556–1562.

60. Bucelli, R.C., Arhzaouy, K., Pestronk, A. et al. (2015). SQSTM1 splice site mutation in distal myopathy with rimmed vacuoles. *Neurology* 85 (8): 665–674.

61. Laurin, N., Brown, J.P., Morissette, J., and Raymond, V. (2002). Recurrent mutation of the gene encoding sequestosome 1 (SQSTM1/p 62) in paget disease of bone. *Am J Hum Genet* 70 (6): 1582–1588.

62. Maruyama, H., Morino, H., Ito, H. et al. (2010). Mutations of optineurin in amyotrophic lateral sclerosis. *Nature* 465 (7295): 223–226.

63. Pottier, C., Bieniek, K.F., Finch, N. et al. (2015). Whole-genome sequencing reveals important role for TBK1 and OPTN mutations in frontotemporal lobar degeneration without motor neuron disease. *Acta Neuropathol* 130 (1): 77–92.

64. Ayaki, T., Ito, H., Komure, O. et al. (2018). Multiple proteinopathies in familial ALS cases with optineurin mutations. *J Neuropathol Exp Neurol* 77 (2): 128–138.

65. Albagha, O.M., Visconti, M.R., Alonso, N. et al. (2010). Genome-wide association study identifies variants at CSF1, OPTN and TNFRSF11A as genetic risk factors for paget's disease of bone. *Nat Genet* 42 (6): 520–524.

66. Nicolas, A., Kenna, K.P., Renton, A.E. et al. (2018). Genome-wide analyses identify KIF5A as a novel ALS gene. *Neuron* 97 (6): 1268–1283.e6.

67. van der Zee, J., Pirici, D., Van Langenhove, T. et al. (2009). Clinical heterogeneity in 3 unrelated families linked to VCP p.Arg159His. *Neurology* 73 (8): 626–632.

68. van Blitterswijk, M., van Es, M.A., Hennekam, E.A. et al. (2012). Evidence for an oligogenic basis of amyotrophic lateral sclerosis. *Hum Mol Genet* 21 (17): 3776–3784.

69. van Blitterswijk, M., Baker, M.C., DeJesus-Hernandez, M. et al. (2013). C9ORF72 repeat expansions in cases with previously identified pathogenic mutations. *Neurology* 81 (15): 1332–1341.

70. Giannoccaro, M.P., Bartoletti-Stella, A., Piras, S. et al. (2017). Multiple variants in families with amyotrophic lateral sclerosis and frontotemporal dementia related to C9orf72 repeat expansion: further observations on their oligogenic nature. *J Neurol* 264 (7): 1426–1433.

71. Restagno, G., Lombardo, F., Sbaiz, L. et al. (2008). The rare G93D mutation causes a slowly progressing lower motor neuron disease. *Amyotroph Lateral Scler* 9 (1): 35–39.

72. Luigetti, M., Conte, A., Madia, F. et al. (2009). Heterozygous SOD1 D90A mutation presenting as slowly progressive predominant upper motor neuron amyotrophic lateral sclerosis. *Neurol Sci* 30 (6): 517–520.

73. Georgoulopoulou, E., Gellera, C., Bragato, C. et al. (2010). A novel SOD1 mutation in a young amyotrophic lateral sclerosis patient with a very slowly progressive clinical course. *Muscle Nerve* 42 (4): 596–597.

74. Del Grande, A., Conte, A., Lattante, S. et al. (2011). D11Y SOD1 mutation and benign ALS: a consistent genotype-phenotype correlation. *J Neurol Sci* 309 (1–2): 31–33.

75. Juneja, T., Pericak-Vance, M.A., Laing, N.G. et al. (1997). Prognosis in familial amyotrophic lateral sclerosis: progression and survival in patients with glu100gly and ala-4val mutations in Cu, Zn superoxide dismutase. *Neurology* 48 (1): 55–75.

76. Takazawa, T., Ikeda, K., Hirayama, T. et al. (2010). Familial amyotrophic lateral sclerosis with a novel G85S mutation of superoxide dismutase 1 gene: clinical features of lower motor neuron disease. *Intern Med* 49 (2): 183–186.

77. Conte, A., Lattante, S., Zollino, M. et al. (2012). P525L FUS mutation is consistently associated with a severe form of juvenile amyotrophic lateral sclerosis. *Neuromuscul Disord* 22 (1): 73–75.

78. Hübers, A., Just, W., Rosenbohm, A. et al. (2015). De novo FUS mutations are the most frequent genetic cause in early-onset German ALS patients. *Neurobiol Aging* 36 (11): 3117.

79. Leblond, C.S., Webber, A., Gan-Or, Z. et al. (2016). De novo FUS P525L mutation in Juvenile amyotrophic lateral sclerosis with dysphonia and diplopia. *Neurol Genet* 2 (2): e63.

80. Oskarsson, B., Gendron, T.F., and Staff, N.P. (2018). Amyotrophic lateral sclerosis: an update for 2018. *Mayo Clin Proc* 93 (11): 1617–1628.

81. Kabashi, E., Champagne, N., Brustein, E., and Drapeau, P. (2010). In the swim of things: recent insights to neurogenetic disorders from zebrafish. *Trends Genet* 26 (8): 373–381.

82. Babin, P.J., Goizet, C., and Raldúa, D. (2014). Zebrafish models of human motor neuron diseases: advantages and limitations. *Prog Neurobiol* 118: 36–58.

83. De Giorgio, F., Maduro, C., Fisher, E.M.C., and Acevedo-Arozena, A. (2019). Transgenic and physiological mouse models give insights into different aspects of amyotrophic lateral sclerosis. *Dis Model Mech* 12 (1).

84. Gurney, M.E., Pu, H., Chiu, A.Y. et al. (1994). Motor neuron degeneration in mice that express a human Cu, Zn superoxide dismutase mutation. *Science* 264 (5166): 1772–1775.

85. Crociara, P., Chieppa, M.N., Vallino Costassa, E. et al. (2019). Motor neuron degeneration, severe myopathy and TDP-43 increase in a transgenic pig model of SOD1-linked familiar ALS. *Neurobiol Dis* 124: 263–275.

86. Benatar, M. (2007). Lost in translation: treatment trials in the SOD1 mouse and in human ALS. *Neurobiol Dis* 26 (1): 1–13.

87. Sullivan, P.M., Zhou, X., Robins, A.M. et al. (2016). The ALS/FTLD associated protein C9orf72 associates with SMCR8 and WDR41 to regulate the autophagy-lysosome pathway. *Acta Neuropathol Commun* 4 (1): 51.

88. Chew, J., Gendron, T.F., Prudencio, M. et al. (2015). Neurodegeneration. C9ORF72 repeat expansions in mice cause TDP-43 pathology, neuronal loss, and behavioral deficits. *Science* 348 (6239): 1151–1154.

89. Liu, Y., Pattamatta, A., Zu, T. et al. (2016). C9orf72 BAC mouse model with motor deficits and neurodegenerative features of ALS/FTD. *Neuron* 90 (3): 521–534.

90. Cook, C. and Petrucelli, L. (2019). Genetic convergence brings clarity to the enigmatic red line in ALS. *Neuron* 101 (6): 1057–1069.

91. Zhang, X., Yamashita, S., Hara, K. et al. (2019). Mutant MATR3 mouse model to explain multisystem proteinopathy. *J Pathol* 249 (2): 182–192.

92. Duan, W., Guo, M., Yi, L. et al. (2019). Deletion of Tbk1 disrupts autophagy and reproduces behavioral and locomotor symptoms of FTD-ALS in mice. *Aging (Albany NY)* 11 (8): 2457–2476.

93. Takahashi, K., Tanabe, K., Ohnuki, M. et al. (2007). Induction of pluripotent stem cells from adult human fibroblasts by defined factors. *Cell* 131 (5): 861–872.

94. Son, E.Y., Ichida, J.K., Wainger, B.J. et al. (2011). Conversion of mouse and human fibroblasts into functional spinal motor neurons. *Cell Stem Cell* 9 (3): 205–218.

CHAPTER 2

Genetic Basis of ALS

Jay P. Ross[1,2], Patrick A. Dion[2,3], and Guy A. Rouleau[1,2,3]

[1] Department of Human Genetics, McGill University, Montréal, Québec, Canada
[2] Montreal Neurological Institute and Hospital, McGill University, Montréal, Québec, Canada
[3] Department of Neurology and Neurosurgery, McGill University, Montréal, Québec, Canada

INTRODUCTION

The recent study of amyotrophic lateral sclerosis (ALS) has generally been driven by its associated genes. While there seems to be a strong environmental component to ALS risk, the heritability of ALS has been estimated to range between 0.523 and 0.61 [1, 2], which suggests a substantial genetic contribution. As the number of cases currently explained by known genetics variants is relatively small, there are likely many genetic contributors yet to be discovered. Further complicating ALS genetics is the distinction between familial and sporadic cases: those with a family history of ALS or frontotemporal dementia, and those without, respectively.

One of the first goals of ALS genetic research has been to identify variants in genes and to fit these genes into our current understanding of ALS biology. Over the years, various methods of gene discovery have been applied. Over time, studies focused on familial linkage, as well as screening of candidate genes encoding a protein with known biological relevance, were replaced by whole-exome (WES) and whole-genome sequencing (WGS) studies; such advances have led to the identification of variants more frequently observed in ALS patients than unaffected individuals.

This chapter will review genes for which there is consistent strong evidence and genes that were recently discovered, explore aspects of inheritance for ALS-associated variants, and consider regulatory and epigenetic variants.

Spectrums of Amyotrophic Lateral Sclerosis: Heterogeneity, Pathogenesis and Therapeutic Directions,
First Edition. Edited by Christopher A. Shaw and Jessica R. Morrice.
© 2021 John Wiley & Sons Ltd. Published 2021 by John Wiley & Sons Ltd.

GENES CAUSING ALS

The following four genes are described in order of discovery and are highlighted due to their importance in ALS. Dysfunction and dysregulation of these genes cause ALS, but even for conclusively causal variants in these genes, the most critical disease mechanisms are still under investigation.

Superoxide Dismutase 1 (SOD1)

The first gene in which variants were associated with ALS pathology was superoxide dismutase 1 (*SOD1*) [3]. First discovered following a polymerase chain reaction (PCR) mutation screening approach of the gene closest to a prior linkage signal, *SOD1* variants remained one of the only known genetic causes of ALS for 15 years. Most *SOD1* variants lead to a highly penetrant, familial, and dominant presentation of ALS [4], and they are observed in approximately 12% of familial and 1% of sporadic ALS cases [4]. Certain variants (p.D90A, for example) are associated with either dominant or recessive inheritance depending on the population [5, 6]. While *SOD1* variants occur in any exon, the frequency of specific *SOD1* variants is associated with different ethnicities [5, 7]. For example, *SOD1* variants are relatively rare in European cohorts but are the most frequent cause of familial ALS in Asian cohorts [7]. Variant penetrance can be as high as 90–95% by the age of 80 [8], suggesting that the encoded SOD1 protein is intolerant to protein-altering variants [9] and that most variants are probably associated with familial ALS given sufficient age.

Despite decades of research, the mechanism of SOD1 toxicity in ALS is still not definite. Aggregation of the SOD1 protein is observed with nearly all protein-altering *SOD1* variants [9–11]. Nonetheless, it is uncertain how these SOD1-positive aggregates are related to the onset and progression of the disease. Variant SOD1 also leads to cell death in the form of excitotoxicity, in which glutamate activity causes prolonged calcium influx and subsequent mitochondrial dysfunction [12]. However, there is evidence that spinal cords with the highest level of SOD1 aggregates are those of longer-survival ALS [13]. One explanation is that the level of SOD1 aggregates increases in response to normal cellular processes that sequester SOD1 and lower their toxicity. Another potential mechanism for SOD1-related cell death could be a loss-of-function model, in which variants in *SOD1* result in a lack of functional SOD1 protein, although such a mechanism has not been convincingly linked to ALS. SOD1 aggregates can recruit wild-type SOD1 protein [12, 14], leading to a lack of functional SOD1 in the cell. A reduction in SOD1 normal activity, that of a dismutase lowering the number of superoxide radicals, is observed in *SOD1* variant carriers [14]. The resulting increase of free radicals in cells has direct negative effects on mitochondrial function and survival. While this observation does not prove that loss of function is the model by which *SOD1* variants cause ALS, it does suggest that the mechanism is more complicated than simply SOD1 aggregates causing motor neuron death.

TAR DNA-Binding Protein 43 (TDP-43)

Informed by prior observations of transactivation response (TAR) DNA binding protein 43 (TDP-43) aggregates in neurons of ALS patients, the gene that encodes TDP-43 (*TARDBP*) was screened for the presence of protein-altering variants in simultaneous studies [15, 16]. Variants in *TARDBP* are a rare cause of ALS and are mainly clustered in the C-terminal low-complexity domain [17]. *TARDBP* variants account for 1–4% of familial ALS and are very rare in sporadic ALS [18], suggesting that altered TDP-43 is a penetrant mechanism for ALS. *TARDBP* variants generally cause a dominant familial ALS [17] and are observed across ethnicities [7]. Certain founder populations can lead to a significantly increased incidence of *TARDBP* variants; for example, between 20 and 30% of Sardinian ALS patients carry the p.A382T variant [19, 20]. Despite the rarity of *TARDBP* variants, the implication of this gene has opened several avenues in ALS research.

TDP-43 is an RNA binding protein, and it has specific transcript targets, which it binds and modifies [21, 22]. Normal TDP-43 function involves repressing cryptic exons in mRNA, as variant (and silenced) *TARDBP* results in exons arising from intronic regions [23–25]. These cryptic exons are generally in nonconserved genomic regions [25]. Transcripts with cryptic exons tend to be processed through nonsense-mediated decay, and lower expression of normal transcripts therefore results from altered TDP-43 [24]. A loss-of-function model for TDP-43 implicates not only mis-spliced targets but also a lower expression of these targets. Conversely, conserved exons that should be included in properly-spliced transcripts are skipped (*skiptic*) in cells with TDP-43 variants [26]. In mice carrying certain variants in either the RNA-binding or low-complexity domains, exons were either aberrantly included (cryptic) or excluded (skiptic), respectively [26].

Cytoplasmic TDP-43–containing inclusions are a common hallmark of ALS, appearing in as many as 97% of ALS cases [27] and in all but *SOD1* variant carriers [28]. There is still debate about whether the aggregates are toxic *per se*. First, while most ALS-causing variants occur in the C-terminal region of the *TARDBP* transcript, aggregated C-terminal TDP-43 fragments do not appear to be the driving force of the pathology [29]. Second, the N-terminus of TDP-43 appears to strongly affect cell pathology and aggregation [30], although ALS-associated variants are not often observed in the first exons of *TARDBP*. Lastly, the normal function of the RNA-binding domains of TDP-43 appears to prevent the aggregation of the protein: when RNA targets of TDP-43 are not available to bind, aggregation of TDP-43 increases [31]. Supporting the involvement of RNA-binding for ALS pathology, *TARDBP* variants require intact TDP-43 RNA-binding domains to exert neurotoxic effects [32].

Fused in Sarcoma (FUS)

Using loss-of-heterozygosity mapping in a consanguineous family, variants in a region of chromosome 16 were identified to be linked with ALS [33]. Simultaneously, a separate group found fused in sarcoma (*FUS*) variants segregating dominantly in several pedigrees after screening a similar linkage region [34]. Protein-altering variants have been observed across the *FUS* coding sequence, but the most penetrant variants (not in unaffected controls) are clustered in the nuclear localization signal (*NLS*) domain of the last exon [17]. *FUS* variants have been linked to strongly penetrant and dominantly inherited forms of ALS. Indeed, variants in *FUS* have been consistently associated with earlier onset and even juvenile cases of ALS, with age at onset generally below the disease average [35]. While this is a rare cause of both familial and sporadic ALS (approximately 4% of familial ALS and less than 1% of sporadic [4]), the discovery of another aggregating RNA-binding protein in ALS strengthened the themes of protein aggregation, RNA metabolism, and nuclear trafficking [17].

FUS and TDP-43 are similar in that they localize in the nucleus under normal conditions, regulate splicing of pre-mRNA, transport transcripts from the nucleus, and form cytoplasmic aggregates in the presence of specific ALS-associated variants [36, 37]. However, FUS is also a transcription factor, binding to open chromatin to regulate transcription of RNA [38]. FUS directly binds to RNA on long introns but also interacts with splicing machinery to affect RNA processing indirectly [37]. FUS has a different RNA sequence recognition motif compared to TDP-43 and does not bind the same set of transcripts [36]. Further, FUS also binds a specific secondary structure of RNA in addition to its sequence motif [35]. Cytoplasmic FUS aggregates might suggest a loss of these specific RNA binding functions as FUS is sequestered [39], and it is unclear whether FUS aggregates are toxic or an indication of lowered FUS activity.

Chromosome 9 Open Reading Frame 72 (C9orf72)

A hexanucleotide repeat expansion (HRE) of GGGGCC in the first intron of chromosome 9 open reading frame 72 *(C9orf72)* was discovered by two simultaneous studies [40, 41]. The locus containing *C9orf72* was identified in linkage scans in large families with multiple ALS cases [42], but the actual variant was elusive due to the contemporary paradigm of searching for single nucleotide exonic variants. The *C9orf72* HRE was the first noncoding variant with a substantial impact on ALS genetic research [4]. Currently the most common genetic cause of ALS, the *C9orf72* HRE explains about 10% of all ALS cases (approximately 40% of familial and 7% of sporadic) [4]. The frequency of the *C9orf72* HRE is strongly dependent on population, ranging from 20% of Finnish ALS cases to very rare in Asian populations [7]. Alleles in the range of 2 to 20 repeats are considered normal and non-pathogenic, with repeat lengths above 30 being strongly penetrant for ALS. Indeed, repeat lengths of several thousand have been reported, with a potential correlation between disease severity and length [43]. Intermediate lengths between 20 and 30 repeats have been observed and have recently been recognized as associated with ALS, although with a lower risk than expanded alleles [44]. The *C9orf72* HRE is unstable at very large repeat lengths [43], but somatic expansion of normal length does not likely occur [45].

Adding to the evidence that RNA metabolism is a significant factor in ALS pathology, *C9orf72* HRE carriers show RNA foci and aberrant RNA translation. RNA foci result when HRE transcripts amass together and subsequently sequester RNA-binding proteins [46]. For example, RNA-binding proteins such as hnRNPA2B1 and hnRNPA1, as well as splicing factors SRSF1 and SRSF2, are also colocalized in RNA foci [46]. TDP-43 has been observed to bind G-quadruplex structures containing the GGGGCC repeat, implicating a loss of TDP-43 function in *C9orf72* ALS [47]. These sequestered proteins could have an impact on proper RNA splicing, and indeed transcriptomic aberrations have been observed in *C9orf72* HRE patient cerebellums [48]. RNA foci are likely not toxic *per se*, as expressions of RNA containing only very long repeats (without the *C9orf72* transcript) do not cause acute toxicity in *Drosophila* neurons [49]. While the *C9orf72* HRE is in an intronic region of the pre-spliced *C9orf72* transcript, the repeat itself can be translated into dipeptide repeat proteins (DPRs) [50]. Through a process known as *repeat-associated non-ATG-initiated (RAN) translation*, five different DPRs with two repeating amino acids each (depending on direction and reading frame) are generated. DPRs might affect ALS pathology in several ways. First, zebrafish models have demonstrated that expressing DPR without the *C9orf72* HRE results in motor deficits and morphological defects [51]. Second, poly-Gly-Arg and poly-Pro-Arg DPR are toxic in *Drosophilia* neurons, and a mass spectrometry screen of proteins bound to DPR showed enrichment of ribosomal proteins, potentially linking translational inhibition [52]. Third, the poly-Pro-Arg DPR might alter proper nuclear pore function and affect nuclear import and export [53]. The direct effects of DPR on cell function and survival are still debated, and more study will be needed to determine whether the levels generated by inherited *C9orf72* HRE are related to ALS progression.

RECENTLY DISCOVERED GENES

The rate of gene discovery appears linear, with new ALS genes discovered each year (Figure 2.1a). However, newly discovered genes tend to explain very few ALS cases; and despite the constant discovery rate of genes, the percent of genetically explained cases appears to have plateaued (Figure 2.1b). Nonetheless, there are genes for which there is significant evidence of their involvement and through which we can expand the scope of ALS cell biology theory. Below we discuss three recent gene discoveries, chosen because they were replicated in multiple cohorts or pedigrees.

Annexin A11 (ANXA11)

By examining families with multiple affected individuals, Smith et al. observed the Annexin A11 *(ANXA11)* p.D40G variant segregating with ALS [62]. In a replication cohort, additional variants were observed; and while more than half were in the N-terminus, no functional domain was enriched for variants. These variants may account for as much as 1–2% of ALS, whether sporadic or familial. Variants in *ANXA11* in ALS patients were quickly replicated in Chinese cohorts [63–65], with results

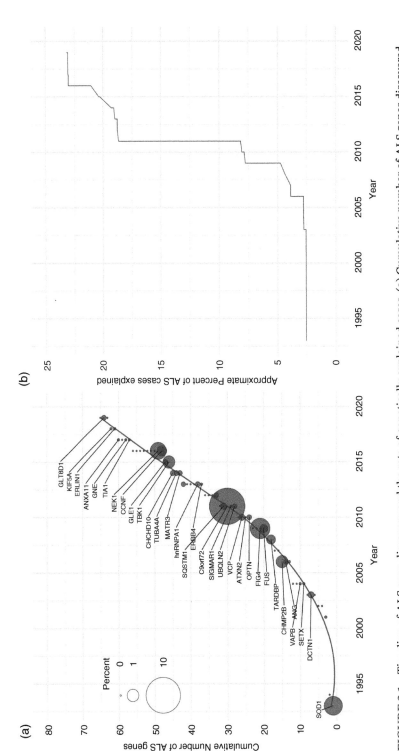

FIGURE 2.1 Timeline of ALS gene discovery and the rate of genetically explained cases. (a) Cumulative number of ALS genes discovered. Each circle represents a single gene reported to cause or predispose to ALS, with the size of the circle representing the approximate proportion of cases explained. The smallest size (0%) represents genes with very rare variants or those that are not genetically implicated. (b) Total percent of ALS cases explained by variation in ALS genes over time. The cumulative percent was calculated per year corresponding to gene discovery. Estimated percent is approximate and informed by published reviews [4, 54–61].

ranging from *ANXA11* variants being a frequently altered gene in sporadic ALS patients [65] to *ANXA11* variants being rare and of uncertain impact [64]. As variants will be found at varying frequencies in different cohorts, more studies will be needed to assess whether any given variant is coincidental or an actual cause of disease. Similar to some RNA-binding proteins and SOD1 [17], *ANXA11* variants appear to cause its encoded protein to aggregate when overexpressed, and in turn these ANXA11 aggregates can recruit the wild-type form of the protein [62]. ANXA11 binds phospholipids in vesicles and may interact with calcyclin in apoptosis and exocytosis pathways [62]. These pathways involve other ALS-associated genes such as *FIG 4*, *OPTN*, and *SQSTM1* [66].

Glycosyltransferase 8 Domain Containing 1 (GLT8D1)

In an experimental paradigm similar to *ANXA11*, variants in *GLT8D1* were observed in familial ALS cases [67]. Exome sequencing was used to identify rare and predicted deleterious variants that segregated well with the disease phenotype, resulting in candidate genes *GLT8D1* and *ARPP21*. Several patients carried both the *ARPP21* p.P529L and *GLT8D1* p.R92C variants, each of which could have been the causal factor. However, an examination of variants identified by the large-scale ALS Project MinE [68] revealed a larger number of ALS cases carrying the *GLT8D1* variant without any *ARPP21* variants than the same variant with the *ARPP21* variant. The gene *GLT8D1* encodes a glycosyltransferase protein, which the authors note is not typically implicated in ALS and might represent a new avenue to investigate for ALS neurodegeneration [67].

Stathmin-2 (STMN2)

The loss-of function hypothesis for TDP-43 has led to the examination of transcripts that are dysregulated following *TARDBP* knockdown. In separate studies, *TARDBP* was silenced in human motor neurons derived from iPSC as well as in *TARDBP* variant carrier cell lines [69, 70]. The primary objective of both studies was to identify transcripts that showed significant expression differences after *TARDBP* depletion; while the overlap of transcripts between the studies has not been examined, both studies identified Stathmin-2 (*STMN2*). The studies further show that certain *TARDBP* variants also cause a similar downregulation of *STMN2* compared to unaffected controls. Moreover, an aberrant exon and subsequent truncation were observed in *STMN2* transcripts following *TARDBP* silencing, further supporting the cryptic exon mechanism of TDP-43 dysregulation in ALS.

As a component of microtubule dynamics, *STMN2* adds to a group of genes implicated in the regulation of assembly and disassembly of tubulin (*TUBA4A* [71]) and movement of molecular cargo along microtubule networks (*KIF5A* [72, 73] and *DCTN1* [71]). While no publications have shown variants in *STMN2* associated with ALS, *STMN2* dysregulation expands our knowledge about TDP-43 binding pre-mRNA transcripts in the nucleus. Both studies identified *STMN2* as a TDP-43 target using motor neuron cultures, demonstrating the necessity of specific cellular models.

ASPECTS OF ALS HERITABILITY

Despite the number of genes associated with ALS, a very low percentage of patients carry a variant in one of these genes. As many as 30% of familial and 90% of sporadic ALS cases can be deemed as "no known genetic cause" [4] – either their disease was caused primarily by environmental factors, or they carry a not-yet-identified causal variant (or variants).

Sporadic vs. Familial

Historically, a patient without a family history of ALS was designated as *sporadic*, while those with at least one relative with ALS were *familial* cases. Despite different genetic backgrounds, sporadic and familial ALS patients have the same spectrum of signs and symptoms. For a disease that has a very low prevalence and a short duration (onset to death), accurate family history likely is not recorded for many sporadic ALS patients [74–76]. Further, while the population risk of ALS in relatives of sporadic ALS patients is up to eight times greater than the general population, an individual has a far greater chance of having a fatal heart condition or cancer [77] and would therefore never be considered in an ALS pedigree.

It might be possible to re-classify ALS into either known-genetic or unknown-genetic causes. Causal variants are found in similar genes in both familial and sporadic ALS [4]. This overlap is more pertinent to the penetrance or average age at onset of specific variants than it is for whether a variant leads to sporadic or familial ALS. However, the distinction between familial and sporadic has been historically helpful in finding new genes. Families with autosomal-dominant ALS and sufficiently early age at onset to avoid unaffected carriers have allowed the discovery of the most penetrant and severe variants. Conversely, the sporadic model of ALS has allowed the discovery of *de novo* variants, those that arise from the germline cells of the parents [78]. While a very rare cause of sporadic ALS, validated and repeatedly observed *de novo* variants in *FUS* (primarily the p.P525L variant) [79, 80] have been reported. Whether familial/sporadic or known/unknown cause is the better choice to describe ALS inheritance will require more genetic research.

Penetrance and the Oligogenic Hypothesis

A small percentage of ALS cases carry more than one variant of an ALS gene [81–83]. Moreover, while the penetrance of *SOD1*, *TARDBP*, *FUS*, and *C9orf72* variant carriers can reach upward of 95% [84], there are always rare asymptomatic carriers [85]. Often, variants that arise in ALS genes of uncertain penetrance are extremely rare, and it is difficult to calculate the penetrance of a variant that has been observed in a single patient or family [4]. Such observations led to the *oligogenic hypothesis* in ALS: multiple variants in multiple ALS genes are necessary for ALS.

The oligogenic hypothesis is useful to frame the genetic discussion about ALS, but it should be used in specific circumstances. In patients carrying several variants in ALS genes, the age of symptom onset tends to be significantly earlier [81]. The rapidity and severity of symptoms are also increased with each additional variant observed in ALS genes. However, considering that cases with multiple ALS variants constitute a low percentage (approximately 1%) of all ALS patients [86], and because variants in ALS genes tend to have high predicted severity and effects on cellular function, it is likely that a single variant is sufficient to instigate the disease in most cases. Further, as most oligogenic cases are those with *C9orf72* HRE [86, 87], and the HRE is highly penetrant at later ages [84], oligogenic ALS cases likely explain disease severity rather than necessity. To better explore the oligogenic hypothesis, variant penetrance and severity should be considered before labeling a multi-variant case as oligogenic.

Multistep Model

In comparison with the oligogenic model, a *multistep* model posits that ALS can be considered in terms of discrete etiological steps that each sequentially contributes to disease [8, 88]. Similar to cancer models, a single germline variant may be tolerated and not directly result in disease, but coupled with environmental exposure, additional variants, age-related cellular damage, or yet unknown factors, ALS may rapidly occur once a *step* threshold has been reached [8, 88]. Because ALS has a strong association with increasing age [89], the multistep model is a logical framework to account for cell stress due to either long-term environmental exposure or the ability of neurons to resist a variant's effect.

NONCODING VARIATION

Investigation of variants associated with ALS has been mainly limited to coding regions. As genomic research progresses, more is known about noncoding regions, allowing a larger scope of inquiry.

Regulatory and Intronic Variants

Although most variants currently associated with ALS are in coding regions of genes, some discoveries of noncoding regions have been made. Variants in the untranslated regions of transcripts are generally regulatory, affecting the level and localization of transcripts [90], while intronic variants might affect splicing and nuclear export of transcripts [91]. While a rare variant is not causal simply because it is in a known ALS gene, at least some noncoding variants in these genes are likely implicated in disease risk. As the association of noncoding variants with ALS has not often been replicated or expressly studied, these variants may represent a significant proportion of missing heritability, and genetically explained cases could be higher than currently reported.

While it is rare that a single variant has a strong effect on ALS risk, ALS cases appear to have a higher burden of rare variants in the 3'UTR region of known ALS genes [86]. For example, variants in the 3'UTR of *FUS* gave elevated *FUS* expression and higher risk for ALS [92] and were observed in 1.2% of ALS cases in a study cohort [92]. Several ALS-associated genes encode for RNA binding proteins [17, 21, 36], which could interact with these untranslated regions of ALS genes. As an example, TDP-43 binding to intronic and 3'UTR regions of its RNA targets is one of its normal functions, and without proper binding, TDP-43 has a significantly higher tendency to form cytoplasmic aggregates [31].

Epigenetics

Epigenetic modifications, such as post-translational histone modifications and DNA methylation, are a mostly unexplored area of ALS genetic etiology. These modifications tend to increase or decrease the expression of genes, rather than alter the function of the gene directly. Because these marks can be impermanent, modulation of these modifications might lead to new therapeutics. However, because post-transcriptional and post-translational modifications tend to be ubiquitous and varied in usage across the genome and cell types, it will require a targeted and informed approach to manipulate these modifications. Two examples of epigenetic study are those of CpG islands in and around the *C9orf72* HRE and genome-wide histone acetylation.

Penetrance of the *C9orf72* HRE is strongly age-dependent, ranging from 60% at 60 years old to over 90% at 80 years old [8]. If cellular modulation could lower the expression of the *C9orf72* HRE, perhaps this would explain the large variance in age at symptom onset for HRE carriers. Since promoter methylation allows for the restricted expression of the downstream gene, several studies have shown a link between methylation of a promoter sequence upstream of the *C9orf72* gene and lowered transcription of the HRE [93–95]. The promoter is only hypermethylated in *cis* with the HRE [93], and non-carriers show little to no methylation [94].

The *C9orf72* HRE is a repeat of $(GGGGCC)_n$ and is therefore composed of several potential CpG sites. Whether this is of consequence to ALS genetic etiology is still in question. Early reports did not observe methylation of the HRE itself [93], but later experiments demonstrated size-dependent methylation of the HRE [96, 97]. Since the *C9orf72* HRE shows somatic instability when expanded [43], the methylation status of the HRE itself could be of interest in terms of cell-specific effects and time/age-dependent aspects. Indeed, both repeat dipeptide proteins and RNA foci are reduced in cell models of methylated HRE [97]. Whether this differential methylation is modifiable is another important consideration, since methylation patterns and age are closely correlated [98]; whether aging changes methylation patterns and therefore gene expression, or whether changes in methylation patterns result in increased aging, is unknown (for a thorough review on genomic considerations of epigenetic changes and aging, refer to Pal and Tyler [99]).

Another level of epigenetic regulation of gene expression is that of histone modifications or post-translational modifications. Observations of an upregulated microRNA (miR-206) in a transgenic h*SOD1* p.G93A mouse model led to speculation that its target mRNA, histone deacetylase 4 (*HDAC4*), could implicate chromatin remodeling in ALS [100]. Further, in ALS patients with more rapid symptom progression, *HDAC4* expression was found to be upregulated, and muscle reinnervation was lessened [101]. If miR206 targets and lowers the expression of the muscle-specific *HDAC4*, and HDAC4 decreases muscle reinnervation, it would follow that the protective effects of miR206 could be reproduced by inhibiting the action of HDAC4. Broadly inhibiting Class II HDAC proteins was found not to be effective in increasing ALS survival in hemizygous h*SOD1* p.G93A mice, although glutamate receptor uptake was restored [102]. Inhibiting HDAC4 directly in mouse skeletal muscles through knockout led to worsened symptoms and disease severity [103]. Even though increased expression of *HDAC4* correlates with ALS symptoms, its inhibition also leads to worsened symptoms [103, 104]. Unfortunately, although current research can identify modified pathways and responses to ALS cellular pathology, a clear picture of epigenetic regulation is not yet available for ALS, and further research will be needed before inhibitors can be used therapeutically [104].

CONCLUSIONS

Genetic research of ALS focuses on what causes the disease, but also on the biological implications of carrying associated variants. Many of the variants associated with ALS lead to protein misfolding or aggregation. However, it is uncertain whether misfolding and subsequent aggregation is a cause of disease or a hallmark of normal cellular response to abnormal proteins. As more biological pathways such as RNA metabolism, mitochondrial function and survival, nuclear-cytoplasmic trafficking, and synaptic transmission are being implicated in ALS, a more complete schema will emerge. One variant may be important to ALS, but as so many ALS cases are without penetrant inherited variants that it is likely a larger-scale consideration of the genome will lead to better understanding of the disease process.

ACKNOWLEDGMENTS

We thank Cal Liao, Cynthia Bourassa, Fulya Akçimen, and Zoe Schmilovich for reviewing the manuscript. JPR has received a doctoral student fellowship from the ALS Society of Canada and currently receives a Canadian Institutes of Health Research Frederick Banting and Charles Best Canada Graduate Scholarship (FRN 159279).

CONFLICT OF INTEREST

The authors declare no potential conflict of interest with respect to research, authorship, and/or publication of this manuscript.

COPYRIGHT AND PERMISSION STATEMENT

To the best of our knowledge, the materials included in this chapter do not violate copyright laws. All original sources have been appropriately acknowledged and/or referenced. Where relevant, appropriate permissions have been obtained from the original copyright holder(s).

REFERENCES

1. Ryan, M., Heverin, M., McLaughlin, R.L., and Hardiman, O. (2019). Lifetime risk and heritability of amyotrophic lateral sclerosis. *JAMA Neurol* 76 (11): 1367–1374.

2. Al-Chalabi, A., Fang, F., Hanby, M.F. et al. (2010). An estimate of amyotrophic lateral sclerosis heritability using twin data. *J Neurol Neurosurg Psychiatry* 81 (12): 1324–1326.

3. Rosen, D.R., Siddique, T., Patterson, D. et al. (1993). Mutations in Cu/Zn superoxide dismutase gene are associated with familial amyotrophic lateral sclerosis. *Nature* 362 (6415): 59–62.

4. Renton, A.E., Chio, A., and Traynor, B.J. (2014). State of play in amyotrophic lateral sclerosis genetics. *Nat Neurosci* 17 (1): 17–23.

5. Kaur, S.J., McKeown, S.R., and Rashid, S. (2016). Mutant SOD1 mediated pathogenesis of amyotrophic lateral sclerosis. *Gene* 577 (2): 109–118.

6. Parton, M.J., Broom, W., Andersen, P.M. et al. (2002). D90A-SOD1 mediated amyotrophic lateral sclerosis: a single founder for all cases with evidence for a Cis-acting disease modifier in the recessive haplotype. *Hum Mutat* 20 (6): 473.

7. Zou, Z.Y., Zhou, Z.R., Che, C.H. et al. (2017). Genetic epidemiology of amyotrophic lateral sclerosis: a systematic review and meta-analysis. *J Neurol Neurosurg Psychiatry* 88 (7): 540–549.

8. Chio, A., Mazzini, L., D'Alfonso, S. et al. (2018). The multistep hypothesis of ALS revisited: the role of genetic mutations. *Neurology* 91 (7): e635–e642.

9. Prudencio, M., Hart, P.J., Borchelt, D.R., and Andersen, P.M. (2009). Variation in aggregation propensities among ALS-associated variants of SOD1: correlation to human disease. *Hum Mol Genet* 18 (17): 3217–3226.

10. Polymenidou, M. and Cleveland, D.W. (2011). The seeds of neurodegeneration: prion-like spreading in ALS. *Cell* 147 (3): 498–508.

11. Prudencio, M. and Borchelt, D.R. (2011). Superoxide dismutase 1 encoding mutations linked to ALS adopts a spectrum of misfolded states. *Mol Neurodegener* 6: 77.

12. Hayashi, Y., Homma, K., and Ichijo, H. (2016). SOD1 in neurotoxicity and its controversial roles in SOD1 mutation-negative ALS. *Adv Biol Regul* 60: 95–104.

13. Gill, C., Phelan, J.P., Hatzipetros, T. et al. (2019). SOD1-positive aggregate accumulation in the CNS predicts slower disease progression and increased longevity in a mutant SOD1 mouse model of ALS. *Sci Rep* 9 (1): 6724.

14. Saccon, R.A., Bunton-Stasyshyn, R.K., Fisher, E.M., and Fratta, P. (2013). Is SOD1 loss of function involved in amyotrophic lateral sclerosis? *Brain* 136 (Pt 8): 2342–2358.

15. Sreedharan, J., Blair, I.P., Tripathi, V.B. et al. (2008). TDP-43 mutations in familial and sporadic amyotrophic lateral sclerosis. *Science* 319 (5870): 1668–1672.

16. Kabashi, E., Valdmanis, P.N., Dion, P. et al. (2008). TARDBP mutations in individuals with sporadic and familial amyotrophic lateral sclerosis. *Nat Genet* 40 (5): 572–574.

17. Harrison, A.F. and Shorter, J. (2017). RNA-binding proteins with prion-like domains in health and disease. *Biochem J* 474 (8): 1417–1438.

18. Van Deerlin, V.M., Leverenz, J.B., Bekris, L.M. et al. (2008). TARDBP mutations in amyotrophic lateral sclerosis with TDP-43 neuropathology: a genetic and histopatho-logical analysis. *Lancet Neurol* 7 (5): 409–416.

19. Borghero, G., Pugliatti, M., Marrosu, F. et al. (2014). Genetic architecture of ALS in Sardinia. *Neurobiol Aging* 35 (12): 2882 e7–e12.

20. Orru, S., Manolakos, E., Orru, N. et al. (2012). High frequency of the TARDBP p.Ala 382Thr mutation in Sardinian patients with amyotrophic lateral sclerosis. *Clin Genet* 81 (2): 172–178.

21. Tollervey, J.R., Curk, T., Rogelj, B. et al. (2011). Characterizing the RNA targets and position-dependent splicing regulation by TDP-43. *Nat Neurosci* 14 (4): 452–458.

22. Van Nostrand, E.L.V., Freese, P., Pratt, G.A., et al. (2020). A large-scale binding and functional map of human RNA binding proteins. *Nature* 583: 711–719. 2018.

23. Deshaies, J.E., Shkreta, L., Moszczynski, A.J. et al. (2018). TDP-43 regulates the alter-native splicing of hnRNP A1 to yield an aggregation-prone variant in amyotrophic lateral sclerosis. *Brain* 141 (5): 1320–1333.

24. Humphrey, J., Emmett, W., Fratta, P. et al. (2017). Quantitative analysis of cryptic splicing associated with TDP-43 depletion. *BMC Med Genet* 10 (1): 38.

25. Ling, J.P., Pletnikova, O., Troncoso, J.C., and Wong, P.C. (2015). TDP-43 repression of nonconserved cryptic exons is compromised in ALS-FTD. *Science* 349 (6248): 650–655.

26. Fratta, P., Sivakumar, P., Humphrey, J. et al. (2018). Mice with endogenous TDP-43 mutations exhibit gain of splicing function and characteristics of amyotrophic lateral sclerosis. *EMBO J* 37 (11): e98684.

27. Chou, C.C., Zhang, Y., Umoh, M.E. et al. (2018). TDP-43 pathology disrupts nuclear pore complexes and nucleocytoplasmic transport in ALS/FTD. *Nat Neurosci* 21 (2): 228–239.

28. Mackenzie, I.R., Bigio, E.H., Ince, P.G. et al. (2007). Pathological TDP-43 distin-guishes sporadic amyotrophic lateral sclerosis from amyotrophic lateral sclerosis with SOD1 mutations. *Ann Neurol* 61 (5): 427–434.

29. Berning, B.A. and Walker, A.K. (2019). The pathobiology of TDP-43 C-terminal frag-ments in ALS and FTLD. *Front Neurosci* 13: 335.

30. Sasaguri, H., Chew, J., Xu, Y.F. et al. (2016). The extreme N-terminus of TDP-43 medi-ates the cytoplasmic aggregation of TDP-43 and associated toxicity in vivo;. *Brain Res* 1647: 57–64.

31. Mann, J.R., Gleixner, A.M., Mauna, J.C. et al. (2019). RNA binding antagonizes neu-rotoxic phase transitions of TDP-43. *Neuron* 102 (2): 321–338. e8.

32. Voigt, A., Herholz, D., Fiesel, F.C. et al. (2010). TDP-43-mediated neuron loss in vivo; requires RNA-binding activity. *PLoS One* 5 (8): e12247.

33. Kwiatkowski, T.J. Jr., Bosco, D.A., Leclerc, A.L. et al. (2009). Mutations in the FUS/TLS gene on chromosome 16 cause familial amyotrophic lateral sclerosis. *Science* 323 (5918): 1205–1208.

34. Vance, C., Rogelj, B., Hortobagyi, T. et al. (2009). Mutations in FUS, an RNA processing protein, cause familial amyotrophic lateral sclerosis type 6. *Science* 323 (5918): 1208–1211.

35. Shang, Y. and Huang, E.J. (2016). Mechanisms of FUS mutations in familial amyotrophic lateral sclerosis. *Brain Res* 1647: 65–78.

36. Colombrita, C., Onesto, E., Megiorni, F. et al. (2012). TDP-43 and FUS RNA-binding proteins bind distinct sets of cytoplasmic messenger RNAs and differently regulate their post-transcriptional fate in motoneuron-like cells. *J Biol Chem* 287 (19): 15635–15647.

37. Ederle, H. and Dormann, D. (2017). TDP-43 and FUS en route from the nucleus to the cytoplasm. *FEBS Lett* 591 (11): 1489–1507.

38. Schwartz, J.C., Ebmeier, C.C., Podell, E.R. et al. (2012). FUS binds the CTD of RNA polymerase II and regulates its phosphorylation at Ser 2. *Genes Dev* 26 (24): 2690–2695.

39. Shiihashi, G., Ito, D., Yagi, T. et al. (2016). Mislocated FUS is sufficient for gain-of-toxic-function amyotrophic lateral sclerosis phenotypes in mice. *Brain* 139 (Pt 9): 2380–2394.

40. Renton, A.E., Majounie, E., Waite, A. et al. (2011). A hexanucleotide repeat expansion in C9ORF72 is the cause of chromosome 9p21-linked ALS-FTD. *Neuron* 72 (2): 257–268.

41. DeJesus-Hernandez, M., Mackenzie, I.R., Boeve, B.F. et al. (2011). Expanded GGGGCC hexanucleotide repeat in noncoding region of C9ORF72 causes chromosome 9p-linked FTD and ALS. *Neuron* 72 (2): 245–256.

42. Morita, M., Al-Chalabi, A., Andersen, P.M. et al. (2006). A locus on chromosome 9p confers susceptibility to ALS and frontotemporal dementia. *Neurology* 66 (6): 839–844.

43. Nordin, A., Akimoto, C., Wuolikainen, A. et al. (2015). Extensive size variability of the GGGGCC expansion in C9orf72 in both neuronal and non-neuronal tissues in 18 patients with ALS or FTD. *Hum Mol Genet* 24 (11): 3133–3142.

44. Iacoangeli, A., Al Khleifat, A., Jones, A.R. et al. (2019). C9orf72 intermediate expansions of 24–30 repeats are associated with ALS. *Acta Neuropathol Commun* 7 (1): 115.

45. Ross, J.P., Leblond, C.S., Catoire, H. et al. (2019). Somatic expansion of the C9orf72 hexanucleotide repeat does not occur in ALS spinal cord tissues. *Neurol Genet* 5 (2): e317.

46. Babic Leko, M., Zupunski, V., Kirincich, J. et al. (2019). Molecular mechanisms of neurodegeneration related to C9orf72 hexanucleotide repeat expansion. *Behav Neurol* 2019: 2909168.

47. Ishiguro, A., Kimura, N., Watanabe, Y. et al. (2016). TDP-43 binds and transports G-quadruplex-containing mRNAs into neurites for local translation. *Genes Cells* 21 (5): 466–481.

48. Prudencio, M., Belzil, V.V., Batra, R. et al. (2015). Distinct brain transcriptome profiles in C9orf72-associated and sporadic ALS. *Nat Neurosci* 18 (8): 1175–1182.

49. Moens, T.G., Mizielinska, S., Niccoli, T. et al. (2018). Sense and antisense RNA are not toxic in drosophila models of C9orf72-associated ALS/FTD. *Acta Neuropathol* 135 (3): 445–457.

50. Mori, K., Weng, S.M., Arzberger, T. et al. (2013). The C9orf72 GGGGCC repeat is translated into aggregating dipeptide-repeat proteins in FTLD/ALS. *Science* 339 (6125): 1335–1338.

51. Swaminathan, A., Bouffard, M., Liao, M. et al. (2018). Expression of C9orf72-related dipeptides impairs motor function in a vertebrate model. *Hum Mol Genet* 27 (10): 1754–1762.

52. Moens, T.G., Niccoli, T., Wilson, K.M. et al. (2019). C9orf72 arginine-rich dipeptide proteins interact with ribosomal proteins in vivo; to induce a toxic translational arrest that is rescued by eIF1A. *Acta Neuropathol* 137 (3): 487–500.

53. Shi, K.Y., Mori, E., Nizami, Z.F. et al. (2017). Toxic PRn poly-dipeptides encoded by the C9orf72 repeat expansion block nuclear import and export. *Proc Natl Acad Sci U S A* 114 (7): E1111–E1117.

54. Taylor, J.P., Brown, R.H. Jr., and Cleveland, D.W. (2016). Decoding ALS: from genes to mechanism. *Nature* 539 (7628): 197–206.

55. Brenner, D. and Weishaupt, J.H. (2019). Update on amyotrophic lateral sclerosis genetics. *Curr Opin Neurol* 32 (5): 735–739.

56. Corcia, P., Couratier, P., Blasco, H. et al. (2017). Genetics of amyotrophic lateral sclerosis. *Rev Neurol (Paris)* 173 (5): 254–262.

57. Leblond, C.S., Kaneb, H.M., Dion, P.A., and Rouleau, G.A. (2014). Dissection of genetic factors associated with amyotrophic lateral sclerosis. *Exp Neurol* 262 (Pt B): 91–101.

58. Mathis, S., Couratier, P., Julian, A. et al. (2017). Current view and perspectives in amyotrophic lateral sclerosis. *Neural Regen Res* 12 (2): 181–184.

59. Zufiria, M., Gil-Bea, F.J., Fernandez-Torron, R. et al. (2016). ALS: a bucket of genes, environment, metabolism and unknown ingredients. *Prog Neurobiol* 142: 104–129.

60. MacNair, L., Xiao, S., Miletic, D. et al. (2016). MTHFSD and DDX58 are novel RNA-binding proteins abnormally regulated in amyotrophic lateral sclerosis. *Brain* 139 (Pt 1): 86–100.

61. Chia, R., Chiò, A., and Traynor, B.J. (2018). Novel genes associated with amyotrophic lateral sclerosis: diagnostic and clinical implications. *Lancet Neurol* 17 (1): 94–102.

62. Smith, B.N., Topp, S.D., Fallini, C. et al. (2017). Mutations in the vesicular trafficking protein annexin A11 are associated with amyotrophic lateral sclerosis. *Sci Transl Med* 9 (388): eaad9157.

63. Liu, X., Wu, C., He, J. et al. (2019). Two rare variants of the ANXA11 gene identified in Chinese patients with amyotrophic lateral sclerosis. *Neurobiol Aging* 74: 235 e9–e12.

64. Tsai, P.C., Liao, Y.C., Jih, K.Y. et al. (2018). Genetic analysis of ANXA11 variants in a Han Chinese cohort with amyotrophic lateral sclerosis in Taiwan. *Neurobiol Aging* 72: 188 e1–e2.

65. Zhang, K., Liu, Q., Liu, K. et al. (2018). ANXA11 mutations prevail in Chinese ALS patients with and without cognitive dementia. *Neurol Genet* 4 (3): e237.

66. Ferrara, D., Pasetto, L., Bonetto, V., and Basso, M. (2018). Role of extracellular vesicles in amyotrophic lateral sclerosis. *Front Neurosci* 12: 574.

67. Cooper-Knock, J., Moll, T., Ramesh, T. et al. (2019). Mutations in the glycosyltransferase domain of GLT8D1 are associated with familial amyotrophic lateral sclerosis. *Cell Rep* 26 (9): 2298–2306. e5.

68. Consortium PMAS (2018). Project MinE: study design and pilot analyses of a large-scale whole-genome sequencing study in amyotrophic lateral sclerosis. *Eur J Hum Genet* 26 (10): 1537–1546.

69. Melamed, Z., Lopez-Erauskin, J., Baughn, M.W. et al. (2019). Premature polyadenylation-mediated loss of stathmin-2 is a hallmark of TDP-43-dependent neurodegeneration. *Nat Neurosci* 22 (2): 180–190.

70. Klim, J.R., Williams, L.A., Limone, F. et al. (2019). ALS-implicated protein TDP-43 sustains levels of STMN2, a mediator of motor neuron growth and repair. *Nat Neurosci* 22 (2): 167–179.

71. Clark, J.A., Yeaman, E.J., Blizzard, C.A. et al. (2016). A case for microtubule vulnerability in amyotrophic lateral sclerosis: altered dynamics during disease. *Front Cell Neurosci* 10: 204.

72. Brenner, D., Yilmaz, R., Muller, K. et al. (2018). Hot-spot KIF5A mutations cause familial ALS. *Brain* 141 (3): 688–697.

73. Nicolas, A., Kenna, K.P., Renton, A.E. et al. (2018). Genome-wide analyses identify KIF5A as a novel ALS gene. *Neuron* 97 (6): 1268–1283. e6.

74. McCann, E.P., Williams, K.L., Fifita, J.A. et al. (2017). The genotype-phenotype landscape of familial amyotrophic lateral sclerosis in Australia. *Clin Genet* 92 (3): 259–266.

75. Gibson, S.B., Figueroa, K.P., Bromberg, M.B. et al. (2014). Familial clustering of ALS in a population-based resource. *Neurology* 82 (1): 17–22.

76. Ryan, M., Heverin, M., Doherty, M.A. et al. (2018). Determining the incidence of familiality in ALS: a study of temporal trends in Ireland from 1994 to 2016. *Neurol Genet* 4 (3): e239.

77. Hanby, M.F., Scott, K.M., Scotton, W. et al. (2011). The risk to relatives of patients with sporadic amyotrophic lateral sclerosis. *Brain* 134 (Pt 12): 3454–3457.

78. Chesi, A., Staahl, B.T., Jovicic, A. et al. (2013). Exome sequencing to identify de novo mutations in sporadic ALS trios. *Nat Neurosci* 16 (7): 851–855.

79. Conte, A., Lattante, S., Zollino, M. et al. (2012). P525L FUS mutation is consistently associated with a severe form of juvenile amyotrophic lateral sclerosis. *Neuromuscul Disord* 22 (1): 73–75.

80. Leblond, C.S., Webber, A., Gan-Or, Z. et al. (2016). De novo FUS P525L mutation in Juvenile amyotrophic lateral sclerosis with dysphonia and diplopia. *Neurol Genet* 2 (2): e63.

81. Cady, J., Allred, P., Bali, T. et al. (2015). Amyotrophic lateral sclerosis onset is influenced by the burden of rare variants in known amyotrophic lateral sclerosis genes. *Ann Neurol* 77 (1): 100–113.

82. Giannoccaro, M.P., Bartoletti-Stella, A., Piras, S. et al. (2017). Multiple variants in families with amyotrophic lateral sclerosis and frontotemporal dementia related to C9orf72 repeat expansion: further observations on their oligogenic nature. *J Neurol* 264 (7): 1426–1433.

83. van Blitterswijk, M., van Es, M.A., Hennekam, E.A. et al. (2012). Evidence for an oligogenic basis of amyotrophic lateral sclerosis. *Hum Mol Genet* 21 (17): 3776–3784.

84. Murphy, N.A., Arthur, K.C., Tienari, P.J. et al. (2017). Age-related penetrance of the C9orf72 repeat expansion. *Sci Rep* 7 (1): 2116.

85. McGoldrick, P., Zhang, M., van Blitterswijk, M. et al. (2018). Unaffected mosaic C9orf72 case: RNA foci, dipeptide proteins, but upregulated C9orf72 expression. *Neurology* 90 (4): e323–e331.

86. Morgan, S., Shatunov, A., Sproviero, W. et al. (2017). A comprehensive analysis of rare genetic variation in amyotrophic lateral sclerosis in the UK. *Brain* 140 (6): 1611–1618.

87. Lattante, S., Ciura, S., Rouleau, G.A., and Kabashi, E. (2015). Defining the genetic connection linking amyotrophic lateral sclerosis (ALS) with frontotemporal dementia (FTD). *Trends Genet* 31 (5): 263–273.

88. Al-Chalabi, A., Calvo, A., Chio, A. et al. (2014). Analysis of amyotrophic lateral sclerosis as a multistep process: a population-based modelling study. *Lancet Neurol* 13 (11): 1108–1113.

89. Niccoli, T., Partridge, L., and Isaacs, A.M. (2017). Ageing as a risk factor for ALS/FTD. *Hum Mol Genet* 26 (R2): R105–R113.

90. Wanke, K.A., Devanna, P., and Vernes, S.C. (2018). Understanding neurodevelopmental disorders: the promise of regulatory variation in the 3'UTRome. *Biol Psychiatry* 83 (7): 548–557.

91. Shaul, O. (2017). How introns enhance gene expression. *Int J Biochem Cell Biol* 91 (Pt B): 145–155.

92. Sabatelli, M., Moncada, A., Conte, A. et al. (2013). Mutations in the 3' untranslated region of FUS causing FUS overexpression are associated with amyotrophic lateral sclerosis. *Hum Mol Genet* 22 (23): 4748–4755.

93. Liu, E.Y., Russ, J., Wu, K. et al. (2014). C9orf72 hypermethylation protects against repeat expansion-associated pathology in ALS/FTD. *Acta Neuropathol* 128 (4): 525–541.

94. Xi, Z., Zinman, L., Moreno, D. et al. (2013). Hypermethylation of the CpG island near the G4C2 repeat in ALS with a C9orf72 expansion. *Am J Hum Genet* 92 (6): 981–989.

95. McMillan, C.T., Russ, J., Wood, E.M. et al. (2015). C9orf72 promoter hypermethylation is neuroprotective neuroimaging and neuropathologic evidence. *Neurology* 84 (16): 1622–1630.

96. Xi, Z., Zhang, M., Bruni, A.C. et al. (2015). The C9orf72 repeat expansion itself is methylated in ALS and FTLD patients. *Acta Neuropathol* 129 (5): 715–727.

97. Bauer, P.O. (2016). Methylation of C9orf72 expansion reduces RNA foci formation and dipeptide-repeat proteins expression in cells. *Neurosci Lett* 612: 204–209.

98. Zhang, M., Tartaglia, M.C., Moreno, D. et al. (2017). DNA methylation age-acceleration is associated with disease duration and age at onset in C9orf72 patients. *Acta Neuropathol* 134 (2): 271–279.

99. Pal, S. and Tyler, J.K. (2016). Epigenetics and aging. *Sci Adv* 2 (7): e1600584.

100. Williams, A.H., Valdez, G., Moresi, V. et al. (2009). Micro RNA-206 delays ALS progression and promotes regeneration of neuromuscular synapses in mice. *Science* 326 (5959): 1549–1554.

101. Bruneteau, G., Simonet, T., Bauche, S. et al. (2013). Muscle histone deacetylase 4 upregulation in amyotrophic lateral sclerosis: potential role in reinnervation ability and disease progression. *Brain* 136 (Pt 8): 2359–2368.

102. Lapucci, A., Cavone, L., Buonvicino, D. et al. (2017). Effect of class II HDAC inhibition on glutamate transporter expression and survival in SOD1-ALS mice. *Neurosci Lett* 656: 120–125.

103. Pigna, E., Simonazzi, E., Sanna, K. et al. (2019). Histone deacetylase 4 protects from denervation and skeletal muscle atrophy in a murine model of amyotrophic lateral sclerosis. *EBioMedicine* 40: 717–732.

104. Boutillier, A.L., Tzeplaeff, L., and Dupuis, L. (2019). The dark side of HDAC inhibition in ALS. *EBioMedicine* 41: 38–39.

CHAPTER 3

Susceptibility Genes and Epigenetics in Sporadic ALS

Jessica R. Morrice[1], Christopher A. Shaw[1,2,3,4], and
Cheryl Y. Gregory-Evans[1,2,4]

[1] Experimental Medicine Program, University of British Columbia, Vancouver, British Columbia, Canada
[2] Department of Ophthalmology and Visual Sciences, University of British Columbia, Vancouver, British Columbia, Canada
[3] Department of Pathology, University of British Columbia, Vancouver, British Columbia, Canada
[4] Program in Neuroscience, University of British Columbia, Vancouver, British Columbia, Canada

INTRODUCTION

Amyotrophic lateral sclerosis (ALS) is an adult-onset neurodegenerative disease characterized by the progressive degeneration of both upper and lower motor neurons. ALS is considered as being either familial or sporadic in origin; however, familial amyotrophic lateral sclerosis (fALS) and sporadic amyotrophic lateral sclerosis (sALS) patients are clinically indistinguishable [1]. A patient is diagnosed as having fALS if there is a familial history of disease, and a number of causal genes have been identified [2]. Approximately 90% of all ALS cases are considered sporadic in origin, meaning there is no clear family history of disease [1]. However, history of familial inheritance may be affected by factors such as premature death from unrelated causes prior to diagnosis, misdiagnosis, or comorbidities [1], which at times makes differentiating sALS from fALS ambiguous.

ENVIRONMENTAL ASSOCIATIONS IN sALS

Many groups have assumed that sALS is not purely genetic in origin [3–7]. The evidence supporting this view is largely based on a lack of a clear inheritance pattern evident in sALS cases and on documented trends of increased incidence relative to a specific geographical location [4, 5], lifestyle [8], or occupation type [3, 9–12]. In this chapter, we discuss noteworthy examples supporting a role for the environment in sALS etiology. For a comprehensive review of this subject, see Al-Chalabi and Hardiman [13] and Riancho et al. [14].

The best-supported examples demonstrating the involvement of environmental factors in sALS are geographical clusters of increased disease incidence on the island of Guam, in Irian Jaya, and on the Kii Peninsula of Japan. These clusters demonstrated a clear increased disease incidence during a limited period. Specifically, an estimated 40× increase incidence of disease was evident in the native Chamorro population on the island of Guam during the 1950s, which rapidly declined after the 1960s [15] (see Chapter 4 for further information), and up to a 5× increased disease incidence was documented on the Kii Peninsula [16]. These disease clusters prompted an investigation into causal factors for disease, including genetic and environmental agents [17, 18]. Initial genetic analysis revealed no causative gene [19, 20], and further investigation has focused primarily on causal environmental factors such as lifestyle [21–23]. It is important to note that a more recent and robust study indicates that up to three loci may be associated with ALS-parkinsonism-dementia complex (ALS-PDC) in the Chammoro population [24]. However, diet-associated toxins emerged as being the most likely trigger, such as those contained in cycad seeds: steryl glucosides or cyanotoxins [25, 26], although this latter toxic factor has been disputed [27].

These studies provided a framework for further investigation of how the environment can contribute to the motor neuron degeneration that characterizes ALS, and this concept has been further exemplified in specific cases with common lifestyle factors or exposures. An example implicating high-level sports includes studies of Italian football (soccer) players who demonstrated a 6.5–11.6 fold excess risk of death from ALS [28, 29]. These types of commonalities between patients have led to the investigation of specific external factors such as pesticide exposure from the playing field [29], high-level athleticism [30], body mass index [31], and traumatic brain injury [32].

Experimentally, it has been demonstrated that certain candidate environmental toxins can cause motor neuron degeneration both *in vitro* [33, 34] and *in vivo* [33, 35]. Yet despite many efforts, a clear conclusion has yet to emerge on the causal role of these various exposures, as some of these findings are not reproducible in different exposure populations [36, 37] or cannot demonstrate motor neuron degeneration *in vivo* [38]. Thus, while it is evident that the environment is associated with sALS, clear causality has yet to be demonstrated. One potential explanation is that an individual has infinite environmental exposures throughout their lifetime, termed an *exposome* [39]. Each individual's particular exposome is unique, and different

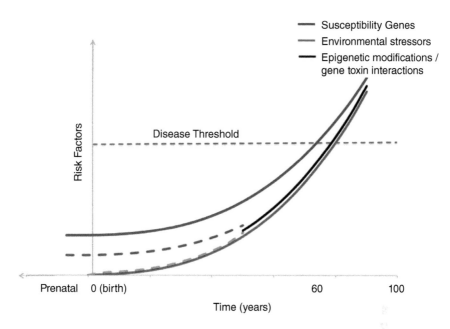

FIGURE 3.1   Risk factors in proposed etiologies for sALS. Susceptibility genes, environmental stressors, and epigenetic modifications are represented by blue, magenta, and black in the graph, respectively. The Y-axis represents the accumulation of sALS risk factors through an individual's lifespan, where some individuals are born with genetic and epigenetic susceptibility to disease, and the X-axis represents age. The red dotted line represents the disease threshold of cellular dysfunction resulting from susceptibility genes and/or environmental stressors that an individual can tolerate until a patient presents with clinical signs of disease. Blue line: Multiple susceptibility genes may have an additive effect on sALS predisposition. Black line: The presence of sALS susceptibility genes may put an individual at an increased risk of developing disease, which is triggered by sufficient exposure to environmental stressors. The green dashed line represents gene-toxin interactions, and the purple dashed line represents epigenomic alterations *in utero*. Magenta line: Extensive exposure to environmental stressor(s) may be sufficient to cause disease onset.

environmental stressors may have a cumulative effect on neuronal dysfunction (Figure 3.1). As implied, this concept is immensely challenging to investigate with current technology, methods, and computational challenges and heavily relies on recall bias [13].

Another potential explanation is that individuals have an inherently vulnerable predisposition to certain environmental stressors, such as through genetic risk factors. Different gene variants may put one at risk for disease development, which can be triggered by sufficient exposure to stressors. Organophosphates are a widely used pesticide to which humans are exposed through diet and occupational exposure. These pesticides are known to inhibit acetylcholinesterase, which causes an accumulation of acetylcholine at the synapse, and to modulate the inflammatory response [40].

Epidemiological studies have described pesticides, in particular organophosphates, as an environmental risk factor for sALS [3, 6]. Organophosphates are hydrolyzed by paraoxonase-1 (PON1), and polymorphisms in this gene are known to affect its enzymatic activity [41]. PON1 is a hydrolytic enzyme that has peroxidase activity important for oxidative stress [42]. Clinical studies show that *PON1* variants are associated with sALS patients [43] and in etiologically grouped ALS patients [44]. However, this finding has not been replicated in other studies [45]. This discrepancy may suggest that more careful inclusion criteria are needed in gene-toxin studies, as a patient cohort with a mixed genetic background may confound results. Further, these studies rely on recall bias and may not reflect reliable exposure doses, and do not consider interactions of different toxins and/or genes. Taken together, while these studies may suggest a gene-toxin interaction in sALS, this complex subject warrants further careful investigation.

GENETIC BASIS OF sALS

Despite a substantial body of evidence suggesting a role for environmental factors in sALS, the lack of clear causal evidence suggests that the etiology may be more complex than solely being driven by environmental factors alone. Specifically, it appears that exposure to environmental stressors may not be sufficient to cause sALS, as not all individuals exposed to similar doses of a specific environmental factor develop disease. This highlights sALS etiology as likely to be multifactorial and complex in origin, and suggests that some individuals may be genetically predisposed to sALS if provided the necessary genetic background.

This concept of a genetic predisposition to sALS is further supported by studies of sALS discordance in monozygotic (MZ) twins. MZ twins share the same genome; therefore, a strong correlation of disease concordance in twins indicates that sALS has a substantial genetic component [46], although we note that early-life environmental factors are also shared. A meta-analysis using 49 MZ twins showed that 10.2% were sALS concordant and 89.8% were discordant [46]; this indicates strong environmental involvement yet also provides evidence for a genetic predisposition for sALS. Further, twin studies estimate sALS heritability to be 61%, nominating this as a complex genetic disease [46]. Together, twin studies provide strong evidence for the involvement of environmental stressors and also support a genetic basis for sALS.

The genetic contribution to sALS is becoming widely accepted [11, 13, 14, 47], and technological advances in genetic analyses are leading to the discovery of many gene variants in sALS patients [48–53]. Gibson et al. found that 10% of sALS patients carried a known causal variant or repeat expansion in known ALS genes, despite lacking a family history of disease [1]. Further, 18 potentially novel rare variants were identified in known ALS genes, and 17.2% of sALS patients had at least one rare variant or repeat expansion in ALS-associated genes [1]. These known ALS genes are the only reliable genes that have consistently been replicated in patient cohorts [46], and many studies have implicated novel susceptibility genes, as discussed below [54–56]. Of note, population studies show that novel susceptibility genes may occur more frequently in specific ethnic populations than others [52, 57–59]. For example, sALS patients with European ancestry are more likely to carry single nucleotide polymorphisms (SNPs) in certain genes than sALS patients of Chinese ancestry [52, 57, 59].

Indeed, a number of gene mutations are found more frequently in sALS patients than unaffected controls [60, 61], and the contribution of genetic variants to sALS patients with European ancestry is estimated between 14.9 and 21.8% [1]. Currently, a hexanucleotide repeat expansion in chromosome 9 open reading frame 72 (*C9orf72*) accounts for the majority of genetic risk for sALS [62, 63], and others such as *UNC13A*, *DPP6*, and *C21orf2* have been identified [51, 55, 56], as discussed below.

Given the classical definition of sALS and fALS, a new perspective on the genetic basis of sALS is emerging. There is an argument that the designation of sALS from fALS is arbitrary, and instead, a classification of ALS patients as either having a clear family history of disease or not is more accurate [46, 64]. ALS can therefore be described as a disease with or without a dominant genetic basis following Mendelian heritability. The latter regards this as a complex genetic disease likely with the environment playing a role. There is also emerging evidence for non-Mendelian heritability in sALS. One study showed that the heritability of sALS in siblings and offspring of a proband has been estimated to be a 9 and 17 times increased risk of developing disease, respectively [65].

Considering that sALS is a relatively rare disease, it may be likely that a single gene variant alone is insufficient to drive an increased risk of disease development, proposing an oligogenic basis of disease [61, 66], where candidate genetic variants may act synergistically to drive sALS susceptibility. Indeed, data suggest that sALS has a polygenic rare variant architecture, where low-frequency SNPs contribute to disease variance and sub-genome-wide significant SNPs may account for the bulk of heritability [51]. This type of complex disease may not display a clear Mendelian pattern of inheritance [61]. Therefore, future genetic studies in sALS may be well advised to focus on low-frequency alleles and non-penetrant genes, and perhaps investigate genetic pleiotropy as the basis for etiology [67].

IDENTIFICATION OF sALS SUSCEPTIBILITY GENES

Together with advances in genome sequencing technology, the use of genome-wide association studies (GWASs) has created a new era for identifying novel susceptibility genes. Since ALS is an adult-onset disease of low prevalence, large GWASs are particularly valuable to investigate the complex genetic structure underlying sALS. Indeed, a number of GWASs have been invaluable for identifying novel gene variants in both fALS and sALS [48, 49, 51, 54–56, 68] and also proposing specific variants as candidate disease modifiers (as reviewed in Ghasemi and Brown [61]). However, GWASs should be interpreted cautiously, particularly if the study was underpowered or had flaws in study design. Of note, it is essential to consider population ethnicity in designing and interpreting results from GWASs as genetic heterogeneity is an important factor in the frequency of genetic sALS susceptibility [69], as discussed above.

CANDIDATE sALS SUSCEPTIBILITY GENES

A number of genes have been implicated in both fALS and sALS, yet it has proven difficult to predict a gene's connection to ALS based on gene function alone [47]. However, when considering the biological processes of many genes implicated in both fALS and sALS, specific biological processes emerge as a common theme: protein homeostasis, RNA processing, and cytoskeletal dynamics [47]. An increasingly prominent perspective is that disruption in these biological processes triggers a secondary downstream dysfunction, including mitochondrial dysfunction, oxidative stress, RNA aggregates, and neuronal excitability [47, 61]. Many different genes can affect these processes, yet these data suggest a common pathway of sensitivity for motor neuron degeneration that can be used as support when interpreting candidate sALS susceptibility genes proposed by findings from GWAS.

An important resource for identifying novel susceptibility genes common to sALS patients is the Project MiNE database, a worldwide repository working to sequence at least 15 000 whole genomes from ALS patients, with a heavy focus on sALS genomes (Project MinE Data Browser, http://databrowser.projectmine.com). As more robust genome-wide data become available, it is reasonable to expect more susceptibility genes to emerge. Below we have highlighted a short list of top candidate sALS susceptibility genes to date, and this list continues to grow and change with improvements in genome sequencing technology and an increased number of sequenced genomes. Because *C9orf72* has been described in detail in Chapter 2, we do not discuss it here. For a more comprehensive list of genes involved in sALS, see Ghasemi and Brown [61].

UNC13A

A relatively large GWAS performed by van Es et al. identified *UNC13A* as a novel susceptibility gene in sALS patients [55]. UNC13A is a presynaptic protein that functions in neurotransmitter regulation at the neuromuscular synapse. *UNC13A*-deficient mice are born paralyzed and die shortly after birth. Mutant mice showed abnormalities in muscle morphology, spinal motor neuron populations, and the structure of neuromuscular junctions [70]. The association between sALS and *UNC13A* has been replicated in independent studies [51, 71–73]. Of note, studies implicating *UNC13A* as a sALS susceptibility gene were performed in non-Asian populations, and this association is not evident in studies using Chinese and Japanese patients [73].

DPP6

After increasing the sample size, the same group that found an association with *UNC13A* also discovered that a SNP in *DPP6* is associated with increased risk of sALS in European populations [56]. The *DPP6* gene encodes a component of neuronal type-A transmembrane protein that functions to bind and regulate voltage-gated potassium channels. *DPP6* knockout mice show increased motor activity as compared to control animals, as well as impaired learning and memory, and showed defects such as in the hippocampus and reduction in the weight of the brain and total body [74]. *DPP6* has previously been associated with autism spectrum disorder and schizophrenia [75]. Interestingly, there is a genetic overlap between schizophrenia and sALS, with an estimated genetic correlation of 14.3% [76]. Another study using European populations supported the association of *DPP6* with sALS [77], although these results have been challenged [78]. These findings have not been replicated in Asian populations [57, 79], which supports that certain risk variants may be specific to particular genetic ancestries.

C21orf2

Another interesting locus that has been implicated as a sALS susceptibility gene in a large and robust GWAS is *C21orf2* [51]. This study used an ALS-specific custom imputation panel, thereby providing a more accurate imputation of statistically inferring unobserved genotypes. This feature was pivotal for revealing *C21orf2* as a sALS susceptibility gene. C21orf2 is a mitochondrial protein involved in DNA damage repair and cytoskeleton organization. Of note, the C21orf2 protein interacts with NEK1 [80], another fALS- and sALS-associated gene. It has been estimated that 75% of mutations in *C21orf2* are likely to be deleterious [81], and indeed it has been associated with many pathologies, including retinal degeneration [82]. The finding that this gene is associated with sALS remains to be replicated in other GWASs, and whether this variant is also found in Asian populations remains to be determined.

EPIGENETIC MECHANISMS IN sALS

Epigenetic modifications are another possible alteration to the genetic architecture that may confer a risk for developing sALS. The term *epigenetics* means "above" the genome, meaning that the epigenome functions to directly affect the expression of genes [83]. A simplified definition of epigenetic modifications is the heritable alteration to gene expression that occurs in response to environmental stimuli without changes to the nucleotide sequence [83, 84]. Alterations in the epigenome may therefore contribute to disease regardless of the presence of any pathogenic variants.

In sALS, epigenetic studies remain limited as most studies are based on genetic models of disease or mixed sALS and fALS patient cohorts [85–88]. At this time, DNA methylation, miRNA, and histone post-translational modification are the best-characterized epigenetic modifications; therefore, we focus on these mechanisms below in the context of sALS patients, or mutant models non-specific to fALS. For a further review of different mechanisms more broadly in ALS, see Jimenez-Pacheco et al. [89] and Bennett et al. [90].

Methylation in sALS

One of the best-characterized epigenetic mechanisms is DNA methylation. DNA is methylated after a methyl group is transferred by DNA methyltransferase (DNMT), typically to a cysteine residue followed by guanine residues, or CpG site. DNA methylation is known to directly affect gene expression, where methylated DNA is most often associated with repressed transgene expression, generally at the promoter [83]. This methyl group transfer is reversible, resulting in demethylation and therefore activating gene expression [83]. Aging is associated with the aberrant methylation status of DNA, prompting the inquiry into age-related neurodegenerative diseases like ALS [91]. For a comprehensive review on DNA methylation and recent advances in epigenetics, see Cavalli and Heard [92].

The study of epigenetics in sALS has revealed a number of DNA modifications that affect gene expression [93, 94]. Altered methylation status is evident in sALS patients. An epigenome-wide association study observed hypo- or hypermethylated sites in 23 genes and 3 CpG islands. This study found that these genes are involved in calcium homeostasis, neurotransmission, and oxidative stress [95]. Motor neurons lacking nuclear TDP-43 appear to have reduced methylated cysteine residues as compared to motor neurons lacking evident TDP-43 pathology [91]. Another group found that methylation and hydroxymethylation of immune and inflammatory genes are altered in sALS patients [93]. This finding is consistent with previous literature demonstrating that microglia and peripheral immune cells display an altered inflammatory state during pathogenesis [96], suggesting an epigenetic basis for this pathologic feature. Interestingly, Appleby-Mallinder et al. found that glial cells collected from the spinal cord tissue of sALS patients have no significant difference in cysteine methylation [91].

Further studies have shown that DNMTs may be involved in ALS pathogenesis (further reviewed in Martin and Wong [97]), providing additional evidence of aberrant methylation status in sALS [95]. Notably, sALS patients with a hexanucleotide repeat expansion in *C9orf72* show hypermethylation in the repeat expansion itself and at the 5′ CpG island [98, 99]. Correspondingly, reduced expression of *C9orf72* is evident [100, 101], suggesting that loss of protein function is a potential pathogenic mechanism. However, a more convincing body of evidence implicates a gain of toxic function in driving neurodegeneration [102], and this methylation of *C9orf72* may be more compensatory than causative to the disease state.

miRNAs in sALS

Many other types of heritable modifications are known to affect gene expression, such as post-translational histone modifications like histone methylation, phosphorylation, and ubiquitination; changes in nucleosome positioning; transcription factors such as polycomb proteins; and noncoding RNAs (as further reviewed in Hwang et al. [83] and Cavalli and Heard [92]). There are different categories of noncoding RNAs, such as long and short noncoding RNAs. MicroRNAs are a type of short noncoding RNA that have a significant role in gene regulation, such as RNA silencing, and regulating post-transcriptional processes by destabilizing mRNA or impairing translation efficiency [89, 92, 103]. MicroRNAs are essential for gene network responses in neurons and can affect neuronal plasticity and survival [89, 90].

Recently, miRNAs have been implicated in sALS and are being pursued for their role both in disease and as potential biomarkers [103–105]. miRNAs have been found largely down-regulated in the post mortem spinal cord [103] and in blood samples [104, 105] of sALS patients. Waller et al. found that differentially expressed miRNAs are involved in glucose metabolism and oxidative stress regulation [106]. Of note, TDP-43 and fused in sarcoma (FUS) are involved in miRNAs biogenesis [103], and the nuclear loss and cytoplasmic pathological aggregation of TDP-43, which is evident in approximately 98% of sALS patients (as further described in Chapter 6), may be an essential mechanism underlying miRNA involvement in sALS. However, it is important to consider that findings from post mortem samples may be more reflective of outcomes rather than causes of upstream pathogenic mechanisms. A primary advantage of pursuing these differentially expressed noncoding RNAs is to gain insight not only into the pathophysiology of sALS, but also into their role as potential diagnostic and progression biomarkers [104, 105]. This is particularly true of blood samples, which may not be representative of epigenetic alterations in the central nervous system (CNS) [91] and may be better suited in the clinic to serve to advance diagnostic and progression accuracy.

Post-Translational Histone Modification in sALS

Histones function to organize DNA into chromatin, which is made up of DNA wrapped around the core histones H2A, H2B, H3, and H4. Histone N-terminal tails and structured globular domains are susceptible to epigenetic modifications [107]. The post-translational modification of histones, such as through the addition and removal of acetyl groups through histone acetyltransferases (HATs) and histone deacetyltransferases (HDACs), respectively, is an important epigenetic modification that alters the stability of interactions between DNA and histones [90]. Histone methylation can be altered by histone methyltransferases on lysine and arginine residues, where the degree of methylation and also symmetry are known to change the electronic charge of the histone side chain [107]. Many other chemical moieties can modify the N-terminal tails of histones, such as through phosphorylation by kinases such as AMP kinase (see Lennartsson and Ekwall [108] for further review). Such modifications can remodel chromatin to active or repressive states, thus influencing gene transcription and expression [90].

Enzymes that alter histone modifications are also implicated in sALS. Elongator protein 3 (ELP3) is a catalytic subunit of the HAT complex. Loss-of-function *ELP3* variants are associated with sALS and were validated to cause a defective motor neuron phenotype *in vivo* [109]. In a mouse model overexpressing human TDP-43, reduced levels and activity of HDAC1 were evident in the nucleus, which correlated with TDP-43 proteinopathy. The neurodegenerative phenotype was ameliorated after inducing HDAC1 activity [110]. Further, levels of HDAC 11 were reduced and levels of HDAC2 were elevated, respectively, in the sALS brain and spinal cord [111]. Berson et al. demonstrated that the chromatin remodeling enzymes chromodomain helicase DNA binding protein 1 (CHD1) modifies TDP-43 proteinopathy, and CHD2 interacts with TDP-43 [112]. Together, these studies support the role of post-translational modifications to histones and chromatin remodeling in sALS.

As post-mitotic cells, neurons do not propagate epigenetic modifications to progeny cells as dividing cells do, making the classical definition of epigenetics unique for the CNS [83]. However, gene transcription in neurons is affected by equivalent epigenetic modifications peripherally, proposing that dysregulation is an important contributing factor for neurological diseases such as sALS [83].

Epigenetic Analysis in Monozygotic sALS Twins

Studies based on MZ twins are particularly useful for investigating the epigenetic basis of disease as these individuals share the same genome and have been exposed to equivalent *in utero* and frequently similar early life *ex utero* exposures [113]. Analysis of the methylation pattern in MZ twins discordant for sALS was found to be distinct across the genome, where the sALS-affected twin displayed an older age epigenetically than the unaffected twin [113, 114]. However, many of these aberrantly methylated regions were found to be non-overlapping between the sALS-affected twins [113]. These non-overlapping regions had a common ontology of sequence-specific DNA binding, implicating transcription as a potential pathogenic feature of sALS [113]. Affected twins had aberrant methylation in genes involved in pathways signaling the γ-aminobutyric acid (GABA) receptor [113], an early pathogenic feature evident in patients. Of note, there was no abnormal methylation pattern in the promoter regions of known ALS genes [113]. It is important to consider that this was a relatively small study based on blood samples, which may not be representative of the epigenetic signature of the CNS. It remains to be seen if other types of epigenetic modifications are evident in discordant MZ twins and also whether epigenetic modifications are a cause or result of disease. To further characterize the role of the epigenome, larger sALS MZ twin studies would prove useful.

MODIFICATIONS TO THE EPIGENOME BY ENVIRONMENTAL FACTORS

Both natural and environmental factors can induce mutations in each individual genome, which can be transmitted to offspring [92]. Although most of these mutations are predicted to have a null protein-coding effect, sequence variations can have a more direct effect on modifying epigenomic landscapes. Different environmental stimuli known to directly affect epigenetics include temperature, metabolism, starvation, and viral infection [92, 115, 116]. The effect of how the environment can alter the epigenome has been well established in plants, and it is expected that similar effects occur in animal species [92]. The environment can induce mutations in the genome, termed *de novo* mutations, which in turn can modify the epigenome (Figure 3.1). As this field further progresses, it is important to consider that in the case of both a gene and an epigenome variant, this may mistakenly be viewed as an *epimutation* if the mutation is overlooked. However, advances in sequences methods for the genome and epigenome will tease out this subtlety in future research [92].

In Utero Environmental Exposures

The *in utero* maternal environment is particularly important for development [117–119] and exposure to certain environmental factors is known to be critical for brain health and the susceptibility to disease [120]. The developing brain is known to be more sensitive to environmental factors than the fully developed brain is, highlighting that *in utero* conditions are of critical importance for fetal brain health [120]. Studies have demonstrated that stressors in the maternal environment such as heavy metal exposure, diet, and pesticides can cause brain defects in offspring [120]. Maternal exposure to heavy metals can alter womb integrity and interact with antioxidants, causing oxidative stress in offspring [120]. Indeed, oxidative stress is a hallmark feature of ALS, yet the relationship between maternal exposure to heavy metal and sALS in offspring remains unknown.

Environmental in Utero Epigenomic Alterations

In humans, the epigenome is naturally reprogrammed early in development [121]. An early potential mechanism for the *in utero* epigenetic basis of disease is that a number of loci associated with disease, including neurodegenerative diseases, appear to be resistant to remethylation in human primordial germ cells [121]. An important consideration for the transmission of epigenetic inheritance is when environmental exposures lead to germline changes to the epigenome which can happen *in utero* by modifications to the fetus subsequent to maternal exposure to environmental stressors [92]. The best-described examples of transgenerational epigenetic inheritance occur with *in utero* exposure to toxins and parental trauma [122–124]. The offspring's epigenome can be modified at later developmental stages [125], highlighting the complex relationship between maternal exposures and disease in offspring.

The concept of fetal developmental basis of disease (termed FeBAD) is not new to the field of ALS. Eisen and colleagues have described a developmental basis of ALS based on disrupted signaling in the GABA-ergic system [126, 127]. The excitatory to inhibitory switch of GABA takes place very early in development, and disruption in this period can lead to neuronal over-excitability with have lasting effects in later life, including neurodegeneration [127]. Indeed, hyper-excitability is a pathological hallmark in sALS preceding clinical onset [128], and this remains an intriguing subject for further studies.

Post Utero Exposures

Similar to maternal exposures *in utero*, postnatal exposures are also critical for brain health. It has long been described that the time from conception to two years of age has a direct impact on lifelong health [129]. As mentioned above, many environmental factors have been associated with sALS; however, there is less evidence for the role of early life exposures, perhaps due to the inherent challenge of performing such retrospective studies. The role of early life exposures has been investigated in terms of susceptibility to Parkinson's and Alzheimer's disease [129], suggesting a plausible role in sALS.

Lead (Pb) exposure is considered an environmental risk factor for sALS [130–133]. This heavy metal is known to cause modifications to the epigenome by DNA methylation and hydroxymethylation, miRNA expression, and histone modifications, among others [134]. Importantly, sub-"toxic" exposures to Pb can drive latent modifications to the epigenome [134]. For example, early life exposure to Pb at levels that do not show apparent evidence of toxicity in early life has been associated with Alzheimer's disease [135]. A tragic example of environmental Pb exposure was the recent Pb contamination in drinking water in Flint, Michigan, which was declared a federal emergency in 2014. This will be an important population to investigate for epigenetic effects in the future. Whether these changes will be passed on to the offspring of affected individuals, thus qualifying this as a true epigenetic effect, remains to be seen. While the result of early life exposure to toxins such as Pb is not well understood in the field of ALS epigenomics, it has been shown that toxins associated with sALS like heavy metals alter miRNA expression [4, 136], making this an important subject for future studies.

CONCLUSION

Despite decades of research efforts, the etiology underlying sALS remains elusive. The lack of clear evidence for a single causal environmental or genetic factor underlying sALS, in combination with the identification of many different susceptibility genes, supports the view that sALS is a complex, multifactorial disease. It is thus likely that sALS may be driven by multiple susceptibility genes, a manifestation of accumulated environmental stressors, or a combination of both. Gene-toxin interactions remain intriguing for further investigation of sALS etiology, either driven by a genetic predisposition incurred by low-frequency sALS susceptibility genes and disease onset triggered by environmental stressors. Another possible gene-toxin basis for disease is that epigenetic modifications from environmental exposures, either through maternal *in utero* or *ex utero* exposures, drives susceptibility. Targeting the epigenome is an appealing therapeutic option as these modifications can be reversible. As the traditional distinction between sALS and fALS becomes blurred, it remains a priority to consider sALS as a complex disease, which may not follow an equivalent pathological mechanism to fALS or be appropriate for the therapeutics developed for fALS.

CONFLICT OF INTEREST

The authors declare no potential conflict of interest with respect to research, authorship, and/or publication of this manuscript.

COPYRIGHT AND PERMISSION STATEMENT

REFERENCES

1. Gibson, S.B., Downie, J.M., Tsetsou, S. et al. (2017). The evolving genetic risk for sporadic ALS. *Neurology* 89 (3): 226–233.

2. Chia, R., Chio, A., and Traynor, B.J. (2018). Novel genes associated with amyotrophic lateral sclerosis: diagnostic and clinical implications. *The Lancet Neurology* 17 (1): 94–102.

3. Merwin, S.J., Obis, T., Nunez, Y., and Re, D.B. (2017). Organophosphate neurotoxicity to the voluntary motor system on the trail of environment-caused amyotrophic lateral sclerosis: the known, the misknown, and the unknown. *Archives of Toxicology* 91 (8): 2939–2952.

4. Ahmed, A. and Wicklund, M.P. (2011). Amyotrophic lateral sclerosis: what role does environment play? *Neurologic Clinics* 29 (3): 689–711.

5. Torbick, N., Hession, S., Stommel, E., and Caller, T. (2014). Mapping amyotrophic lateral sclerosis lake risk factors across northern New England. *International Journal of Health Geographics* 13: 1.

6. Kamel, F., Umbach, D.M., Bedlack, R.S. et al. (2012). Pesticide exposure and amyotrophic lateral sclerosis. *Neurotoxicology* 33 (3): 457–462.

7. Bello, A., Woskie, S.R., Gore, R. et al. (2017). Retrospective assessment of occupational exposures for the GENEVA study of ALS among military veterans. *Annals of Work Exposures and Health* 61 (3): 299–310.

8. Filippini, T., Fiore, M., Tesauro, M. et al. (2020). Clinical and lifestyle factors and risk of amyotrophic lateral sclerosis: a population-based case-control study. *International Journal of Environmental Research and Public Health* 17 (3): 857.

9. Mostafalou, S. and Abdollahi, M. (2017). Pesticides: an update of human exposure and toxicity. *Archives of Toxicology* 91 (2): 549–599.

10. Oskarsson, B., Horton, D.K., and Mitsumoto, H. (2015). Potential environmental factors in amyotrophic lateral sclerosis. *Neurologic Clinics* 33 (4): 877–888.

11. Bozzoni, V., Pansarasa, O., Diamanti, L. et al. (2016). Amyotrophic lateral sclerosis and environmental factors. *Functional Neurology* 31 (1): 7–19.

12. Plato, C.C., Garruto, R.M., Fox, K.M., and Gajdusek, D.C. (1986). Amyotrophic lateral sclerosis and parkinsonism-dementia on Guam: a 25-year prospective case-control study. *American Journal of Epidemiology* 124 (4): 643–656.

13. Al-Chalabi, A. and Hardiman, O. (2013). The epidemiology of ALS: a conspiracy of genes, environment and time. *Nature Reviews Neurology* 9 (11): 617–628.

14. Riancho, J., Bosque-Varela, P., Perez-Pereda, S. et al. (2018). The increasing importance of environmental conditions in amyotrophic lateral sclerosis. *International Journal of Biometeorology* 62 (8): 1361–1374.

15. Galasko, D., Salmon, D.P., Craig, U.-K. et al. (2002). Clinical features and changing patterns of neurodegenerative disorders on Guam, 1997–2000. *Neurology* 58 (1): 90–97.

16. Kihira, T., Yoshida, S., Kondo, T. et al. (2012). An increase in ALS incidence on the Kii Peninsula, 1960–2009: a possible link to change in drinking water source. *Amyotrophic Lateral Sclerosis: Official Publication of the World Federation of Neurology Research Group on Motor Neuron Diseases* 13 (4): 347–350.

17. Reed, D.M., Torres, J.M., and Brody, J.A. (1975). Amyotrophic lateral sclerosis and parkinsonism-dementia on Guam, 1945–1972. II. Familial and genetic studies. *American Journal of Epidemiology* 101 (4): 302–310.

18. Reed, D.M. and Brody, J.A. (1975). Amyotrophic lateral sclerosis and parkinsonism-dementia on Guam, 1945–1972. I. Descriptive epidemiology. *American Journal of Epidemiology* 101 (4): 287–301.

19. Harlin, M.C., Crawford, F., Perl, D.P. et al. (1993). Sequencing of exons 16 and 17 of the beta-amyloid precursor protein gene reveals the beta-amyloid sequence to be normal in cases of the parkinson dementia complex of Guam. *Journal of Neural Transmission Parkinson's Disease and Dementia Section* 5 (1): 63–65.

20. Waring, S.C., O'Brien, P.C., Kurland, L.T. et al. (1994). Apolipoprotein E allele in Chamorros with amyotrophic lateral sclerosis/parkinsonism-dementia complex. *Lancet (London, England)* 343 (8897): 611.

21. Iwata, S. (1977). Study of the effects of environmental factors on the local incidence of amyotrophic lateral sclerosis. *Ecotoxicology and Environmental Safety* 1 (3): 297–303.

22. Crapper McLachlarf, D.R., McLachlan, C.D., Krishnan, B. et al. (1989). Aluminium and calcium in soil and food from Guam, Palau and Jamaica: implications for amyotrophic lateral sclerosis and parkinsonism-dementia syndromes of Guam. *Environmental Geochemistry and Health* 11 (2): 45–53.

23. Kurland, L.T. (1972). An appraisal of the neurotoxicity of cycad and the etiology of amyotrophic lateral sclerosis on Guam. *Federation Proceedings* 31 (5): 1540–1542.

24. Sieh, W., Choi, Y., Chapman, N.H. et al. (2009). Identification of novel susceptibility loci for Guam neurodegenerative disease: challenges of genome scans in genetic isolates. *Human Molecular Genetics* 18 (19): 3725–3738.

25. Kurland, L.T. (1988). Amyotrophic lateral sclerosis and Parkinson's disease complex on Guam linked to an environmental neurotoxin. *Trends in Neurosciences* 11 (2): 51–54.

26. Wilson, J.M., Khabazian, I., Wong, M.C. et al. (2002). Behavioral and neurological correlates of ALS-parkinsonism dementia complex in adult mice fed washed cycad flour. *Neuromolecular Medicine* 1 (3): 207–221.

27. Torres, J., Iriarte, L.L., and Kurland, L.T. (1957). Amyotrophic lateral sclerosis among Guamanians in California. *California Medicine* 86 (6): 385–388.

28. Beretta, S., Carri, M.T., Beghi, E. et al. (2003). The sinister side of Italian soccer. *The Lancet Neurology* 2 (11): 656–657.

29. Chiò, A., Benzi, G., Dossena, M. et al. (2005). Severely increased risk of amyotrophic lateral sclerosis among Italian professional football players. *Brain: A Journal of Neurology* 128 (Pt 3): 472–476.

30. Turner, M.R. (2017). Is cardiovascular fitness a risk factor for ALS? *Journal of Neurology, Neurosurgery, and Psychiatry* 88 (7): 538.

31. Ning, P., Yang, B., Li, S. et al. (2019). Systematic review of the prognostic role of body mass index in amyotrophic lateral sclerosis. *Amyotrophic Lateral Sclerosis & Frontotemporal Degeneration* 20 (5–6): 356–367.

32. Wright, D.K., Liu, S., van der Poel, C. et al. (2017). Traumatic brain injury results in cellular, structural and functional changes resembling motor neuron disease. *Cerebral Cortex (New York, NY: 1991)* 27 (9): 4503–4515.

33. Tabata, R.C., Wilson, J.M.B., Ly, P. et al. (2008). Chronic exposure to dietary sterol glucosides is neurotoxic to motor neurons and induces an ALS–PDC phenotype. *Neuromolecular Medicine* 10 (1): 24–39.

34. Kumawat, K.L., Kaushik, D.K., Goswami, P., and Basu, A. (2014). Acute exposure to lead acetate activates microglia and induces subsequent bystander neuronal death via caspase-3 activation. *Neurotoxicology* 41: 143–153.

35. Morrice, J.R., Gregory-Evans, C.Y., and Shaw, C.A. (2018). Modeling environmentally-induced motor neuron degeneration in zebrafish. *Scientific Reports* 8 (1): 4890.

36. Vinceti, M., Violi, F., Tzatzarakis, M. et al. (2017). Pesticides, polychlorinated biphenyls and polycyclic aromatic hydrocarbons in cerebrospinal fluid of amyotrophic lateral sclerosis patients: a case-control study. *Environmental Research* 155: 261–267.

37. Gresham, L.S., Molgaard, C.A., Golbeck, A.L., and Smith, R. (1986). Amyotrophic lateral sclerosis and occupational heavy metal exposure: a case-control study. *Neuroepidemiology* 5 (1): 29–38.

38. Perry, T.L., Bergeron, C., Biro, A.J., and Hansen, S. (1989). Beta-N-methylamino-L-alanine. Chronic oral administration is not neurotoxic to mice. *Journal of the Neurological Sciences* 94 (1–3): 173–180.

39. Wild, C.P. (2005). Complementing the genome with an "exposome": the outstanding challenge of environmental exposure measurement in molecular epidemiology. *Cancer Epidemiology, Biomarkers & Prevention: A Publication of the American Association for Cancer Research, Cosponsored by the American Society of Preventive Oncology* 14 (8): 1847–1850.

40. Sánchez-Santed, F., Colomina, M.T., and Herrero, H.E. (2016). Organophosphate pesticide exposure and neurodegeneration. *Cortex* 74: 417–426.

41. Dardiotis, E., Aloizou, A.M., Siokas, V. et al. (2019). Paraoxonase-1 genetic polymorphisms in organophosphate metabolism. *Toxicology* 411: 24–31.

42. Menini, T. and Gugliucci, A. (2014). Paraoxonase 1 in neurological disorders. *Redox Report: Communications in Free Radical Research* 19 (2): 49–58.

43. Cronin, S., Greenway, M.J., Prehn, J.H., and Hardiman, O. (2007). Paraoxonase promoter and intronic variants modify risk of sporadic amyotrophic lateral sclerosis. *Journal of Neurology, Neurosurgery, and Psychiatry* 78 (9): 984–986.

44. Verde, F., Tiloca, C., Morelli, C. et al. (2019). PON1 is a disease modifier gene in amyotrophic lateral sclerosis: association of the Q192R polymorphism with bulbar onset and reduced survival. *Neurological Sciences* 40 (7): 1469–1473.

45. Lee, Y.H., Kim, J.H., Seo, Y.H. et al. (2015). Paraoxonase 1 Q192R and L55M polymorphisms and susceptibility to amyotrophic lateral sclerosis: a meta-analysis. *Neurological Sciences: Official Journal of the Italian Neurological Society and of the Italian Society of Clinical Neurophysiology* 36 (1): 11–20.

46. Al-Chalabi, A., Fang, F., Hanby, M.F. et al. (2010). An estimate of amyotrophic lateral sclerosis heritability using twin data. *Journal of Neurology, Neurosurgery, and Psychiatry* 81 (12): 1324–1326.

47. Brown, R.H. and Al-Chalabi, A. (2017). Amyotrophic lateral sclerosis. *The New England Journal of Medicine* 377 (2): 162–172.

48. Osmanovic, A., Rangnau, I., Kosfeld, A. et al. (2017). FIG 4 variants in central European patients with amyotrophic lateral sclerosis: a whole-exome and targeted sequencing study. *European Journal of Human Genetics: EJHG* 25 (3): 324–331.

49. Williams, K.L., Topp, S., Yang, S. et al. (2016). CCNF mutations in amyotrophic lateral sclerosis and frontotemporal dementia. *Nature Communications* 7: 11253.

50. Mitropoulos, K., Merkouri Papadima, E., Xiromerisiou, G. et al. (2017). Genomic variants in the FTO gene are associated with sporadic amyotrophic lateral sclerosis in Greek patients. *Human Genomics* 11 (1): 30.

51. van Rheenen, W., Shatunov, A., Dekker, A.M. et al. (2016). Genome-wide association analyses identify new risk variants and the genetic architecture of amyotrophic lateral sclerosis. *Nature Genetics* 48 (9): 1043–1048.

52. Liu, X., Yang, L., Tang, L. et al. (2017). DCTN1 gene analysis in Chinese patients with sporadic amyotrophic lateral sclerosis. *PLOS One* 12 (8): e0182572.

53. Kim, H., Lim, J., Bao, H. et al. (2019). Rare variants in MYH15 modify amyotrophic lateral sclerosis risk. *Human Molecular Genetics* 28 (14): 2309–2318.

54. van Es, M.A., Van Vught, P.W., Blauw, H.M. et al. (2007). ITPR2 as a susceptibility gene in sporadic amyotrophic lateral sclerosis: a genome-wide association study. *The Lancet Neurology* 6 (10): 869–877.

55. van Es, M.A., Veldink, J.H., Saris, C.G. et al. (2009). Genome-wide association study identifies 19p13.3 (UNC13A) and 9p21.2 as susceptibility loci for sporadic amyotrophic lateral sclerosis. *Nature Genetics* 41 (10): 1083–1087.

56. van Es, M.A., van Vught, P.W., Blauw, H.M. et al. (2008). Genetic variation in DPP6 is associated with susceptibility to amyotrophic lateral sclerosis. *Nature Genetics* 40 (1): 29–31.

57. Chen, Y., Zeng, Y., Huang, R. et al. (2012). No association of five candidate genetic variants with amyotrophic lateral sclerosis in a Chinese population. *Neurobiology of Aging* 33 (11): 2721.e3–2721.e5.

58. Wei, Q., Chen, X., Chen, Y. et al. (2019). Unique characteristics of the genetics epidemiology of amyotrophic lateral sclerosis in China. *Science China Life Sciences* 62 (4): 517–525.

59. He, J., Tang, L., Benyamin, B. et al. (2015). C9orf72 hexanucleotide repeat expansions in Chinese sporadic amyotrophic lateral sclerosis. *Neurobiology of Aging* 36 (9): 2660. e1–2660.e8.

60. Marangi, G. and Traynor, B.J. (1607). Genetic causes of amyotrophic lateral sclerosis: new genetic analysis methodologies entailing new opportunities and challenges. *Brain Research* 2015: 75–93.

61. Ghasemi, M. and Brown, R.H. Jr. (2018). Genetics of amyotrophic lateral sclerosis. *Cold Spring Harbor Perspectives in Medicine* 8 (5): a024125.

62. DeJesus-Hernandez, M., Mackenzie, I.R., Boeve, B.F. et al. (2011). Expanded GGGGCC hexanucleotide repeat in noncoding region of C9ORF72 causes chromosome 9p-linked FTD and ALS. *Neuron* 72 (2): 245–256.

63. Sabatelli, M., Conforti, F.L., Zollino, M. et al. (2012). C9ORF72 hexanucleotide repeat expansions in the Italian sporadic ALS population. *Neurobiology of Aging* 33 (8): 1848. e15–1848.e20.

64. Ajroud-Driss, S. and Siddique, T. (2015). Sporadic and hereditary amyotrophic lateral sclerosis (ALS). *Biochimica et Biophysica Acta (BBA) - Molecular Basis of Disease* 1852 (4): 679–684.

65. Fang, F., Kamel, F., Lichtenstein, P. et al. (2009). Familial aggregation of amyotrophic lateral sclerosis. *Annals of Neurology* 66 (1): 94–99.

66. Renton, A.E., Chio, A., and Traynor, B.J. (2014). State of play in amyotrophic lateral sclerosis genetics. *Nature Neuroscience* 17 (1): 17–23.

67. van Es, M.A., Hardiman, O., Chio, A. et al. (2017). Amyotrophic lateral sclerosis. *Lancet (London, England)* 390 (10107): 2084–2098.

68. Kenna, K.P., van Doormaal, P.T., Dekker, A.M. et al. (2016). NEK1 variants confer susceptibility to amyotrophic lateral sclerosis. *Nature Genetics* 48 (9): 1037–1042.

69. He, J., Mangelsdorf, M., Fan, D. et al. (2015). Amyotrophic lateral sclerosis genetic studies: from genome-wide association mapping to genome sequencing. *The Neuroscientist: A Review Journal Bringing Neurobiology, Neurology and Psychiatry* 21 (6): 599–615.

70. Varoqueaux, F., Sons, M.S., Plomp, J.J., and Brose, N. (2005). Aberrant morphology and residual transmitter release at the Munc13-deficient mouse neuromuscular synapse. *Molecular and Cellular Biology* 25 (14): 5973–5984.

71. Gaastra, B., Shatunov, A., Pulit, S. et al. (2016). Rare genetic variation in UNC13A may modify survival in amyotrophic lateral sclerosis. *Amyotrophic Lateral Sclerosis & Frontotemporal Degeneration* 17 (7–8): 593–599.

72. Diekstra, F.P., Van Deerlin, V.M., van Swieten, J.C. et al. (2014). C9orf72 and UNC13A are shared risk loci for amyotrophic lateral sclerosis and frontotemporal dementia: a genome-wide meta-analysis. *Annals of Neurology* 76 (1): 120–133.

73. Yang, B., Jiang, H., Wang, F. et al. (2019). UNC13A variant rs12608932 is associated with increased risk of amyotrophic lateral sclerosis and reduced patient survival: a

meta-analysis. *Neurological Sciences: Official Journal of the Italian Neurological Society and of the Italian Society of Clinical Neurophysiology* 40 (11): 2293–2302.

74. Lin, L., Murphy, J.G., Karlsson, R.M. et al. (2018). DPP6 loss impacts hippocampal synaptic development and induces behavioral impairments in recognition. *Learning and Memory. Frontiers in Cellular Neuroscience* 12: 84.

75. Lin, L., Sun, W., Throesch, B. et al. (2013). DPP6 regulation of dendritic morphogenesis impacts hippocampal synaptic development. *Nature Communications* 4: 2270.

76. McLaughlin, R.L., Schijven, D., van Rheenen, W. et al. (2017). Genetic correlation between amyotrophic lateral sclerosis and schizophrenia. *Nature Communications* 8: 14774.

77. Cronin, S., Berger, S., Ding, J. et al. (2008). A genome-wide association study of sporadic ALS in a homogenous Irish population. *Human Molecular Genetics* 17 (5): 768–774.

78. Cronin, S., Tomik, B., Bradley, D.G. et al. (2009). Screening for replication of genome-wide SNP associations in sporadic ALS. *European Journal of Human Genetics: EJHG* 17 (2): 213–218.

79. Li, X.G., Zhang, J.H., Xie, M.Q. et al. (2009). Association between DPP6 polymorphism and the risk of sporadic amyotrophic lateral sclerosis in Chinese patients. *Chinese Medical Journal* 122 (24): 2989–2992.

80. Fang, X., Lin, H., Wang, X. et al. (2015). The NEK1 interactor, C21ORF2, is required for efficient DNA damage repair. *Acta Biochimica et Biophysica Sinica* 47 (10): 834–841.

81. Iyer, S., Acharya, K.R., and Subramanian, V. (2019). Prediction of structural consequences for disease causing variants in C21orf2 protein using computational approaches. *Journal of Biomolecular Structure & Dynamics* 37 (2): 465–480.

82. Gustafson, K., Duncan, J.L., Biswas, P. et al. (2017). Whole genome sequencing revealed mutations in two independent genes as the underlying cause of retinal degeneration in an Ashkenazi Jewish Pedigree. *Genes* 8 (9): 210.

83. Hwang, J.Y., Aromolaran, K.A., and Zukin, R.S. (2017). The emerging field of epigenetics in neurodegeneration and neuroprotection. *Nature Reviews Neuroscience* 18 (6): 347–361.

84. Reinberg, D. and Vales, L.D. (2018). Chromatin domains rich in inheritance. *Science (New York, NY)* 361 (6397): 33–34.

85. Masala, A., Sanna, S., Esposito, S. et al. (2018). Epigenetic changes associated with the expression of amyotrophic lateral sclerosis (ALS) causing genes. *Neuroscience* 390: 1–11.

86. Coppedè, F., Stoccoro, A., Mosca, L. et al. (2018). Increase in DNA methylation in patients with amyotrophic lateral sclerosis carriers of not fully penetrant SOD1 mutations. *Amyotrophic Lateral Ssclerosis & Frontotemporal Degeneration* 19 (1–2): 93–101.

87. Stoccoro, A., Mosca, L., Carnicelli, V. et al. (2018). Mitochondrial DNA copy number and D-loop region methylation in carriers of amyotrophic lateral sclerosis gene mutations. *Epigenomics* 10 (11): 1431–1443.

88. Van Acker, Z.P., Declerck, K., Luyckx, E. et al. (2019). Non-methylation-linked mechanism of REST-induced neuroglobin expression impacts mitochondrial phenotypes in a mouse model of amyotrophic lateral sclerosis. *Neuroscience* 412: 233–247.

89. Jimenez-Pacheco, A., Franco, J.M., Lopez, S. et al. (2017). Epigenetic mechanisms of gene regulation in amyotrophic lateral sclerosis. *Advances in Experimental Medicine and Biology* 978: 255–275.

90. Bennett, S.A., Tanaz, R., Cobos, S.N., and Torrente, M.P. (2019). Epigenetics in amyotrophic lateral sclerosis: a role for histone post-translational modifications in neurodegenerative disease. *Translational Research: The Journal of Laboratory and Clinical Medicine* 204: 19–30.

91. Appleby-Mallinder, C., Schaber, E., Kirby, J. et al. (2020). TDP43 proteinopathy is associated with aberrant DNA methylation in human amyotrophic lateral sclerosis. *Neuropathology and Applied Neurobiology*.

92. Cavalli, G. and Heard, E. (2019). Advances in epigenetics link genetics to the environment and disease. *Nature* 571 (7766): 489–499.

93. Figueroa-Romero, C., Hur, J., Bender, D.E. et al. (2012). Identification of epigenetically altered genes in sporadic amyotrophic lateral sclerosis. *PLOS One* 7 (12): e52672.

94. Tarr, I.S., McCann, E.P., Benyamin, B. et al. (2019). Monozygotic twins and triplets discordant for amyotrophic lateral sclerosis display differential methylation and gene expression. *Scientific Reports* 9 (1): 8254.

95. Morahan, J.M., Yu, B., Trent, R.J., and Pamphlett, R. (2009). A genome-wide analysis of brain DNA methylation identifies new candidate genes for sporadic amyotrophic lateral sclerosis. *Amyotrophic Lateral Sclerosis: Official Publication of the World Federation of Neurology Research Group on Motor Neuron Diseases* 10 (5–6): 418–429.

96. Cartier, N., Lewis, C.A., Zhang, R., and Rossi, F.M. (2014). The role of microglia in human disease: therapeutic tool or target? *Acta Neuropathologica* 128 (3): 363–380.

97. Martin, L.J. and Wong, M. (2013). Aberrant regulation of DNA methylation in amyotrophic lateral sclerosis: a new target of disease mechanisms. *Neurotherapeutics: The Journal of the American Society for Experimental NeuroTherapeutics* 10 (4): 722–733.

98. Xi, Z., Zhang, M., Bruni, A.C. et al. (2015). The C9orf72 repeat expansion itself is methylated in ALS and FTLD patients. *Acta Neuropathologica* 129 (5): 715–727.

99. Gijselinck, I., Van Mossevelde, S., van der Zee, J. et al. (2016). The C9orf72 repeat size correlates with onset age of disease, DNA methylation and transcriptional downregulation of the promoter. *Molecular Psychiatry* 21 (8): 1112–1124.

100. Belzil, V.V., Bauer, P.O., Gendron, T.F. et al. (2014). Characterization of DNA hypermethylation in the cerebellum of c9FTD/ALS patients. *Brain Research* 1584: 15–21.

101. Waite, A.J., Baumer, D., East, S. et al. (2014). Reduced C9orf72 protein levels in frontal cortex of amyotrophic lateral sclerosis and frontotemporal degeneration brain with the C9ORF72 hexanucleotide repeat expansion. *Neurobiology of Aging* 35 (7): 1779.e5–e13.

102. Taylor, J.P., Brown, R.H. Jr., and Cleveland, D.W. (2016). Decoding ALS: from genes to mechanism. *Nature* 539 (7628): 197–206.

103. Figueroa-Romero, C., Hur, J., Lunn, J.S. et al. (2016). Expression of microRNAs in human post-mortem amyotrophic lateral sclerosis spinal cords provides insight into disease mechanisms. *Molecular and Cellular Neurosciences* 71: 34–45.

104. Chen, Y., Wei, Q., Chen, X. et al. (2016). Aberration of miRNAs expression in leukocytes from sporadic amyotrophic lateral sclerosis. *Frontiers in Molecular Neuroscience* 9: 69.

105. Waller, R., Goodall, E.F., Milo, M. et al. (2017). Serum miRNAs miR-206, 143-3p and 374b-5p as potential biomarkers for amyotrophic lateral sclerosis (ALS). *Neurobiology of Aging* 55: 123–131.

106. Waller, R., Wyles, M., Heath, P.R. et al. (2017). Small RNA sequencing of sporadic amyotrophic lateral sclerosis cerebrospinal fluid reveals differentially expressed miRNAs related to neural and glial activity. *Frontiers in Neuroscience* 11: 731.

107. Hyun, K., Jeon, J., Park, K., and Kim, J. (2017). Writing, erasing and reading histone lysine methylations. *Experimental & Molecular Medicine* 49 (4): e324-e.

108. Lennartsson, A. and Ekwall, K. (2009). Histone modification patterns and epigenetic codes. *Biochimica et Biophysica Acta* 1790 (9): 863–868.

109. Simpson, C.L., Lemmens, R., Miskiewicz, K. et al. (2009). Variants of the elongator protein 3 (ELP3) gene are associated with motor neuron degeneration. *Human Molecular Genetics* 18 (3): 472–481.

110. Wu, C.C., Jin, L.W., Wang, I.F. et al. (2020). HDAC1 dysregulation induces aberrant cell cycle and DNA damage in progress of TDP-43 proteinopathies. *EMBO Molecular Medicine* 12 (6): e10622.

111. Janssen, C., Schmalbach, S., Boeselt, S. et al. (2010). Differential histone deacetylase mRNA expression patterns in amyotrophic lateral sclerosis. *Journal of Neuropathology and Experimental Neurology* 69 (6): 573–581.

112. Berson, A., Sartoris, A., Nativio, R. et al. (2017). TDP-43 promotes neurodegeneration by impairing chromatin remodeling. *Current Biology: CB* 27 (23): 3579–90.e6.

113. Young, P.E., Kum Jew, S., Buckland, M.E. et al. (2017). Epigenetic differences between monozygotic twins discordant for amyotrophic lateral sclerosis (ALS) provide clues to disease pathogenesis. *PLOS One* 12 (8): e0182638.

114. Zhang, M., Xi, Z., Ghani, M. et al. (2016). Genetic and epigenetic study of ALS-discordant identical twins with double mutations in SOD1 and ARHGEF28. *Journal of Neurology, Neurosurgery, and Psychiatry* 87 (11): 1268–1270.

115. Rechavi, O., Houri-Ze'evi, L., Anava, S. et al. (2014). Starvation-induced transgenerational inheritance of small RNAs in C. elegans. *Cell* 158 (2): 277–287.

116. Rechavi, O., Minevich, G., and Hobert, O. (2011). Transgenerational inheritance of an acquired small RNA-based antiviral response in C. elegans. *Cell* 147 (6): 1248–1256.

117. Chen, P., Piaggi, P., Traurig, M. et al. (2017). Differential methylation of genes in individuals exposed to maternal diabetes in utero. *Diabetologia* 60 (4): 645–655.

118. Tanwar, V., Gorr, M.W., Velten, M. et al. (2017). In utero particulate matter exposure produces heart failure, electrical remodeling, and epigenetic changes at adulthood. *Journal of the American Heart Association* 6 (4): e005796.

119. Chatterton, Z., Hartley, B.J., Seok, M.H. et al. (2017). In utero exposure to maternal smoking is associated with DNA methylation alterations and reduced neuronal content in the developing fetal brain. *Epigenetics & Chromatin* 10: 4.

120. Modgil, S., Lahiri, D.K., Sharma, V.L., and Anand, A. (2014). Role of early life exposure and environment on neurodegeneration: implications on brain disorders. *Translational Neurodegeneration* 3: 9.

121. Tang, W.W., Dietmann, S., Irie, N. et al. (2015). A unique gene regulatory network resets the human germline epigenome for development. *Cell* 161 (6): 1453–1467.

122. Anway, M.D., Cupp, A.S., Uzumcu, M., and Skinner, M.K. (2005). Epigenetic transgenerational actions of endocrine disruptors and male fertility. *Science (New York, NY)* 308 (5727): 1466–1469.

123. Gapp, K., van Steenwyk, G., Germain, P.L. et al. (2020). Alterations in sperm long RNA contribute to the epigenetic inheritance of the effects of postnatal trauma. *Molecular Psychiatry* 25 (9): 2162–2174.

124. Dias, B.G. and Ressler, K.J. (2014). Parental olfactory experience influences behavior and neural structure in subsequent generations. *Nature Neuroscience* 17 (1): 89–96.

125. Lahiri, D.K., Maloney, B., and Zawia, N.H. (2009). The LEARn model: an epigenetic explanation for idiopathic neurobiological diseases. *Molecular Psychiatry* 14 (11): 992–1003.

126. Eisen, A., Kiernan, M., Mitsumoto, H., and Swash, M. (2014). Amyotrophic lateral sclerosis: a long preclinical period? *Journal of Neurology, Neurosurgery, and Psychiatry* 85 (11): 1232–1238.

127. Kiernan, M.C., Ziemann, U., and Eisen, A. (2019). Amyotrophic lateral sclerosis: origins traced to impaired balance between neural excitation and inhibition in the neonatal period. *Muscle & Nerve* 60 (3): 232–235.

128. Vucic, S., Ziemann, U., Eisen, A. et al. (2013). Transcranial magnetic stimulation and amyotrophic lateral sclerosis: pathophysiological insights. *Journal of Neurology, Neurosurgery, and Psychiatry* 84 (10): 1161–1170.

129. Barker, D.J. and Osmond, C. (1986). Infant mortality, childhood nutrition, and ischaemic heart disease in England and Wales. *Lancet (London, England)* 1 (8489): 1077–1081.

130. Dickerson, A.S., Hansen, J., Kioumourtzoglou, M.A. et al. (2018). Study of occupation and amyotrophic lateral sclerosis in a Danish cohort. *Occupational and Environmental Medicine* 75 (9): 630–638.

131. Wang, M.D., Gomes, J., Cashman, N.R. et al. (2014). A meta-analysis of observational studies of the association between chronic occupational exposure to lead and amyotrophic lateral sclerosis. *Journal of Occupational and Environmental Medicine* 56 (12): 1235–1242.

132. Campbell, A.M., Williams, E.R., and Barltrop, D. (1970). Motor neurone disease and exposure to lead. *Journal of Neurology, Neurosurgery, and Psychiatry* 33 (6): 877–885.

133. Zahran, S., Laidlaw, M.A., Rowe, D.B. et al. (2017). Motor neuron disease mortality and lifetime petrol lead exposure: evidence from national age-specific and state-level age-standardized death rates in Australia. *Environmental Research* 153: 181–190.

134. Maloney, B., Bayon, B.L., Zawia, N.H., and Lahiri, D.K. (2018). Latent consequences of early-life lead (Pb) exposure and the future: addressing the Pb crisis. *Neurotoxicology* 68: 126–132.

135. Wu, J., Basha, M.R., Brock, B. et al. (2008). Alzheimer's disease (AD)-like pathology in aged monkeys after infantile exposure to environmental metal lead (Pb): evidence for a developmental origin and environmental link for AD. *The Journal of Neuroscience: The Official Journal of the Society for Neuroscience* 28 (1): 3–9.

136. Callaghan, B., Feldman, D., Gruis, K., and Feldman, E. (2011). The association of exposure to lead, mercury, and selenium and the development of amyotrophic lateral sclerosis and the epigenetic implications. *Neuro-Degenerative Diseases* 8 (1–2): 1–8.

CHAPTER 4

The Lessons of ALS-PDC – Environmental Factors in ALS Etiology

Christopher A. Shaw[1,2,3,4] and Thomas E. Marler[5]

[1] Experimental Medicine Program, University of British Columbia, Vancouver, British Columbia, Canada
[2] Department of Ophthalmology and Visual Sciences, University of British Columbia, Vancouver, British Columbia, Canada
[3] Department of Pathology, University of British Columbia, Vancouver, British Columbia, Canada
[4] Program in Neuroscience, University of British Columbia, Vancouver, British Columbia, Canada
[5] College of Natural and Applied Sciences, University of Guam, Mangilao, Guam, USA

INTRODUCTION

The search for environmental factors leading to motor neuron degeneration in sporadic ALS (sALS) has proven to be a daunting task for two main reasons. First, many toxic substances exist that can destroy motor neurons, but demonstrating that they are toxic *in vivo* in a way that satisfies the key criteria of model validity – face, construct, and predictive – has proven difficult. For example, Morrice et al. have demonstrated that Bisphenol A (BPA) can cause motor neuron death in a zebrafish model [1], but BPA is a molecule of relatively recent origin and thus cannot account for sALS historically. The second reason is that there have been at most two clusters of sALS hotspots, one of which is discussed below, which does not account for the majority of cases worldwide. A second possible cluster, the forms of ALS associated with Gulf War Syndrome, are not considered here. This latter observation suggests that sALS arises from chronic, low-level exposure to environmental stressors that requires some sort of co-factor, either genetic or environmental, to trigger disease initiation and progression. The likelihood of the need for additional factors together in a perfect storm[i] makes the search even more challenging. Chapter 3 explores such interactions in this book in a discussion of possible sALS susceptibility genes.

Some of following discussion of one of the key ALS clusters, amyotrophic lateral sclerosis-parkinsonism dementia complex (ALS-PDC) was originally presented in a previous book [2], and portions of several chapters in that book have been used in this expanded chapter.

KOCH'S POSTULATES IN THE SEARCH OF ETIOLOGICAL ALS FACTORS

In the field of infectious disease, Koch's postulates are criteria aimed at establishing a causal relationship between a microorganism and disease. These criteria often find their counterparts in the search for the etiology of ALS or other neurological diseases. Koch's postulates have the following general features, which, notably, have variations and may not always be met: (i) the microorganism (bacterial or viral) will be found in those suffering from the disease, but not in healthy individuals; (ii) the microorganism can be isolated from diseased persons and grown in cell culture; (iii) the cultured microorganism should induce the same disease if given to a healthy individual; and (iv) the microorganism can be isolated again from the latter infected individual and used again to induce the disease in the same way as in postulate 3.

Following from this scientifically testable perspective, it is often assumed that the sporadic forms of the disease will arise from a single toxic agent. Researchers focused on familial ALS (fALS) often argue for a particular dominant gene mutation.

However, in the search for causal factors in all ALS, it has been clear for many years that a number of toxins and toxicants, such as those described below, can lead to motor neuron dysfunction and/or degeneration. Similarly, different gene mutations can trigger a similar pathologic loss of motor neurons and motor function at disease end state. This point has been well made by Ross and Abbott [3].

A broader view of sALS, but still relying on Koch's postulates, is the notion that even if there are multiple toxicants or genes all involved individually and synergistically in ALS, these factors will converge on a common stage that, when activated, triggers the progressive disease cascade. A growing realization in the field, however, is that there may be many such toxins/toxicants and genes and an even greater number of additive or synergistic interactions between toxicants and between genes, and even more when toxicant-gene interactions are considered. A less mainstream view is that there are multiple ways for toxicants, genes, and toxicant-gene interactions to deliver an individual to the ALS end state [2]. This last view would, in fact, predict the spectrum nature of ALS that is beginning to emerge as a more likely prospect than that of ALS being a single disease state – and that is reflected in the title of this book.

The attraction of a single-factor model, sometimes called a *one-hit* model, is that it fits neatly with Koch's postulates and offers the hope, as for infectious diseases, that preventing a particular factor can prevent the disease. The notion of many disease paths leading to a common end state is less attractive because it makes the notion of disease prevention or treatment difficult or perhaps even impossible to achieve – a point to which we will return later in this chapter.

NEUROLOGICAL DISEASE CLUSTERS

One solution to the problem of too many potential causal factors (see Al-Chalabi and Hardiman [4] for further review) is to try to identify a disease cluster. A *cluster* is a relatively large number of similar cases of a disease constrained by time and geographical space. In principle, if enough people show the related signs and symptoms of a disease in a small enough area in a limited period of time, the search for the disease culprit(s), either genes, toxicants, or their interactions, becomes far more tractable. This is not to say it necessarily becomes uncomplicated, as the history of ALS-PDC, discussed below, will indicate (see also Shaw [2]).

Disease clusters are often associated with epidemics of infectious diseases to which Koch's postulates can relatively readily be applied. However, clusters of neurological diseases are rarer, such as lathyrism in World War II prisoner-of-war-camps [5], the Minamata methylmercury contamination cluster [6], and a case of domoic acid–induced neurological deficits [7]. However, most age-related neurological diseases have not proven to be so straightforward. In fact, with the exception of the above examples and a few others [2], when seeking causal factors for most cases of neurological disease – especially regarding toxicants – it seems that we are witnessing chronic, rather than acute, toxicant exposures occurring at relatively low levels. Since the level of the toxicant(s) appears to be low, relatively few people go on to show obvious neurological signs or symptoms in any designated time frame. Instead, whatever toxicants might be contributing to neurological diseases may take years or decades to manifest clinically obvious signs of their cumulative damage [2].

The impact of low-level toxicity thus affects the rate at which both individuals and populations express the disease state. One consequence of this type of environmental exposure is that real disease clusters do not form. Add to this the additional well-known variables of age, sex, other trauma to the nervous system, heterogeneity of genetic susceptibility, and individual microbiomes, and it becomes perhaps clearer why such disease clusters are the exception rather than the rule.

Another complication is that in the modern world, people are mobile in a way that is vastly different from our ancestors only a few generations past. For example, a person may grow up in one part of the country – or even a different country – go to school in a separate location, follow a career or partner/spouse elsewhere, and finally retire in still another place.

The multitude of environmental stressors an individual is exposed to over a life span is thus potentially unlimited. The lack of geographical consistency and our lack of understanding of when the disease process begins vastly complicate the already complex problems of sifting for answers against a backdrop of low-level toxicant exposure.

Sporadic ALS in North America and Europe may thus fall into a category of nearly unsolvable epidemiological mysteries, at least at present. This point was typified in a series of 18 epidemiological reports compiled by the Public Health Service of Canada in 2014 that failed to find a clear etiology for ALS or Parkinson's and Alzheimer's diseases [8].

However, if at least one real cluster for ALS existed, researchers would have a place to start the process of sorting through the myriad possible genetic and toxic/environmental factors. The success or failure in teasing out possible contributing factors in neurological disease etiologies would have dramatic and far-reaching implications for a better understanding of disease etiology – and related diseases – in general.

Fortunately, known clusters of ALS exist, the primary one being ALS-PDC in Guam and the Western Pacific [9–11].

THE NATURAL HISTORY OF ALS-PDC

Guam is the southernmost island of the Marianas chain located between the Philippines and Hawaii, which was originally settled about 1500 BCE by a Malay people now called Chamorros. In addition to Guam, the Chamorro people historically inhabited a string of islands further north, including Rota, Tinian, and Saipan.

Two key features of Chamorro history are important to consider in the origins of ALS-PDC. First, during the initial colonization of Guam by the Spanish in the 1600s, the Chamorro population of Guam was significantly reduced by both disease and war, with the result that the population likely became more genetically homogeneous. Second, during World War II, many Chamorros were put into labor camps by the Japanese, leading to widespread malnutrition. Malnutrition has an impact on dysbiosis in the microbiome [12]. In addition, the conditions in the camps, like water scarcity, likely changed the way the Chamorros processed the main putative culprit – the seeds of the cycad tree – by repeated rinsing in water.

A neurological disorder resembling ALS-PDC had been documented on Guam by early Spanish colonizers [2]. This disorder was "rediscovered" as a significant neurological disorder after World War II by American Navy doctors. Initially, the focus was on what appeared to be a typical ALS presentation [9–11, 13]. The Chamorros called this condition *lytico*, a variant of the Spanish word *paralytico*, or *paralyzed* (Figure 4.1). Signs included muscular weakness, often beginning unilaterally in the legs or, less often, in the arms, and then spreading to the contralateral limbs. The initial unilateral presentation resembled ALS elsewhere. However, lytico was unique in that it typically showed an ascending pattern, moving upward in the body to produce prominent neurological signs such as dysphagia and dysarthria, in contrast to a bulbar onset form of the disease elsewhere [14]. As typical in ALS, death was usually due to respiratory failure and often associated with pneumonia.

(a)

(b)

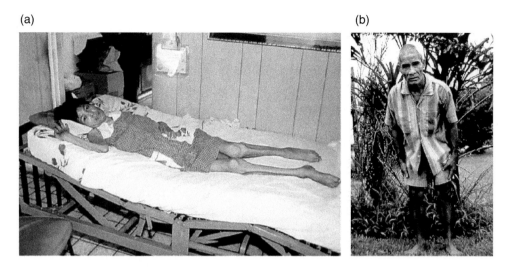

FIGURE 4.1 People with lytico (ALS) and bodig (PDC) on Guam. (a) A woman bed-bound with advanced ALS; (b) a man with parkinsonism and dementia. *Source*: Used with permission from Dr. John Steele.

Post mortem analysis of the nervous system showed the loss of motor neurons in the spinal cord. Curiously, lytico also showed non-typical features of ALS, including some features characteristic of Alzheimer's disease, such as the presence of neurofibrillary tangles (NFTs) composed of hyperphosphorylated tau protein inside neurons in the hippocampus and frontal cortex [10]. These features were later found in frontotemporal dementia (FTD) [15].

Lytico on Guam affected men to a greater degree than women, with symptom onset at an average age of 45. The age of onset was particularly notable, since at the time, and to a lesser extent now, this was 10–20 years younger than for ALS in North America and Europe [16].

The appearance of a second neurological disorder in Guam was soon described. This was termed *parkinsonism dementia complex* (PDC), and it resembled a cross between Parkinson's and Alzheimer's diseases, or *bodig* in Chamorro [2, 17].

In both lytico and bodig, the presence of widespread NFTs was one of the more surprising and intriguing facets of ALS-PDC's pattern of expression. In ALS-PDC, NFTs were found not only in those who had the disease, but also in those who appeared to be disease-free at the time of death [10]. For those who had ALS-PDC, the distribution of the tangles within the cortex was quite different from that of Alzheimer's disease, involving the upper rather than the lower layers of the cortex [10].

In addition to NFTs, other peculiar structures were found. One was initially thought to be unique to ALS-PDC: odd, rod-shaped structures called *Hirano bodies* after neurologist Asao Hirano, who first described them.

Together with Hirano [18], Kurland and Mulder came to believe that these diseases were not entirely distinct entities but formed an extremely wide-ranging disease spectrum, with often overlapping symptoms, signs, and pathologies. About 10% of those initially presenting with lytico could eventually develop bodig as well. The reverse also applied but was less common.

Kurland later estimated that Guamanian ALS and PDC were both 50–100 times more prevalent than in North America. In villages such as Umatac in Southern Guam, disease incidence may have been closer to 400 times greater [10]. As documented by later investigators, the numbers were quite telling, as was the changing incidence pattern over time. Guamanian ALS had an incidence of 140 per 100 000 in 1950, dropping to 7 per 100 000 in 1989 and then to only 10 patients in total from 1997 to 2000. PDC showed similar patterns of decline [16].

The diseases of the ALS-PDC spectrum tended to cluster in Chamorro families, with some members having one or the other disease, and some having both (Figure 4.2). Within families in which there were multiple cases of the spectrum, birth order and birth year did not affect the disease phenotype, duration of illness, or age of onset [17]. This led to the hypothesis that environmental factors were involved in disease etiology. Adding further to the complexity of the spectrum was the extremely unusual observation that there might be a huge latency between environmental exposure and the expression of clinical signs, which in one case occurred 46 years after the patient left Guam. A study of Chamorros who had migrated to California suggested that previous exposure to something during childhood years on Guam resulted in a higher rate of ALS-PDC in Chamorro expatriates than among Californians in general. Regarding the age of onset for those remaining on Guam, the youngest documented case of ALS was at age 20 [20].

After the 1960s, when disease rates started to decline sharply (Figure 4.3), lytico did so more rapidly than bodig [21]. What made the ALS-PDC cluster most appealing from a neuro-epidemiology perspective was that the historical and ethnic circumstances on Guam vastly limited the number of possible causal factors. Genetic studies in the 1950s and 1960s had been carried out on a relatively homogeneous ethnic population, and environmental studies in those early years had fewer toxic factors to contend with than might be found in the more industrialized countries.

As with the age-related neurological diseases, including classical ALS, ALS-PDC showed the involvement of other organ systems. For those with Guamanian ALS, a skin disorder was described in the form of collagen disorganization similar to that already observed with ALS [22]. Another involved diaphyseal aclasis or cartilage-capped benign bone tumors (exostoses) [23]. Still another involved retinal "tracks" that appeared in the pigment epithelial cell layer of the retina [19, 24], but which did not seem to impact visual function.

INVESTIGATING ETIOLOGICAL FACTORS

Kurland, Mulder, and many others began an intensive search for potential causal factors, and the list, short as it was in comparison to North America's, was still large. A dominant genetic basis for the disease was considered and then discarded for lack of evidence, a conclusion largely the same after more than 60 years [25, 26]. The disease

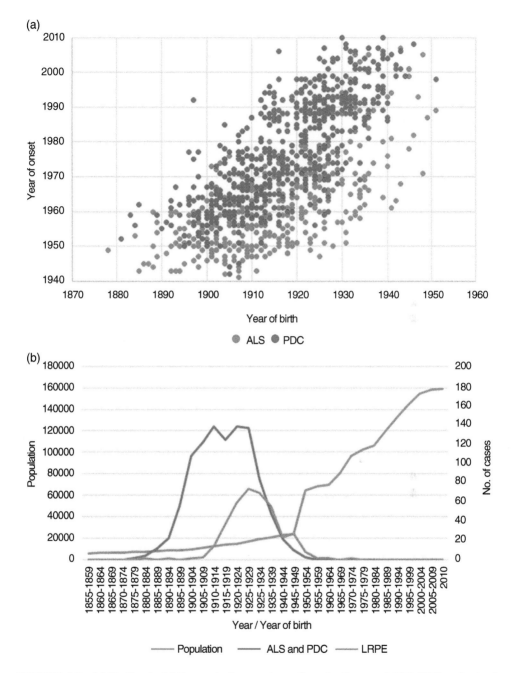

FIGURE 4.2 (a) Decline by birth year in the numbers of newly diagnosed ALS, PDC, and mixed ALS/PDC cases in 1195 Chamorros from 1956 to 2014; the numbers by birth year of those diagnosed with linear retinal pigment epitheliopathy (LRPE) after 1989, when its association with ALS/PDC was first made [19]; and the increasing population of the Mariana Islands after 1855. (b) Changing prevalence rates of ALS–PDC, leading to the end of the disease spectrum. This scattergram of 1195 Chamorros identified with ALS and PDC from 1956 to 2014 shows the ending of both phenotypes in those born after 1952. The year of onset of PDC is later than ALS. *Source:* Both figure panels and captions courtesy of Dr. John Steele.

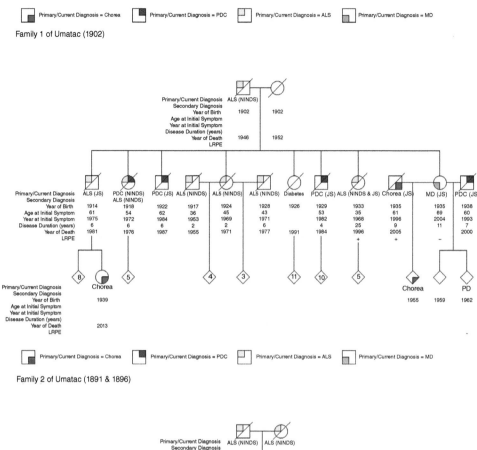

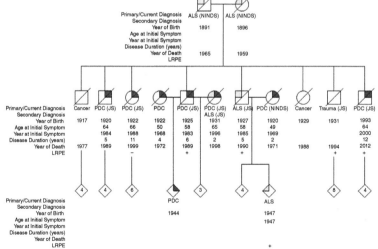

FIGURE 4.3   Pedigrees of four typical, unrelated families of Umatac village in Southern Guam. Note that in families 1 and 2, the generation born in the 1920s and 1930 suffer both ALS and PDC. Twenty of 30 members of the second generation developed ALS and/or PDC. They had 98 children who were all at age risk of ALS or PDC at the time of follow-up in 2014. Two children born in the 1940s developed PDC (1944) and ALS (1947) (family 2), one born in 1962 developed PD, and two had unrelated Huntington's chorea (family 1). None of the 93 remaining children developed ALS or PDC. Source. Graphs and captions courtesy of Dr. John Steele.

clustered within families, but as before, no clearly heritable gene was identified. However, researchers have not yet examined all genetic elements through technology such as whole-genome sequencing, and this may be a fruitful future area of study.

Since families share far more than genes, contributory factors could be anything the family members had in common, such as food, water, infectious disease states, and living conditions, to name only a few of the most obvious examples. Environmental studies looked at various possibilities. Some examined the effects of radiation from nuclear testing in the Pacific, or toxic compounds left behind by the war. Others examined various trace metals in the soil and water and features of the Chamorro diet [2].

Kurland invited Dr. Margaret Whiting, a nutritionist specializing in indigenous plants of the Pacific islands, to come to Guam. Whiting lived with Chamorro families for a number of months, and her time on Guam shifted the focus in the search for the cause of ALS-PDC. On the advice of botanist Dr. F. Raymond Fosberg, Whiting began focusing on the seeds of an indigenous variety of palm-like trees in appearance, the cycad [27], whose Guamanian population is now classified as *Cycas micronesica* KD Hill (Figure 4.4). The link of ALS-PDC to this species of cycad has been supported by a newer epidemiological study [28].

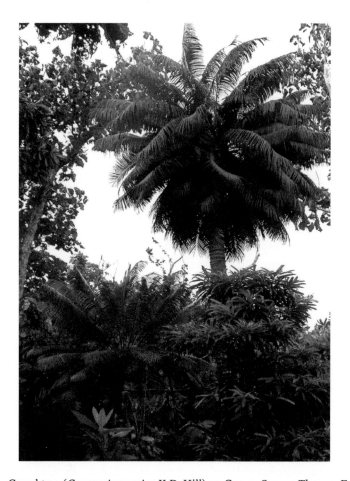

FIGURE 4.4   Cycad tree (*Cycas micronesica* K.D. Hill) on Guam. *Source*: Thomas E. Marler.

On Guam and Rota, different parts of cycads in the wild are often consumed by animals and humans. On Guam, the native species of cycad have numerous animal predators. Feral pigs and deer eat the leaves, the seeds, and sometimes the stalk. Coconut crabs have been known to consume the seeds. Scarab beetles and fruit bats may feed on the outer spongy later of the seed. The observations of animal consumption of cycad eventually led some investigators to suggest a form of biomagnification in which animals later eaten by humans might accumulate potential toxicants. The Chamorros of Guam ate the seeds and had done so for hundreds of years. They also seem to have chewed the sarcotesta, the soft outer portion of the seed, for its liquid content. However, they may not always have used cycad seeds as food, and some reports suggest that cycad consumption did not occur until the Chamorros were taught to wash out suspected toxicants by Mexican natives who came to Guam with the Spanish (Steele, personal communication) [2].

The entire process followed by the Chamorros was to remove the inner gametophyte from the seeds, cut this into strips, wash these for up to eight days in water, dry them, and then grind the "chips" into flour (Steele, personal communication).

Much later, as Guam became Westernized in diet after World War II, cycad consumption declined, but many older Chamorros continued to use and enjoy *fadang* or *federico*, their terms for the flour of the cycad seed. Some Chamorros still do so to the present day, seeing in the use of fadang an affirmation of their cultural identity.

Elsewhere in the Western Pacific, parts of various cycad species were also historically used as a food or medicine, and neurological disease spectrums resembling that of ALS-PDC of Guam were also apparently found in some of these other locales. On the Kii Peninsula of Honshu Island, Japan, seeds of *Cycas revoluta* were used apparently without processing as a miso paste (*sotetsu*) and a medicinal balm [29]. Japanese and Western researchers spent years considering the possible relationships between cycad use in the two loci and the similarities of the disease spectrums. Current researchers in Japan, however, have tended to deny any linkage between the neurological disease-spectrum disorder in Kii and ALS-PDC of Guam. In Irian Jaya of Western New Guinea, the Auyu and Jakai people used *Cycas circinalis* (currently described as *Cycas rumphii*) seed flour (*kurru*) without processing as a medicinal poultice. Among these populations, neurological disease prevalence was even higher than the average on Guam [30]. As on Guam, the prevalence of ALS and PDC gradually declined for unknown reasons [31].

The notion that the consumption of cycad seeds could cause ALS-PDC seemed both attractive and, at the same time, problematic for Kurland and others studying the disease. One of the main attractions of the so-called *cycad hypothesis* was its simplicity, in that a toxin/toxicant contained in a food product could cause neuronal degeneration leading to neurological disease if consumed in sufficient quantity. Much of the then-emerging epidemiology of ALS-PDC seemed to fit this hypothesis. The problem was that there seemed to be numerous potential toxicants in cycad seeds and the environment generally.

In addition to cycad, researchers have speculated on different compositions of ions in the soil and water [32] and/or the presence of other toxic elements, such as aluminum, whose neurotoxic properties are now well established [33–39].

Overall, the epidemiology of ALS-PDC clearly indicated a role for cycad consumption in the disease. However, there were, and remain, problems with this simple interpretation. Other peoples around the world eat tissue from various species of cycad but do not typically show an increased incidence of neurological diseases.

IDENTIFIED CYCAD TOXIN/TOXICANTS

Many questions arose from the early epidemiological studies of cycad on Guam. For example, if cycad consumption indeed causes lytico and bodig, do the seeds have one toxicant that damages all of the neural areas affected in the two diseases, or are multiple toxicants, each with a specific neuronal target, to blame? If multiple toxicants are present in cycad seeds, do they work alone or in synergy? Why were men, on average, usually more affected than women, as in North America [40], and why did ALS-PDC strike at younger ages than the related diseases in North America? The putative link between cycad consumption and ALS-PDC led to a detailed search over a number of years for potential neurotoxins in cycad seeds. These included cycasin, a glycosylated plant amino compound [41]. The same amino compound with two attached glucose molecules forms the toxin macrozamin. Cycasin and macrozamin are not particularly toxic by themselves, but removal of the glucose molecules during digestion transforms both into the deglycosylated form, methylazoxymethanol (MAM). MAM is a relatively potent hepatic toxin that, in animals, causes liver cancer [42]. Various studies have shown that pregnant rats fed MAM give birth to offspring with birth defects, including retinal abnormalities (albeit not pigment epithelial tracks, as already cited in relation to human ALS-PDC) and damage to the cerebellum, the latter inducing fine motor dysfunctions [43]. Regarding those neural subsystems that are damaged in ALS-PDC, investigators investigating the effects of MAM delivered the compound either orally or intravenously in adult animals but failed to find pathologies similar to the human disorders. In addition, the Chamorro practice of washing the seeds removed virtually all the cycasin/MAM present.

The legume that causes lathyrism – *Lathurus sativus* – contains the plant amino acid beta-N-oxalylamino-L-alanine (BOAA), which is also found in some cycad species, including *C. micronesica* on Guam. Although BOAA may be present in foods commonly consumed by humans, at high doses it can be an excitotoxin and cause motor neuron death. The notion that excitotoxicity through over-activation of glutamate receptors leads to motor neuron death has long been one of the major hypotheses for ALS. However, a major difference between lathyrism and ALS is the degree of neuronal dysfunction. In lathyrism, the motor neurons are not typically destroyed; in ALS, motor neuron degeneration is a key end-state feature of the disease. Additionally, BOAA, like cycasin, is washed away by the traditional Chamorro processing of cycad seeds.

Another toxic cycad amino acid is beta-methylamino-L-alanine (BMAA), isolated from cycad in 1967 [44]. At the time, BMAA was considered to be unique to cycad. In the years that followed, various groups, including Spencer and colleagues, began to revisit the cycad hypothesis and in the process took a more detailed look at various cycad-derived excitatory amino acids. Spencer's group initially explored the notion that BOAA could be the cause of ALS-PDC but quickly realized that the signs, symptoms, and pathologies of the two disorders were quite dissimilar [11]. BMAA seemed a more suitable candidate in that it activated both AMPA and NMDA subtypes of the excitatory glutamate receptors [45].

In a series of papers, Spencer's group claimed that feeding BMAA to monkeys reproduced some of the features of ALS-PDC, including muscle wasting and the presence of abnormal, pathological motor neurons [46]. However, the dosages needed to produce these effects were extremely high. Some calculations showed that for the Chamorros to have ingested enough BMAA by eating cycad flour, they would have had to have eaten at least 7 kg of unwashed raw cycad seed per day [47]. Second, the pathological changes in the nervous system of the BMAA-fed monkeys did not completely reproduce the fundamental signs of ALS-PDC. Specifically, while motor neurons did become dysfunctional, they did not actually degenerate. Additionally, once BMAA feeding ceased, the monkeys recovered some motor function, suggesting a transient toxic effect. In tissue-culture studies using isolated neuronal cells, BMAA appears to be a low-potency agonist that can be toxic, but only at relatively high concentrations. Studies performed by various investigators showed that BMAA was rapidly removed from cycad seeds by the washing steps typically performed by the Chamorros, falling to near-trace levels that were far too low to impact neurons in the nervous system [5, 47]. Other groups failed to find ALS-PDC-like outcomes in other experimental animal models [48, 49]. These latter data, along with the failure of the Spencer group and others to replicate the initial findings, led to a weakening of the BMAA hypothesis for ALS-PDC.

In 2002, the notion that BMAA might indeed be the cause of ALS-PDC experienced a resurgence with a study by Cox and Sacks [50]. Various later claims by Cox and colleagues include the assertion that cycads contain BMAA by virtue of the colonization of cycad roots by cyanobacteria of the species *Nostoc*, a view that was not supported by Marler et al. [51]. The elaboration of the Cox hypothesis was that *Nostoc*-derived BMAA makes its way through the cycad and into the seeds to be consumed by fruit bats which then biomagnify the toxic dose when humans eat the bats [48]. The hypothesis also hinges on the notion that BMAA is abnormally incorporated into protein in place of alanine. Newer evidence from the Cox group suggests that vervet monkeys fed BMAA in high doses develop some of the pathological features of ALS-PDC, including NFTs and amyloid plaques, although without any neuronal cell loss or behavioral dysfunction [52].

Our own work on the subject of cycad toxicity in ALS-PDC led to the isolation of several toxic steryl glucosides from cycad seeds [53]. There are now hundreds of plant steryls known to science, many of them glycosylated. The glucose molecule may confer neurotoxic properties to some of these, including digitalis and oleandrin [54]. Removal of the glucose moiety by deglycosylation reactions, as well as the addition of added glucose molecules beyond a single one, renders the molecules less toxic [2]. The mechanism of glucose toxicity of steryl compounds remains to be understood.

Early studies in our laboratory demonstrated that a common steryl has multiple roles in animals. For example, cholesterol can be made toxic by glycosylation. A frequent critique of this work is that the three key toxic steryl glucosides that Khabazian et al. [53] identified are quite common in most plants, although cycad seeds appear to have higher than average levels, which are dependent on the maturity of the seeds [55]; and some largely anecdotal evidence suggested that immature cycad seeds were consumed during World War II due to food shortages. Our additional studies demonstrated neurotoxicity not only *in vitro* but also *in vivo* in both mice and rats. The initial studies by Wilson et al. [56] on cycad and steryl glucosides, notably isolated β-sitosterol-β-D glucoside (BSSG) given to mice by diet at a level concordant with human cycad consumption [57], showed motor neuron loss in various regions of the brain and spinal cord. Although the behavioral deficits were primarily motor in nature, as was the underlying pathology, the mice would progressively show lesions in the *subtantia nigra pars compacta*, hippocampus, and cortex. These studies have now largely been supported by work in other laboratories [58, 59] with links to the liver X receptor as a potential target.

One of the more surprising outcomes is the differences seen with cycad or isolated BSSG in mice compared to rats. In mice, the dominant pathological feature was a progressive ALS phenotype. In rats, the sole phenotype was that of a Lewy body type of parkinsonism [60, 61]. What these results seem to suggest is that the same molecule can drive very different neuronal outcomes that are, in part, species-dependent, in a way that produces the full ALS-PDC spectrum of disorders. Whether this means the molecule is metabolized differently in mice compared to rats or whether it gains preferential access to particular regions of the nervous system in each species remains unknown.

ALUMINUM AND IONIC ETIOLOGIES FOR ALS-PDC

There has been a considerable amount of work attempting to link purportedly high levels of aluminum in the soil and water of parts of Guam to where ALS-PDC–like disorders appear to be particularly prevalent [32]. Supporting this, Garruto et al. [20, 62] noted high levels of calcium and aluminum in NFTs in the post mortem hippocampus of ALS-PDC patients. Similar associations between NFTs and aluminum have been noted by other investigators [63], including for the disease spectrum in Kii, Japan [64]. The investigators looking at high aluminum on Guam and Irian Jaya postulated that a contributing factor was the low concentrations of calcium and magnesium which, in their view, led to a secondary parathyroidism causing aluminum accumulation by neurons. This suggestion was reinforced by studies that found low vitamin D levels in males with ALS on Guam, but these studies also noted that differences in calcium were "subtle" [65]. *In vivo* models using monkeys given a high-aluminum/low-calcium diet support the general hypothesis of an aluminum involvement by showing degenerative changes in the motor neurons of the spinal cord and brain stem, as well as neurons in the SN and cerebrum [62]. Many of the pathological features of these affected neurons resemble those of ALS-PDC. It should be noted that the measured ionic concentrations of calcium and aluminum in the soil and water of Guam were not validated by other researchers [66].

There is, however, another line of evidence for aluminum being involved in motor neuron degeneration. These are studies using injected aluminum hydroxide in mice and sheep that result in motor neuron loss and dramatic alterations in motor behaviors [37–39].

OTHER MOLECULES THAT MIGHT HAVE BEEN INVOLVED IN ALS-PDC

The list of potential toxicants involved in ALS-PDC includes a variety of other molecules of both natural and human origin. These include some toxin/toxicants associated with fishing using powdered *Barringtonia asiatica*, known as "the fish-kill plant" [67], zinc from galvanized pails used for washing cycad seeds [68], and a host of others. Part of the search for additional toxicants results from the very clear observation that none of those described to date can be said to be the definitive toxicant responsible for the disease spectrum on Guam.

Additionally, despite the initial hope of Kurland and others that Guam might serve as a model "geographic isolate," the search among the relatively limited potential causal factors has not proven as straightforward as they might have wished. In reality, Guam in the years during and after World War II was a very toxic environment due to a number of contaminants that came with the war.

This observation highlights that although Guamanian ALS-PDC may arise from a smaller subset of potential toxicants and toxic synergies than is present in North America, the number is still large.

A PUTATIVE VIRAL ETIOLOGY FOR ALS-PDC ON GUAM AND ALS IN GENERAL

The notion that some viral infection may play a distinct role in the etiology of ALS and other neurodegenerative disorders has been speculated about for years, particularly given the observation that an enterovirus such as Poliovirus can clearly induce motor neuron death in polio. Unlike in ALS neural degeneration, however, polio-induced motor neuron death is not progressive [69].

The evidence for various viruses such as enteroviruses, retroviruses, and herpes viruses being involved as causal to ALS is mixed. For example, it remains unclear to what extent any viral infection may be causal to ALS versus a consequence of another process. In the latter case, it is certainly possible that viral infections merely serve as a final insult to cells already suffering from some underlying dysfunctional state. In regard to this point, Celeste and Miller note that ALS features a number of alternations in cellular function, including mitochondrial dysfunction, oxidant stress and the mishandling of calcium, impacts on stress granules and RNA metabolism, inflammation, endoplasmic reticulum stress, and toxic protein aggregation and propagation, all of which have been shown to be triggered by viral infections [70]. In animal models, infection with a cocksackievirus construct caused the pathological translocation of TAR DNA binding protein 43 (TDP-43) from nuclei to cytoplasm in motor neurons, the latter a feature of most forms of ALS [71].

Some of the viruses linked to ALS or in animal models of the disease include human endogenous retrovirus K (HERV K) [72], cocksackievirus [71], and Cas—Br—E murine leukemia virus (*MuLV*) [73].

Linking viral infections to ALS presents a temporal problem in that ALS does not seem to arise in the same time frame as the infection. This general concern may also apply to ALS-PDC on Guam: while Zimmerman [13] had described a larger than expected incidence of ALS on Guam in 1945, studies by Edgren et al. [74, 75] described an outbreak of Japanese encephalitis, a mosquito-borne flavivirus, on Guam in 1947. An analysis of the Japanese encephalitis outbreak by Solomon et al. [75] showed that many of the features of the parkinsonism part of the spectrum, PDC, resembled the neural outcomes of the viral infection. Further, some of the victims showed acute flaccid paralysis with motor neuron degeneration as in ALS. Further linking Japanese encephalitis with ALS-PDC was the observation [20] of the development of ALS-PDC in Chamorros who later migrated to California. Admittedly, the description of at least the ALS portion of the disease prior to the "official" start of the encephalitis outbreak is a problem for such a viral hypothesis as a key etiological factor. However, the later finding of the PDC portion in the early 1950s [18], which more closely resembles outcomes in Japanese encephalitis, is not.

For these reasons, while no definitive conclusions can be reached about a viral etiology for ALS or ALS-PDC, it should be stressed that the possibility of such a link cannot be discounted and remains a possibly fruitful avenue for further research.

THE CONTINUING IMPORTANCE OF ALS-PDC

ALS-PDC has historically elicited a range of opinions among neurologists, neuroscientists, and epidemiologists who either obsessively love or intensely dislike the example set by this cluster [2]. Those who are passionate about ALS-PDC feel that the disease is mysterious, exotic, and still unsolved. With regard to the last, ALS-PDC offers for some the hope of a relatively straightforward universal toxin and/or genetic etiology – or at least process – that may be applicable to ALS and other age-dependent neurological diseases elsewhere.

What are the chief complaints about the use of ALS-PDC as a model neurological disease cluster? First, ALS-PDC is a "messy" neurological disease, combining in families and even in some individuals features of what are traditionally considered very distinct neurological diseases. In some ways, the spectrum of ALS-PDC resembles the overlapping features of ALS and FTD and the often overlapping pathologies of Parkinson's and Alzheimer's diseases [76]. Next, there may also be a temporal lag from exposure to some toxic factor (or the onset of a particular gene product) that makes the correlation to any potential toxin nearly impossible to satisfy using the Hill criteria [77]. In these regards, those seeking a simple etiology for ALS-PDC find that the spectrum does not have one, but rather has a range of likely additive or perhaps synergistic factors.

Next, while there remains an ethnic factor (i.e. Chamorro heritage/ethnicity), no clear genetic mutation or even distinct polymorphism can be linked to the disorder in any of its multiple manifestations [25]. It should be noted that genetic studies in ALS-PDC were based on older technologies than are currently available today, and any underlying genetic contribution may not have been detected, as discussed above. Finally, the various toxin/toxicant studies that have been carried out on ALS-PDC have shown disparate, contradictory, and even biologically implausible outcomes.

Perhaps most definitively, a key reason for dismissing ALS-PDC as still relevant is that it has been disappearing: no one born after the 1960s developed the disease [16], reinforcing the notion that it was, and is, a neurological anomaly with no particular relevance for understanding any of the other age-related, progressive neurological diseases elsewhere, including ALS.

All of these reasons are valid and understandable. And yet, to a large measure, they miss the key point that ALS-PDC remains the sole widely accepted disease cluster of ALS and the other disorders in this spectrum.

The study of ALS-PDC had – and maybe still has – in spite of the disorder's fading away – some key lessons to teach the world of ALS research with the following being the key points to consider. These are:

1. None of the main disorders in the ALS-PDC spectrum are truly independent of the others in that a reasonably large fraction of those with one feature of the neurological disease spectrum have some variation of the others as well. For example, those with ALS and Parkinson's disease often show cognitive dysfunctions as the disease progresses. This is quite obvious for ALS-FTD but occurs in more classical ALS as well.

2. The classical hallmark protein features of Alzheimer's disease, abnormally phosphorylated tau protein and Aβ deposits, however toxic to neurons, are not the key disease triggering factors. This can be concluded from the fact that abnormal tau deposits can be found in individuals unaffected by ALS-PDC [10] and that the amyloid deposits typical in non-Guamanian Alzheimer's are largely absent in ALS-PDC. An argument can, however, be made that both tau and Aβ deposits are "downstream" events that might have occurred at later times in these patients.

3. The neuronal diseases in the spectrum of ALS-PDC can occur in a familial setting, but the expression of one type versus another is apparently dependent on other, still-unknown factors. These factors, given a family setting, are not likely to be solely dietary/waterborne (environmental), sex-linked, or genetic in nature. They might, however, be caused by genetic susceptibility factors – polymorphisms, deletions, expansions, etc. – that both contribute to the onset

of the disorder and further specify which region of the central nervous system (CNS) is affected and thus which subtype of disease will arise.

4. The decline in ALS-PDC incidence suggests that the triggering factor, presumably of environmental origin, has diminished over the same time period. This could display as a direct decline in the triggering factor or as an indirect decrease in environmental exposure due to changes in lifestyle. A second and also likely possibility is that since the Guamanian population is now more genetically heterogeneous due to greater intermarriage with non-Chamorros, genetic susceptibility factors have changed as well.

5. These issues point to gene–toxin/toxicant interactions as key to the etiology of ALS-PDC. This makes it likely that the field could search endlessly (assuming the diseases still exists in a few years) without identifying a clear causal gene mutation, as suggested by Morris et al. [25]. It also means that no one environmental trigger, no matter how toxic in model systems that normally use high doses of putative risk factors, is going to account for the entire disease spectrum.

6. The impact of the microbiome is likely to be seen in the future as having a profound effect on how toxin/toxicant and/or genetic mutations affect disease expression. In the context of Guam, it remains important to remember that the relatively homogeneous genetic population prior to World War II and the impact of widespread starvation during the years of Japanese occupation may have contributed in significant ways to disease rates, as well as possible infectious disease factors, as cited above.

7. A more productive way to think about gene–toxin/toxicant/microbiome interactions might be to try to reverse engineer the entire process. Thus, rather than seeking distinct gene mutations, maybe research should be focused on toxicant-induced pathway signaling and which genes allow the toxin/toxicant to have differential access to regions of the CNS.

SUMMARY AND CONCLUSIONS

In spite of ALS-PDC declining sharply after 1960 from a peak in the 1950s, the study of this disease spectrum may still be critical for understanding the factors leading to ALS elsewhere. Certainly, Leonard Kurland and others thought so, and the enthusiasm Kurland brought to this field of study inspired many others to follow in his footsteps.

Perhaps the clearest lesson to draw from the study of ALS-PDC is that the onset of a complex disease such as this requires that perfect storm of multiple factors: genes, environmental toxins/toxicants or pathogens, and their myriad interactions (Figure 4.5).

The hope still remains that understanding the elements of this storm will, as Kurland suggested, be the neurological "Rosetta Stone" that enables us to finally understand how ALS arises and perhaps, from this, how it can be prevented or halted. A more thorough understanding of ALS-PDC would allow for novel insights into the spectrum nature of not only ALS but neurological diseases in general.

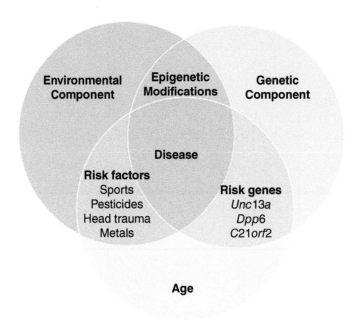

FIGURE 4.5   Venn diagram showing suggested interactions of genes and toxicants leading to sALS. *Source*: Courtesy of Jessica R. Morrice.

ACKNOWLEDGMENTS

The authors thank Dr. John Steele for providing figures, for his advice, and for providing feedback on the chapter. Jess Morrice provided a critical early review of a draft of this chapter, and Michael Kuo obtained the permissions for some of the figures used.

CONFLICT OF INTEREST

The authors declare no potential conflict of interest with respect to research, authorship, and/or publication of this manuscript.

COPYRIGHT AND PERMISSION STATEMENT

To the best of our knowledge, the materials included in this chapter do not violate copyright laws. All original sources have been appropriately acknowledged and/or referenced. Where relevant, appropriate permissions have been obtained from the original copyright holder.

NOTE

1. *Perfect storm*: A particularly violent storm arising from a rare combination of adverse meteorological factors; a particularly bad or critical state of affairs, arising from a number of negative and unpredictable factors (Oxford Definitions).

REFERENCES

1. Morrice, J.R., Gregory-Evans, C.Y., and Shaw, C.A. (2018). Modeling environmentally-induced motor neuron degeneration in zebrafish. *Sci. Rep.* 8 (1): 4890.
2. Shaw, C.A. (2017). *Neural Dynamics of Neurological Disease*. Boston: Wiley.
3. Ross, G.W. and Abbott, R.D. (2014). Living and dying with Parkinson's disease. *Mov. Disord.* 29 (13): 1571–1573.
4. Al-Chalabi, A. and Hardiman, O. (2013). The epidemiology of ALS: a conspiracy of genes, environment and time. *Nat. Rev. Neurol.* 9 (11): 617–628.
5. Kisby, G. (2000). β-N-methylamino-L-alanine. In: *Experimental and Clinical Neurotoxicology*, 2e (eds. P.S. Spencer, H.H. Schaumburg and A.C. Ludolph), 789–794. Oxford: Oxford University Press.
6. Risher, J.F., Murray, H.E., and Prince, G.R. (2002). Organic mercury compounds: human exposure and its relevance to public health. *Toxicol. Ind. Health.* 18 (3): 109–160.
7. Perl, T.M., Bedard, L., Kosatsky, T. et al. (1990). An outbreak of toxic encephalopathy caused by eating mussels contaminated with domoic acid. *N. Engl. J. Med.* 322 (25): 1775–1780.
8. Neurological Health Charities Canada and Public Health Agency of Canada. (2014). Mapping connections: An understanding of neurological conditions in Canada. The National Population Health Study of Neurological Conditions, Ottawa.
9. Kurland, L.T. (1972). An appraisal of the neurotoxicity of cycad and the etiology of amyotrophic lateral sclerosis on Guam. *Fed. Proc.* 31 (5): 1540–1542.
10. Kurland, L.T. (1988). Amyotrophic lateral sclerosis and Parkinson's disease complex on Guam linked to an environmental neurotoxin. *Trends Neurosci.* 11 (2): 51–54.
11. Kurland, L.T. and Mulder, D.W. (1954). Epidemiologic investigations of amyotrophic lateral sclerosis. I. Preliminary report on geographic distribution, with special reference to the Mariana Islands, including clinical and pathologic observations. *Neurology* 4 (5): 355–378.
12. Kane, A.V., Dinh, D.M., and Ward, H.D. (2015). Childhood malnutrition and the intestinal microbiome. *Pediatr. Res.* 77 (1–2): 256–262.
13. Zimmerman, H. (1945). Progress report of work in the laboratory of pathology during May 1945, Guam. US Naval Medical Research Unit, Washington, DC.
14. van Es, M.A., Hardiman, O., Chio, A. et al. (2017). Amyotrophic lateral sclerosis. *Lancet* 390 (10107): 2084–2098.
15. Bang, J., Spina, S., and Miller, B.L. (2015). Frontotemporal dementia. *Lancet* 386 (10004): 1672–1682.

16. Galasko, D., Salmon, D.P., Craig, U.K. et al. (2002). Clinical features and changing patterns of neurodegenerative disorders on Guam, 1997–2000. *Neurology* 58 (1): 90–97.

17. Steele, J.C. (2005). Parkinsonism-dementia complex of Guam. *Mov. Disord.* 20 (Suppl 12): S99–S107.

18. Hirano, A., Kurland, L.T., Krooth, R.S., and Lessell, S. (1961). Parkinsonism-dementia complex, an endemic disease on the island of Guam. I. Clinical features. *Brain* 84: 642–661.

19. Cox, T.A., McDarby, J.V., Lavine, L. et al. (1989). A retinopathy on Guam with high prevalence in Lytico-Bodig. *Ophthalmology* 96 (12): 1731–1735.

20. Garruto, R.M. (1996). Early environment, long latency and slow progression of late onset neuro-degenerative disorders. In: *Long-Term Consequences of Early Environment: Growth, Development, and the Lifespan Developmental Perspective* (eds. C.J.K. Henry and S.J. Ulijaszek), 219. Melbourne: Cambridge University Press.

21. Plato, C.C., Garruto, R.M., Galasko, D. et al. (2003). Amyotrophic lateral sclerosis and parkinsonism-dementia complex of Guam: changing incidence rates during the past 60 years. *Am. J. Epidemiol.* 157 (2): 149–157.

22. Fullmer, H.M., Siedler, H.D., Krooth, R.S., and Kurland, L.T. (1960). A cutaneous disorder of connective tissue in amyotrophic lateral sclerosis. A histochemical study. *Neurology* 10: 717–724.

23. Krooth, R.S., Macklin, M.T., and Hilbish, T.F. (1961). Diaphysial aclasis (multiple exostoses) on Guam. *Am. J. Hum. Genet.* 13: 340–347.

24. Campbell, R.J., Steele, J.C., Cox, T.A. et al. (1993). Pathologic findings in the retinal pigment epitheliopathy associated with the amyotrophic lateral sclerosis/parkinsonism-dementia complex of Guam. *Ophthalmology* 100 (1): 37–42.

25. Morris, H.R., Steele, J.C., Crook, R. et al. (2004). Genome-wide analysis of the parkinsonism-dementia complex of Guam. *Arch. Neurol.* 61 (12): 1889–1897.

26. Steele, J.C., Guella, I., Szu-Tu, C. et al. (2015). Defining neurodegeneration on Guam by targeted genomic sequencing. *Ann. Neurol.* 77 (3): 458–468.

27. Whiting, M.G. (1963). Toxicity of cycads. *Econ. Bot.* 17 (4): 270–302.

28. Borenstein, A.R., Mortimer, J.A., Schofield, E. et al. (2007). Cycad exposure and risk of dementia, MCI, and PDC in the Chamorro population of Guam. *Neurology* 68 (21): 1764–1771.

29. Kobayashi, A. (1972). Cycasin in cycad materials used in Japan. *Fed. Proc.* 31 (5): 1476–1477.

30. Gajdusek, D.C. and Salazar, A.M. (1982). Amyotrophic lateral sclerosis and parkinsonian syndromes in high incidence among the Auyu and Jakai people of West New Guinea. *Neurology* 32 (2): 107–126.

31. Spencer, P.S., Palmer, V.S., and Ludolph, A.C. (2005). On the decline and etiology of high-incidence motor system disease in West Papua (Southwest New Guinea). *Mov. Disord.* 20 (Suppl 12): S119–S126.

32. Garruto, R.M., Yanagihara, R., Gajdusek, D.C., and Arion, D.M. (1984). Concentrations of heavy metals and essential minerals in garden soil and drinking water in the Western Pacific. In: *Amyotrophic Lateral Sclerosis in Asia and Oceania* (eds. K.-M. Chen and Y. Yase), 265–329. Taipei: National Taiwan University.

33. Exley, C., Burgess, E., Day, J.P. et al. (1996). Aluminum toxicokinetics. *J. Toxicol. Environ. Health* 48 (6): 569–584.

34. Exley, C. (2004). The pro-oxidant activity of aluminum. *Free Radic. Biol. Med.* 36 (3): 380–387.

35. Exley, C., Siesjo, P., and Eriksson, H. (2010). The immunobiology of aluminium adjuvants: how do they really work? *Trends Immunol.* 31 (3): 103–109.

36. Exley, C. (2012). The coordination chemistry of aluminium in neurodegenerative disease. *Coordin. Chem. Rev.* 256 (19–20): 2142–2146.

37. Lujan, L., Perez, M., Salazar, E. et al. (2013). Autoimmune/autoinflammatory syndrome induced by adjuvants (ASIA syndrome) in commercial sheep. *Immunol. Res.* 56 (2–3): 317–324.

38. Petrik, M.S., Wong, M.C., Tabata, R.C. et al. (2007). Aluminum adjuvant linked to gulf war illness induces motor neuron death in mice. *Neuromolecular Med.* 9 (1): 83–100.

39. Shaw, C.A. and Petrik, M.S. (2009). Aluminum hydroxide injections lead to motor deficits and motor neuron degeneration. *J. Inorg. Biochem.* 103 (11): 1555–1562.

40. Manjaly, Z.R., Scott, K.M., Abhinav, K. et al. (2010). The sex ratio in amyotrophic lateral sclerosis: a population based study. *Amyotroph Lateral Scler.* 11 (5): 439–442.

41. Matsumoto, H. and Strong, F.M. (1963). The occurrence of methylazoxymethanol in Cycas circinalis L. *Arch. Biochem. Biophys.* 101 (2): 299–310.

42. Fukunishi, R. (1973). Acute hepatic lesions induced by cycasin. *Acta Pathol. Jpn.* 23 (3): 639–646.

43. Spencer, P.S., Kisby, G., Palmer, V., and Obendorf, P. (2000). Cycasin, methylazoxymethanol and related compounds. In: *Experimental and Clinical Neurotoxicology*, 2ee (eds. P.S. Spencer, H.H. Schaumburg and A.C. Ludolph), 436–447.

44. Vega, A. and Bell, E.A. (1967). Alpha-amino-beta-methylaminopropionic acid a new amino acid from seeds of Cycas circinalis. *Phytochemistry* 6 (5): 759–762.

45. Weiss, J.H., Koh, J.Y., and Choi, D.W. (1989). Neurotoxicity of beta-N-methylamino-L-alanine (BMAA) and beta-N-oxalylamino-L-alanine (BOAA) on cultured cortical neurons. *Brain Res.* 497 (1): 64–71.

46. Spencer, P.S., Nunn, P.B., Hugon, J. et al. (1987). Guam amyotrophic lateral sclerosis-parkinsonism-dementia linked to a plant excitant neurotoxin. *Science* 237 (4814): 517–522.

47. Duncan, M.W. (1991). Role of the cycad neurotoxin BMAA in the amyotrophic lateral sclerosis-parkinsonism dementia complex of the Western Pacific. *Adv. Neurol.* 56: 301–310.

48. Cruz-Aguado, R., Winkler, D., and Shaw, C.A. (2006). Lack of behavioral and neuropathological effects of dietary beta-methylamino-L-alanine (BMAA) in mice. *Pharmacol. Biochem. Behav.* 84 (2): 294–299.

49. Perry, T.L., Bergeron, C., Biro, A.J., and Hansen, S. (1989). Beta-N-methylamino-L-alanine. Chronic oral administration is not neurotoxic to mice. *J. Neurol. Sci.* 94 (1–3): 173–180.

50. Cox, P.A. and Sacks, O.W. (2002). Cycad neurotoxins, consumption of flying foxes, and ALS-PDC disease in Guam. *Neurology* 58 (6): 956–959.

51. Marler, T.E., Snyder, L.R., and Shaw, C.A. (2010). Cycas micronesica (Cycadales) plants devoid of endophytic cyanobacteria increase in beta-methylamino-L-alanine. *Toxicon* 56 (4): 563–568.

52. Cox, P.A., Davis, D.A., Mash, D.C. et al. (2016). Dietary exposure to an environmental toxin triggers neurofibrillary tangles and amyloid deposits in the brain. *Proc. Biol. Sci.* 283 (1823).

53. Khabazian, I., Bains, J.S., Williams, D.E. et al. (2002). Isolation of various forms of sterol beta-D-glucoside from the seed of Cycas circinalis: neurotoxicity and implications for ALS-parkinsonism dementia complex. *J. Neurochem.* 82 (3): 516–528.

54. Akihisa, T., Kokke, W.C.M., and Tamura, T. (1991). Naturally occurring sterols and related compounds from plants. In: *Physiology and Biochemistry of Sterols* (eds. G.W. Patterson and W.D. Nes), 172–228. Champaign, IL: American Oil Chemist's Soceity.

55. Marler, T.E., Lee, V., Chung, J., and Shaw, C.A. (2006). Steryl glucoside concentration declines with Cycas micronesica seed age. *Funct. Plant Biol.* 33 (9): 857–862.

56. Wilson, J.M., Khabazian, I., Wong, M.C. et al. (2002). Behavioral and neurological correlates of ALS-parkinsonism dementia complex in adult mice fed washed cycad flour. *Neuromolecular Med.* 1 (3): 207–221.

57. Tabata, R.C., Wilson, J.M., Ly, P. et al. (2008). Chronic exposure to dietary sterol glucosides is neurotoxic to motor neurons and induces an ALS-PDC phenotype. *Neuromolecular Med.* 10 (1): 24–39.

58. Andersson, S., Gustafsson, N., Warner, M., and Gustafsson, J.A. (2005). Inactivation of liver X receptor beta leads to adult-onset motor neuron degeneration in male mice. *Proc. Natl. Acad. Sci. U. S. A.* 102 (10): 3857–3862.

59. Kim, H.J., Fan, X.T., Gabbi, C. et al. (2008). Liver X receptor beta (LXR beta): a link between beta-sitosterol and amyotrophic lateral sclerosis-Parkinson's dementia. *Proc. Natl. Acad. Sci. U. S. A.* 105 (6): 2094–2099.

60. Shen, W.B., McDowell, K.A., Siebert, A.A. et al. (2010). Environmental neurotoxin-induced progressive model of parkinsonism in rats. *Ann. Neurol.* 68 (1): 70–80.

61. Van Kampen, J.M., Baranowski, D.C., Robertson, H.A. et al. (2015). The progressive BSSG rat model of Parkinson's: recapitulating multiple key features of the human disease. *PLoS One* 10 (10): e0139694.

62. Garruto, R.M., Shankar, S.K., Yanagihara, R. et al. (1989). Low-calcium, high-aluminum diet-induced motor neuron pathology in cynomolgus monkeys. *Acta Neuropathol.* 78 (2): 210–219.

63. Perl, D.P., Gajdusek, D.C., Garruto, R.M. et al. (1982). Intraneuronal aluminum accumulation in amyotrophic lateral sclerosis and parkinsonism-dementia of Guam. *Science* 217 (4564): 1053–1055.

64. Kihira, T., Yoshida, S., Mitani, K. et al. (1993). ALS in the Kii Peninsula of Japan, with special reference to neurofibrillary tangles and aluminum. *Neuropathology* 13: 125–136.

65. Yanagihara, R., Garruto, R.M., Gajdusek, D.C. et al. (1984). Calcium and vitamin D metabolism in Guamanian Chamorros with amyotrophic lateral sclerosis and parkinsonism-dementia. *Ann. Neurol.* 15 (1): 42–48.

66. Steele, J.C. and Williams, D.B. (1995). Calcium and aluminium in the Chamorro diet: unlikely causes of Alzheimer-type neurofibrillary degeneration on Guam. In: *Motor Neuron Disease* (eds. P.N. Leigh and M. Swash), 189–200. London: Springer.

67. Cannon, J.G., Burton, R.A., Wood, S.G., and Owen, N.L. (2004). Naturally occurring fish poisons from plants. *J. Chem. Educ.* 81 (10): 1457–1461.

68. Duncan, M.W., Marini, A.M., Watters, R. et al. (1992). Zinc, a neurotoxin to cultured neurons, contaminates cycad flour prepared by traditional guamanian methods. *J. Neurosci.* 12 (4): 1523–1537.

69. Nomoto, A. (2007). Molecular aspects of poliovirus pathogenesis. *Proc. Jpn. Acad. Ser. B Phys. Biol. Sci.* 83 (8): 266–275.

70. Celeste, D.B. and Miller, M.S. (2018). Reviewing the evidence for viruses as environmental risk factors for ALS: a new perspective. *Cytokine* 108: 173–178.

71. Xue, Y.C., Ruller, C.M., Fung, G. et al. (2018). Enteroviral infection leads to transactive response DNA-binding protein 43 pathology *in vivo*. *Am. J. Pathol.* 188 (12): 2853–2862.

72. Douville, R., Liu, J., Rothstein, J., and Nath, A. (2011). Identification of active loci of a human endogenous retrovirus in neurons of patients with amyotrophic lateral sclerosis. *Ann. Neurol.* 69 (1): 141–151.

73. Jolicoeur, P., Rassart, E., DesGroseillers, L. et al. (1991). Retrovirus-induced motor neuron disease of mice: molecular basis of neurotropism and paralysis. *Adv. Neurol.* 56: 481–493.

74. Edgren, D.C., Palladino, V.S., and Arnold, A. (1958). Japanese B and mumps encephalitis: a clinicopathological report of simultaneous outbreaks on the island of Guam. *Am. J. Trop. Med. Hyg.* 7 (5): 471–480.

75. Solomon, T., Dung, N.M., Kneen, R. et al. (2000). Japanese encephalitis. *J. Neurol. Neurosurg. Psychiatry* 68 (4): 405–415.

76. Kurosinski, P., Guggisberg, M., and Gotz, J. (2002). Alzheimer's and Parkinson's disease--overlapping or synergistic pathologies? *Trends Mol. Med.* 8 (1): 3–5.

77. Hill, A.B. (1965). The environment and disease: association or causation? *Proc. R. Soc. Med.* 58: 295–300.

CHAPTER 5

The Microbiome of ALS – Does It Start from the Gut?

Audrey Labarre[1,2] and Alex Parker[1,2]

[1] Department of Neuroscience, University of Montréal, Montréal, Québec, Canada
[2] Centre de recherche du centre hospitalier de l'Université de Montréal (CRCHUM), Montréal, Québec, Canada

INTRODUCTION

Hundreds of bacteria species live in the human body and contribute to general health. These microbes are referred as the *microbiome*. The study of the brain-gut-microbiome axis is an emergent topic in global health and neurodegenerative disorders. Over the last few years, a perturbed microbiome, also called a *dysbiosis*, has been associated with various complex mood disorders and neurological diseases including depression, Parkinson's disease, multiple sclerosis, and Alzheimer's disease [1]. To this day, little evidence has linked amyotrophic lateral sclerosis (ALS) and the microbiome. However, some studies have identified a number of bacteria contributing to dysbiosis that could be linked to ALS pathogenesis [2–5]. Moreover, some studies have identified bacterial products that could potentially be beneficial in the disease course [3, 6]. Nonetheless, the implications of the microbiome for ALS remain a blossoming field that could revolutionize the way the disease is studied.

Even if some cases of ALS are associated with genetic causes, one of the leading hypotheses regarding sporadic ALS etiology remains the implication of environmental factors [7]. These factors, including diet, lifestyle, and exposure to chemicals, can modulate microbiome composition by influencing the bacterial balance in the gut

Spectrums of Amyotrophic Lateral Sclerosis: Heterogeneity, Pathogenesis and Therapeutic Directions,
First Edition. Edited by Christopher A. Shaw and Jessica R. Morrice.
© 2021 John Wiley & Sons Ltd. Published 2021 by John Wiley & Sons Ltd.

as well as the over- or underproduction of some bacterial metabolites, potentially affecting the pathogenesis of ALS.

In this chapter, we will provide an overview of how the microbiome is believed to play a role in ALS pathophysiology and how dysbiosis could influence the central nervous system (CNS). We will also discuss the implication of gut dysbiosis on neuronal health, as well as the models used to study the microbiome in an ALS context. Finally, we will discuss modifications of the gut microbiome as a potential therapeutic tool to help manage ALS symptoms and progression.

RECENT STUDIES

The study of the microbiome is a relatively new topic in the ALS field, with limited accompanying literature. The first manuscript linking the potential effect of the microbiome in ALS was published in 2015, and to date, fewer than a dozen research papers have been published. However, they can mainly be separated into two categories: animal and clinical studies (Table 5.1).

Animal and *in vitro* Studies

The first research paper reporting a link between ALS and the microbiome in an animal model was published in 2015 [8]. The authors demonstrated that SOD1^{G93A} mice display an alternative gut microbiome composition at different stages of the disease. Bacterial profiling of the gut using 16S rRNA sequencing revealed a shifted profile of microbial composition, with reduced levels of *Butyrivibrio fibrisolvens, Escherichia coli*, and *Fermicus* in presymptomatic SOD1^{G93A} mice, as well as a significant decrease in butyrate-producing bacteria. This microbiome profiling focused only on the colon, known to be the part of the intestine containing the most abundant microflora, where the majority of host-bacteria interactions occur. Mice displayed damaged tight junctions and a reduction in the expression levels of tight-junction protein ZO-1 and adherent junction E-cadherin. Distribution of ZO-1 was highly abnormal in the membrane of intestinal epithelial cells, while E-cadherin distribution appeared normal. Moreover, ALS mouse models display increased gut permeability, a digestive condition in which microorganisms, toxins, and bacterial-derived products can leak through the intestinal barrier [13]. All these observations were made on two-month-old mice (presymptomatic stage).

Paneth cells are one of the most important cell types of the small intestine epithelium and are key effectors of innate mucosal defense, as well as essential for host-defense and autophagy activity. Paneth cell secretory granules include lysozymes, α-defensins, and phospholipase [14]. The small intestine epithelium of SOD1^{G93A} animals has an increased number of abnormal Paneth cells, characterized by disorganized or diminished secretory granules with diffuse cytoplasmic lysozyme distribution. Symptomatic mice show a decrease of antimicrobial peptide defensin 5 alpha (DEF5α)

TABLE 5.1 Summary of key findings linking ALS and the microbiome.

References	Experimental model	Key findings
Animal and in vitro studies		
Wu et al. [8]	SOD1^{G93A} mouse (B6/SJL background, no information regarding gender)	Alternative gut microbiome composition at different stages of the disease ↓ B. fibrisolvens, ↓ E. coli, ↓ Fermicus, ↓ butyrate-producing bacteria Damaged tight junctions, ↓ expression levels of ZO-1 and E-cadherin, highly abnormal distribution of ZO-1 ↑ gut permeability, ↑ abnormal Paneth cells ↑ Il-17 (blood and intestines) ↓ intestinal DEF5α and lysozyme1mRNAs
Zhang et al. [3]	SOD1^{G93A} mouse (B6/SJL background, no information regarding gender), HCT116 and HT29C19A cell line	**SOD1^{G93A} mouse** ↓ expression of butyryl-CoA: acetate CoA-transferase mRNA <u>After 2% sodium butyrate treatment</u> Delayed onset and extended lifespan Correction of dysbiosis: ↑ B. fibrisolvens, ↑ F. peptostreptococcus, ↑ Eubacterium, ↑ Odoribacter, ↑ Bacteroides ↑ mRNA expression of butyryl-CoA: acetate CoA-transferase Restoration of ZO-1 levels, ↓ abnormal Paneth cells ↑ lysozyme1 and ↑ DEF5α mRNA levels ↓ intestinal permeability, ↓ intestinal SOD1 aggregation **HCT116 cell line** <u>After 24-hour 2 mM butyrate treatment</u> ↓ SOD1 aggregation **HT29C19A cell line** <u>After butyrate treatment</u> ↑ transepithelial resistance, ↓ permeability

(Continued)

TABLE 5.1 (Continued)

References	Experimental model	Key findings
Figueroa-Romero et al. [9]	SOD1^{G93A} mouse (C57BL/6 background, males and females)	Dysbiosis, variations of α and β microbial diversity ↓ A. muciniphila, ↓ B. caccae ↑ A. muris, ↓ B. vulgatus Differences in KEGG pathways functions: neurodegeneration, immune system function, lipid metabolism and development, and signal transduction ↓ lifespan when housed in a "dirty" animal facility
Blacher et al. [5]	SOD1^{G93A} mouse (C57BL/6 background, males and females)	Dysbiosis through all stages of the disease, including before onset ↑ operational taxonomic units (OTUs) ↓ enzymes participating in tryptophan and NAM metabolism, ↓ A. muciniphila <u>Germ-free rederivation</u> ↑ mortality, phenotype persistent after being colonized with a new microbiome around the onset of disease de novo dysbiosis after spontaneous colonization <u>Broad-spectrum antibiotic treatment</u> ↑ motor symptoms, ↑ loss of spinal cord neurons ↑ brain atrophy and neurodegeneration No alteration of main immune cell populations (spinal cord, small intestine, colon) <u>A. muciniphila inoculation after microbiome depletion</u> ↑ motor function, ↑ lifespan, ↓ brain atrophy No effect on intestinal permeability ↑ phenol sulfate and NAM <u>Treatment with bacterial metabolites</u> Phenol sulfate had no effect NAM ↑ performance on motor tests, ↑ NAM levels (sera, CSF), no lifespan extension

Reference	Model	Findings
Burberry et al. [10]	C9orf72 (loss-of-function, C57BL/6 background, males and females)	Dysbiosis, ↓ of α microbial diversity, variations of β diversity ↑ murine norovirus, *Helicobacter* spp., *P. pneumotropica*, and *T. muris* <u>Rederivation in a new facility</u> Premature mortality, ↑ motor behavior deficit, ↑ autoimmune and inflammatory phenotypes (Harvard facility) No mortality or behavior deficit, ↓ autoimmune and inflammatory phenotypes (Broad facility, after rederivation) <u>Chronic broad-spectrum antibiotic treatment (before onset)</u> ↓ abundance and diversity of bacterial species ↓ inflammation and autoimmunity phenotypes <u>Acute broad-spectrum antibiotic treatment (after onset)</u> ↓ inflammation and autoimmunity phenotypes ↑ rotarod performance <u>Fecal transplantation of pro-survival gut microflora</u> ↓ autoimmune and inflammatory phenotypes
Clinical studies		
Fang et al. [2]	6 ALS patients (5 males and 1 female) and 5 healthy controls (2 males and 3 females). No information on the origin of the disease.	Dysbiosis observed in ALS patients ↓ Firmicutes/Bacteroidetes (F/B) ratio ↓*Oscillibacter*, ↓ *Anaerostipes*, ↓ *Lachnospiraceae* ↑ *Dorea*
Rowin et al. [11]	5 patients (4 ALS and 1 BAD/ ALS variant, 1 male and 4 females) and 96 healthy controls (no information on gender). No information on the origin of the disease.	Dysbiosis, ↓ diversity in microbiome, ↓ *Ruminococcus* spp. ↓ Firmicutes/Bacteroidetes (F/B) ratio (5/5 patients) ↑ intestinal inflammation, ↑ fecal secretory IgA, ↑ calprotectin, ↑ eosinophilic protein X (3/5 patients) ↓ SCFAs in feces (2/5 patients)

(Continued)

TABLE 5.1 (Continued)

References	Experimental model	Key findings
Brenner et al. [12]	25 ALS patients (12 males and 13 females) and 32 healthy controls (16 males and 16 females), matched for gender and age. 2 familial (C9orf72) and 23 sporadic cases.	No substantial alteration of the microbiome
Mazzini et al. [4]	50 ALS patients and 50 healthy controls, matched for gender, age, and origin. Small clinical assay, randomized double-blind treatment of Lactobacillus strains (L. fermentum, L. delbrueckii, L. plantarum, L. salivarius) for 6 mo. Male and female (No information on gender distribution). No information on the origin of the disease.	Modifications of microbiome observed in ALS patients ↑ E. coli and enterobacteria, ↑ total bacterial load 6 mo of Lactobacillus treatment ↓ plasma-inflammatory cytokines, ↓ oxidative stress markers, modification of nutritional status
Blacher et al. [5]	37 ALS patients, 29 healthy BMI- and aged-matched family members as controls. Male and female (No information on gender distribution). No information on the origin of the disease.	Dysbiosis observed in ALS patients Difference in the global bacterial gene content ↓ expression in several key genes implicated in tryptophan and NAM metabolism (sera and CSF)

Note: ALS = amyotrophic lateral sclerosis; BAD = brachial amyotrophic diplegia; CSF = cerebrospinal fluid; NAM = nicotinamide; SCFA = short-chain fatty acid.

mRNA, the most abundant enteric microbial peptide and a key regulator of microbiome homeostasis [15]. mRNA production of lysozyme 1 was also decreased in the intestine. These data suggest that Paneth cell alteration in the intestine of SOD1^{G93A} might be implicated in ALS pathogenesis. Moreover, Interleukin 17 (Il-17), a proinflammatory cytokine, is increased in blood and small intestine tissues, a sign of a preinflammatory state. These differences seem to modulate the production of metabolites as well as intestinal permeability and mostly occur prior to disease onset, implying that microbiome composition can affect ALS pathogenesis before the appearance of the first symptoms.

Butyrate-producing bacteria are underrepresented in the intestine of SOD1^{G93A} presymptomatic mice, and the lack of butyrate production has been identified as a potential factor involved in ALS pathogenesis [8]. Butyrate is a four-carbon short-chain fatty acid (SCFA) produced through microbial fermentation of dietary fibers by anaerobic bacteria through butyryl-CoA: acetate CoA-transferase [16]. Expression of butyryl-CoA: acetate CoA-transferase mRNA is greatly decreased in the SOD1^{G93A} mouse model [3]. Butyrate is now known to positively affect the prognosis of various diseases including obesity, genetic metabolic diseases, hypercholesterolemia, and stroke [17]. In the context of neurodegenerative diseases, and more specifically ALS, butyrate might be of therapeutic interest due to its properties of regulating inflammatory and oxidative status, as well as the immune response [18]. The use of butyrate and its effects as a potential therapeutic avenue have been recently investigated using the SOD1^{G93A} mouse model [3]. Treatment with 2% sodium butyrate delayed disease onset and extended lifespan by 38 days. *B. fibrisolvens* and *Firmicutes peptostreptococcus,* both butyrate-producing bacteria, are increased in the mouse colon after butyrate treatment. mRNA expression of butyryl-CoA: acetate CoA-transferase was increased after treatment, consistent with the restoration of the ratio of butyrate-producing bacteria. Fecal sample 16S rDNA sequencing revealed a correction of dysbiosis, with an increased abundance of other butyrate-producing bacteria including *Eubacterium*, *Odoribacter,* and *Bacteroides* genus.

Butyrate supplementation restored ZO-1 levels and distribution in the intestine. Moreover, it decreased the number of abnormal Paneth cells, and their secretory granules showed restoration of lysozyme1 and DEF5α mRNA levels. Butyrate treatment also decreased intestinal permeability in the SOD1^{G93A} mouse model. The effect of butyrate on intestine permeability was also studied in an *in vitro* model, the HT29C19A cells. HT29C19A is a polarized human intestinal epithelial cell line often used to study the host-defense mechanism and microbiome interaction *in vitro*. Measuring transepithelial resistance is a procedure to assess the integrity and permeability of membranes by assessing the electrical resistance across the cellular membrane [19]. HT29C19A cells showed a higher transepithelial resistance after butyrate treatment, indicating the role of butyrate in restoring permeability through enhancing intestinal epithelial function.

SOD1 aggregation is a key pathological feature in SOD1^{G93A} mice neurons but can occur in other cell types, including intestinal cells [3, 20]. A decrease of SOD1 aggregation was observed in human intestinal epithelial cell line HCT116 and

SOD1^{G93A} mice intestines after butyrate treatment. However, there is no available data on aggregation in the CNS after butyrate treatment. Taken altogether, this evidence suggests that intestinal aggregation of SOD1 can contribute to the disease and can be modulated by microbiome composition.

The exact mechanism of action of butyrate in ALS is not well known. However, it is considered one of the major sources of energy for intestinal epithelial cells and has the ability to decrease oxidative stress in a germ-free intestinal environment [21]. Neuronal cells are known to be highly susceptible to oxidative stress due to their significant oxygen consumption [22]. Moreover, bacterial-produced butyrate is known to act as a histone deacetylase (HDAC) inhibitor [23, 24]. Histone acetylation homeostasis impairment has been previously linked with various neurodegenerative disorders, including ALS, and HDAC inhibitors are known to have neuroprotective properties [25]. Preventing intestinal cell abnormalities through these mechanisms might play a role in gut-brain axis communication by preventing neuronal damage.

A study published recently investigated the direct effect of microbiome depletion in SOD1^{G93A} mice [5]. A broad-spectrum antibiotic cocktail (vancomycin, ampicillin, neomycin, and metronidazole) was administered to remove microbial species from the mouse gut. Antibiotic treatment exacerbated motor symptoms through the disease course in transgenic mice. Partial loss of spinal cord neurons was also higher in microbiome-depleted animals. Magnetic resonance imaging of the mouse brain revealed that chronic administration of antibiotics increased brain atrophy and neurodegeneration in SOD1^{G93A} animals. Antibiotic-treated mice did not show any alterations of the main immune cell populations in the spinal cord, small intestine, or colon, meaning the observed differences in microbiome-depleted animals likely are not due to the involvement of the immune system.

Rederivation of the SOD1^{G93A} mouse colony into a germ-free setting significantly increased mortality rates. This phenotype is persistent even in mice spontaneously colonized with a new microbiome around the onset of disease, leading to the notion that the microbiome can modulate ALS pathogenesis and progression at an early stage of the disease. Moreover, microbiome alteration or absence can enhance symptoms in an ALS context [5].

16S rDNA sequencing of the fecal microbiome revealed a continuous dysbiosis through all stages of the disease, including before onset. Overall, SOD1^{G93A} animals display an increased number of operational taxonomic units (OTUs), which is consistent with what was previously described [3]. Enzymes participating in tryptophan metabolism were underrepresented in SOD1^{G93A} fecal samples, as were enzymes involved in nicotinamide (NAM) metabolism. Metabolism of tryptophan is implicated in neurotransmitter synthesis, including serotonin. The serotonergic neurons are one of the most affected neuronal types in ALS [26]. NAM is metabolized into nicotinamide adenine dinucleotide+ (NAD+), fuel to a large number of key processes in the cells, including energy production through glycolysis, β-oxidation, and oxidative phosphorylation [27].

The spontaneous colonization of germ-free SOD1^{G93A} mice resulted in *de novo* dysbiosis. However, this bacterial imbalance was not observed when animals were held in another animal facility with different conditions regarding pathogen monitoring requirements. Alteration of the microbiome is influenced by a combination of genetic factors and the commensal bacterial species of each facility, thus perhaps contributing to the modulation of ALS phenotypes. Interestingly, there are disparities in the relative abundance of bacterial species identified in the dysbiosis from one animal facility to another, as well as between different studies [5, 8]. Animal microbiome studies are difficult to correlate due to variability of housing conditions, including food type, how often cages are manipulated, and housing in a specific-pathogen free (SPF) facility or not [28]. Housing conditions can influence microbiome composition because animals are not exposed to the same microorganisms throughout their lives. Moreover, genetic backgrounds (C57BL/6, B6/SJL) can affect the disease course, even in animals with identical ALS-associated mutations, and might also contribute to disparities [29].

16S rDNA sequencing and shotgun metagenomic sequencing revealed a progressive decline in the abundance of *Akkermansia muciniphila,* a commensal bacteria, through the disease course in SOD1^{G93A} transgenic mice [5]. Inoculation of antibiotic-treated ALS mouse models with mono-cultured *A. muciniphila* was sufficient to improve motor function while prolonging lifespan and reducing brain atrophy. *A. muciniphila* did not have any effect on intestinal permeability. Untargeted metabolomic serum profiling revealed that 51 metabolites were increased by the treatment, with only 2 having the highest probabilities to be synthesized by the wild type (WT) mouse microbiome: phenol sulfate and NAM. When administered to SOD1^{G93A} mice, phenol sulfate failed to have any effect on the motor phenotype or survival [5]. NAM treatment increased performance on motor tests and contributed to effectively increase NAM levels in sera and cerebrospinal fluid (CSF) of treated mice. However, NAM-treated mice showed no lifespan extension, suggesting that microbiome products might contribute to improved healthspan rather than lifespan. *Healthspan* is defined as the period of time in an organism's life when it is healthy, without any chronic illness. RNA-Seq analysis of *A. muciniphila* and NAM-treated ALS mouse model spinal cord revealed various changes in expression patterns after the treatment. Gene ontology-term analysis showed an enrichment of many pathways, including mitochondrial structure and function, NAD+ homeostasis, and removal of superoxide radicals, pathways already known to be potentially implicated in ALS pathogenesis [30, 31].

Recently, Figueroa-Romero et al. published a longitudinal study of the microbiome over the disease progression [9]. Authors compared SOD1^{G93A} mice housed in a "dirty" facility (i.e. no restrictions on the equipment brought in or animal imports) and in a clean facility (i.e. strict restriction on equipment and animal imports). Animals housed in an older facility, considered dirty, had a shorter lifespan compared to animals held in a newer facility, considered to be clean of several bacterial strains, including various pathogens. Microbial diversity (i.e. the variability of microorganisms composing the microbiome) can be assessed using various measures divided into two categories: alpha and beta diversity. Alpha diversity measures the variability of species in a sample, while beta diversity refers to the diversity of species between samples [32]. The study revealed that SOD1^{G93A} mice have a higher alpha microbial diversity in feces than WT between P37 and P105 (presymptomatic state). Furthermore, beta diversity was also significantly different in feces and intestines (colon, ileum) of SOD1^{G93A} mice starting at days 60 and 90, respectively. Also, dysbiosis is observed long before the onset of the disease, consistent with previous findings [5, 8]. Two bacterial species have been identified as less abundant in SOD1^{G93A} mouse colon and are believed to potentially drive the microbial differences between ALS and healthy mice: *A. muciniphila* and *Bacteroides caccae*. Interestingly *A. muciniphila* has been recently identified as less abundant in SOD1^{G93A} mice in another study, and its reintroduction in the transgenic mouse is sufficient to improve motor phenotype and extend lifespan [5]. *Acetatifactor muris* and *Bacteroides vulgatus* have also been identified as less abundant in SOD1^{G93A} feces pellets. KEGG (Kyoto Encyclopedia of Genes and Genomes) analysis of colon, ileum, and feces samples revealed upregulation of KEGG pathways functions associated with neurodegeneration and immune system function, as well as differences between lipid metabolism and development and signal transduction pathways at day 90 (presymptomatic state).

The recent study of Burberry et al. focused on another ALS mouse model, the *C9orf72*$^{-/-}$ loss-of-function (LOF) model [10]. In this study, the authors wondered if the housing environment can influence the course of the disease, explaining why several teams observed great disparities in terms of survival and other ALS-associated phenotypes when working with *C9orf72* models [33–36]. The authors rederived their *C9orf72* mice (*C9orf72*$^{-/-}$ Harvard) into a new environmental setting at the Broad Institute (*C9orf72*$^{-/-}$ Broad). Rederivation into a new animal facility had the effect of suppressing premature mortality, behavioral deficits, and inflammation phenotypes previously observed at the Harvard facility [34]. 16S rDNA sequencing of *C9orf72*$^{-/-}$ Harvard animals feces revealed increased levels of murine norovirus, *Helicobacter* spp., *Pasteurella pneumotropica* and *Tritrichomonas muris* when compared to *C9orf72*$^{-/-}$ Broad animals. Interestingly, *Helicobacter* spp. are known to participate in various inflammatory responses in the host [37]. A decrease of alpha diversity and variations of beta diversity were also observed in these animals. The study also revealed that a chronic broad-spectrum antibiotic treatment before disease onset is sufficient to decrease inflammation, autoimmune, and cytokine storm phenotypes. Acute suppression of the gut microbiome with antibiotics after disease onset showed a similar effect while improving rotarod performance. Fecal transplantation from a pro-survival gut microflora alleviated inflammation markers in *C9orf72*$^{-/-}$ Harvard animals, showing that disease status can be modulated by the gut microbiome.

So far, most of the animal studies demonstrate that there are significant microbiome differences between SOD1^{G93A} and WT animals, especially regarding the abundance of certain species. Modulation of the animal microbiome, including induced dysbiosis or elimination of existing natural bacterial flora, can directly affect disease phenotypes in SOD1^{G93A} and *C9orf72* LOF mouse models.

Clinical Studies

The intestinal microbiome plays a significant role in maintaining essential gut homeostasis and health in humans and mammals. It constitutes the first barrier against pathogens and supports intestinal barrier integrity [38, 39]. Feces and intestinal microbiome compositions may differ from each other and between individuals, even if their genetics and environment are very similar [40]. The vast majority of human intestinal microbial species belong to four major phyla: *Firmicutes, Actinobacteria, Proteobacteria*, and *Bacteroidetes*. Dysbiosis is often evaluated by the *Firmicutes/Bacteroidetes* ratio and has been associated with neurodegenerative disorders like Parkinson's disease [41].

ALS is believed to be a multisystem disorder affecting the gastrointestinal tract with various symptoms, including constipation, delayed gastric emptying, and longer intestinal transit linked to autonomic nerve dysfunction [42, 43]. Constipation is a major issue in patients with ALS, even prior to the onset of the disease and diagnosis [44]. Constipation alters the natural microbiome composition and can promote intestinal overexposure to bacterial products, including bacterial lipopolysaccharides (LPS). ALS patients show a significant decrease in *Firmicutes/Bacteroidetes* (F/B) ratio along with a reduced relative abundance of beneficial microorganisms *Oscillibacter*, *Anaerostipes,* and *Lachnospiraceae*. An increased abundance of harmful bacteria from the *Dorea* genus has also been identified. These results suggest that dysbiosis could compromise the intestinal epithelial barrier and promote immune and inflammatory responses, with consequent alterations of gut functions [2]. However, there is no evidence of morphological or functional alterations of the intestinal epithelial barrier or intestinal immune-inflammatory responses in ALS patients. Dysbiosis has also been identified in ALS patients by other teams, with a higher abundance of *E. coli* and *enterobacteria* and a low abundance of total yeast [4, 5]. Higher total bacterial load and a decrease of expression in several key genes implicated in tryptophan and NAM metabolism were also observed [5].

A small-scale study, including only five ALS patients, was performed by Rowin et al. to analyze intestinal microbial diversity. Fecal samples were analyzed and showed low diversity in the microbiome, with a low abundance of *Ruminococcus* spp. and a low *Firmicutes/Bacteroidetes* (F/B) ratio in three out of five patients [11]. A majority of the patients had intestinal inflammation, revealed by elevated inflammatory markers, including fecal secretory immunoglobulin A (IgA), calprotectin, and/or eosinophilic protein X. All five patients showed dysbiosis. Two patients had low levels of total SCFAs in their fecal sample, one of the major byproducts secreted by intestinal bacteria. However, no information on SCFAs in plasma or CSF is available.

The fecal microbiome of ALS patients has also been studied by Brenner et al. 16S rRNA gene sequencing analysis of stool revealed that the diversity and abundance of the bacterial taxa and phylogenetic investigation of communities by reconstruction of unobserved states (PCRUSt) predicted metagenomes are almost indistinguishable between ALS patients (2 *C9orf72* and 23 sporadic cases) and healthy individuals [12].

The only significant difference was the abundance of uncultured *Ruminococcaceae*, which is higher in ALS patients. The authors conclude that there are no substantial alterations of gut microbiota composition in their cohort. Despite the absence of significant differences in the composition and predicted metagenome compared to healthy individuals, the authors argue that the intestinal microbiome of ALS patients might still display an altered production of bacterial metabolites such as SCFAs, known for their significant impact on immune cell signaling in health and pathology, including microglial cells [45]. This is the only study reporting no alterations in the gut microbiome of ALS patients.

Modulation of the intestinal microbiome with probiotics has demonstrated a protective role in inflammation and by resolving dysbiosis in human diseases, including neurodegenerative disorders like multiple sclerosis [46]. Recently, probiotics have been used in a small clinical assay [4]. Patients were randomized in double-blind treatment of *Lactobacillus* strains (*Lactobacillus fermentum, Lactobacillus delbrueckii, Lactobacillus plantarum,* and *Lactobacillus salivarius*) for six months. After treatment, patients displayed reduction of plasma-inflammatory cytokines, reduction in oxidative stress markers, and modification of nutritional status. Fecal transplantation has also proved efficient in modulating intestinal microbiome and resolving dysbiosis [47]. A fecal microbial transplantation (FMT) protocol for ALS patients was recently published to study if FMT is effective in modulating immune markers, reversing dysbiosis in patients, and improving symptoms associated with the disease [48]. The results of this clinical trial are set to be published in 2022.

The microbiome is a very diversified system evolving in a complex environment. The human microbiome contains more than 10 trillion commensal microbial cells [49]. Differences in population, age, life habits, nutritional status, and genetic pedigree can all affect intestinal microbiome composition. Clinical studies are not consistent in their conclusions about differences in gut bacterial composition in ALS. However, many factors that could influence microbiome composition usually are not addressed in clinical investigations and can account in part for discrepancies between these studies.

HOW COULD THE MICROBIOME CONTRIBUTE TO ALS?

Even though a high diversity of microbial species is generally linked to a healthy microbiome, some studies suggest that the gain or loss of specific bacteria contributes to aging and disease pathogenesis [50]. But how can these variations influence the CNS? The vagus nerve crosstalk communication between the gut and the brain, along with the transmission of signaling molecules through the circulatory system and across the blood–brain barrier (BBB), might facilitate the contribution of the microbiome to ALS pathogenesis [51, 52]. Thus, four main hypotheses emerge from the literature and may explain how the microbiome could contribute to ALS pathogenesis (Figure 5.1).

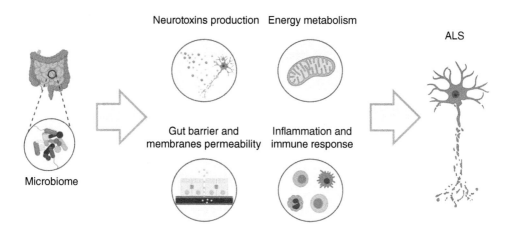

FIGURE 5.1 Main hypotheses explaining the role of the microbiome in ALS. The microbiome might act through various pathways to contribute to disease pathogenesis, including by influencing gut barrier integrity, membrane permeability, inflammation and immune responses, production of neurotoxins, and energy metabolism.

Gut Barrier and Membrane Permeability

The intestinal microbiome has been recognized for its contribution to gastrointestinal development, barrier integrity and function, key metabolic processes, immune responses, and CNS development. An important part of CNS development is the formation of the BBB and the blood-spinal cord barrier (BSCB), which are essential to provide a controlled environment. Imaging studies of the CNS have demonstrated early BBB and BSCB dysfunctions in ALS patients, as well as in animal models, and were confirmed in post mortem tissue analysis [53, 54]. Reduced tight-junction proteins have been identified in the lumbar spinal cord of ALS patients, as well as disruption of tissue barriers like the BBB and gut epithelial barrier [55–57]. Moreover, it has been demonstrated that the absence of a normal intestinal microbiome in germ-free mice is associated with hyperpermeability of the BBB [58].

In the SOD1^{G93A} mouse model, a permeable BSCB is associated with the early stages of the disease. Restoring the permeability of this barrier is sufficient to slow the phenotypes associated with the disease [54]. Studies have demonstrated that there is also increased permeability of the epithelial gut barrier in animal models of ALS and that improvement of impermeability leads to lifespan extension and delayed onset [3, 8]. ZO-1 and claudin-5, tight-junction proteins, have been identified as key proteins influenced by bacterial metabolites and mutations associated with ALS [8, 59]. Impaired integrity of tissue barriers in ALS due to decreased tight junctions in the gut and spinal cord allows larger molecules to diffuse instead of being blocked, including neurotoxins and bacterial LPS. Translocation of Gram-negative bacteria, such as cyanobacteria, across the gut epithelial barrier, is believed to play a role in ALS pathophysiology [60]. The composition of the microbiome plays a crucial role in membrane permeability, especially in a predisposed cellular environment as in ALS. An increase of intestinal or BBB/BSCB permeability can have dramatic consequences and might contribute to the disease pathogenesis.

Inflammation and Immune Response

The gut microbiome has the capacity to influence host immunity [61]. The gut-brain axis communication is bidirectional, which implies that host immunity can also impact gut microbiome composition [62]. Innate immunity and bacterial LPS sensitivity play an important role in ALS pathogenesis [63]. LPS act as extremely strong stimulators of innate immunity and are found in the outer membrane of almost all Gram-negative bacteria. LPS are known to be proinflammatory molecules and are increased in ALS patient serum and CSF, as well as inflammatory cytokines IL-17 and IL-23 [64, 65]. The presence of some intestinal bacteria correlates with microglial activation during disease course in animal models of ALS and can be modulated through antibiotic treatment [9, 10].

Butyrate and propionate are the two main SCFAs produced by gut microflora and are essential signaling molecules for the immune system, like microglia. Dysbiosis can alter levels of immune cells and inflammation [66, 67]. Among the principal players of ALS pathogenesis, microglia and T regulatory lymphocytes (Treg) are candidate cells for modifying the course of the disease. The guts of SOD1^{G93A} mice contain less butyrate-producing bacteria, a product known to induce Treg cell differentiation [8, 68]. The intestinal environment and microbiome composition favor the generation of autoreactive Treg cells with regulatory functions specific to their setting. This production is essential to prevent CNS autoimmunity [69]. Paneth cells also play an important role in the host innate immune system and participate by releasing antimicrobial peptides in response to bacterial pathogens. However, SOD1^{G93A} mice display disrupted Paneth cell homeostasis that is shaped by dysbiosis, while correction of dysbiosis improves negative Paneth cell phenotypes [3].

An increasing number of studies suggest that the immune response can be modulated by the intestinal microbiome through the gut-brain axis, the main communication axis between intestinal microflora and the CNS [66, 70]. Microbial flora is in direct communication with the enteric immune system, molding immune tolerance and therefore contributing to immune reaction cascades during inflammation. It plays an important role in the human body and acts as one of the first checkpoints of the immune system [71]. The resident microbiome acts as a vigilante in the gut and has the ability, upon pathogen presence, marked bacterial imbalance, or barrier alteration, to trigger macrophages and dendritic cells into a proinflammatory cascade, including the production of proinflammatory cytokines. This proinflammatory state leads to a breach in immune homeostasis and the loss of Treg cells. Chronic systemic inflammation can contribute to neuronal death [70].

Gut microbiome variations might have an impact on several CNS biological processes. Germ-free mice, born without a microbiome, display an altered density, morphology, and maturity of microglia. Treatment with SCFAs can restore the density and morphology of brain microglia, implying that the microbiome can shape the development of microglia as well as modify their functions [70, 72]. Intestinal bacteria can contribute to ALS by producing proinflammatory cytokines and inducing microglial inflammation and reactive astrocytosis. However, antibiotic-induced aggravation of motor function in SOD1^{G93A} mice does not correlate with differences in immune system activation, leading to the belief that activation of the immune system through microbiome alteration might not be the only way bacteria can contribute to the disease [5].

Neurotoxins

The environment might play an important role in ALS pathogenesis. Among the environmental sources identified as potentially implicated in ALS, bacterial and fungal neurotoxins have been pinpointed. β-Methylamino-L-alanine (BMAA) is a neurotoxin produced by cyanobacteria, and its action is potentially associated with various neurodegenerative disorders [73, 74]. BMAA levels from various food sources were once higher for residents of Guam, a small US island territory in Micronesia that had a cluster of ALS cases in a general spectrum of neurological disorders termed ALS-parkinsonism dementia complex (ALS-PDC) [75]. Moreover, some ALS patients, even outside Guam, show alteration of LPS and BMAA levels in plasma [64].

Other neurotoxins produced by bacteria have the potential to affect CNS and might participate in ALS pathogenesis. *Listeria monocytogenes* is an intracellular, Gram-positive bacterium that is responsible for listeriosis. In the general population, exposure to *L. monocytogenes* and asymptomatic clearance are believed to occur several times per year. Microbiome composition is believed to play an important role in its elimination by the immune system [76]. *L. monocytogenes* secretes a virulence factor called listeriolysin O (LLO). LLO has the potential to aggregate in infected cells, and the composition of these aggregates is very similar to that found in various neurodegenerative disorders, including ALS [77, 78]. Moreover, *L. monocytogenes* has the ability to infect endothelial cells and cross the BBB to infect the CNS [79]. Also, the fungi *Candida albicans*, a resident species of a healthy microbiome, has the potential to disseminate and produce candidalysin in stressful conditions, including alteration of normal microbiome. Interestingly, fungal peptides and DNA have been found in CSF and brain tissue from ALS patients [80, 81]. Many other commensal bacteria from the healthy intestinal microbiome have the potential to produce toxins affecting the CNS, including *Staphylococcus aureus* and *Clostridium perfringens* [82, 83].

In 2005, Longstreth et al. [84] hypothesized that most cases of sporadic ALS are caused by chronic exposition to toxins produced by clostridial species, like tetanus and botulinum toxins, known for affecting neurons [85, 86]. However, this hypothesis awaits further investigation. Dysbiosis could prompt gut bacteria to produce toxins affecting CNS and contribute to ALS. Despite extensive work and sequencing efforts, the complete bacterial range of the human intestinal microbiome remains undefined, implying that some unknown bacterial species could affect the pathogenesis of the disease [87]. ALS patients might have been chronically exposed to these toxins, making their neurons more vulnerable than the rest of the population.

Energy Metabolism

A growing body of evidence shows that impaired energy homeostasis is a key feature of the ALS course, manifesting even before disease onset. Motoneurons are among the largest cells in the human body and the primary contributors to the massive energy demand of the CNS. They are highly sensitive to variations in adenosine triphosphate (ATP) concentrations [88]. The gut microbiome is a significant source of various energy molecules essential for healthy cells, including ATP, NAM, and SCFAs [89]. NAM is a precursor of NAD+, a vital redox cofactor for the metabolism and ATP production, as well as essential for glycolysis and citric acid cycle (TCA). NAD+ is fundamental for the mitochondria to maintain its energy homeostasis [90]. Interestingly, deficiencies in NAM have been identified in animal models of ALS [5]. Acetate, propionate, and butyrate are the main SCFAs produced by the human microbiome to contribute to energy production through fatty acids β-oxidation and the TCA cycle. SCFAs are a favored energy source of enteric neurons because of their rapid consumption by the mitochondria. All these molecules secreted by intestinal bacteria are essential to ensure cell energy efficiency. Gut dysbiosis may disrupt the equilibrium of molecules available for fuel consumption and, thus, further weaken the motoneurons, which already require more energy than other cells.

MICROBIOME MODULATION AS A POTENTIAL THERAPEUTIC AVENUE

The only approved drugs for ALS are riluzole and edaravone, which have modest effects on survival and symptoms [91–94]. Moreover, Riluzole recently failed to prolong survival in SOD1^{G93A} mice and other mammalian models, while still being widely used to treat ALS, suggesting that lifespan extension might not be the main parameter to consider for moving molecules forward for clinical investigation [95]. Improving healthspan and disease management are of growing interest for various neurodegenerative disorders, including ALS, where drugs have repeatedly failed to cure these diseases.

Prebiotics and probiotics could be used to support bacterial species established in the gut or to reverse the dysbiosis observed by replacing the missing bacteria. Indeed, severe adverse effects are a significant reason for the discontinuation of clinical drug development, often in Phase III trials. Thus, modulation of the microbiome may be an alternative or complementary approach for neurodegenerative diseases since chronic treatment with probiotics is associated with a low risk of side effects. Microbiome products like butyrate have already proved efficient to extend the lifespan and delay disease onset in animal models [3]. Further studies are needed to fully understand the beneficial aspect of the gut microbiome and how alterations associated with the disease can be addressed in a therapeutic manner.

CONCLUSION

Several publications have identified gut dysbiosis in animal models and ALS patients. However, many discrepancies emerge from these studies. A lack of clear evidence of bacterial species potentially implicated in ALS pathogenesis might be due in part to heterogeneity of patients and incomplete information (genotype, origins) used in clinical studies, variability between animal models, and a low number of experimental samples. Various elements can affect gut microbiome flora, including stress, exercise, and food, and this essential information has not been fully reported in various clinical studies. Moreover, gender-specific differences in the immune system and gut microbiota composition have been identified in healthy subjects but not in ALS [96]. Currently, there are no guidelines to standardize microbiome investigations, making it difficult to compare studies. In addition, there is no comparative study linking findings in murine models and humans.

On the other hand, a better understanding of mechanisms implicated in ALS pathophysiology is needed to guide microbiome studies, since a clear link between the microbiome and ALS would be a game-changer. In light of the current evidence, we believe that the microbiome contributes to ALS pathogenesis rather than driving it. Microbiome supplementation is a relatively easy and non-invasive way to influence the health of whole organisms and has potential as a therapeutic approach. The role of the intestinal microbiome is currently understudied in the ALS field and should be the subject of more investigations in the future.

CONFLICT OF INTEREST

The authors declare no potential conflict of interest with respect to research, authorship, and/or publication of this manuscript.

COPYRIGHT AND PERMISSION STATEMENT

To the best of our knowledge, the materials included in this chapter do not violate copyright laws. All original sources have been appropriately acknowledged and/or referenced. Where relevant, appropriate permissions have been obtained from the original copyright holder(s)). Figure 5.1 was created with BioRender. Parts of this work have been submitted in partial fulfillment of the requirements for a PhD at the University of Montreal.

REFERENCES

1. Cryan, J.F., O'Riordan, K.J., Sandhu, K. et al. (2020). The gut microbiome in neurological disorders. *Lancet Neurol.* 19 (2): 179–194.

2. Fang, X., Wang, X., Yang, S. et al. (2016). Evaluation of the microbial diversity in amyotrophic lateral sclerosis using high-throughput sequencing. *Front. Microbiol.* 7 (22): 1479.

3. Zhang, Y.-G., Wu, S., Yi, J. et al. (2017). Target intestinal microbiota to alleviate disease progression in amyotrophic lateral sclerosis. *Clin. Ther.* 39 (2): 322–336.

4. Mazzini, L., Mogna, L., De Marchi, F. et al. (2018). Potential role of gut microbiota in ALS pathogenesis and possible novel therapeutic strategies. *J. Clin. Gastroenterol.* 52 (Suppl 1), Proceedings from the 9th Probiotics, Prebiotics and New Foods, Nutraceuticals and Botanicals for Nutrition & Human and Microbiota Health Meeting, held in Rome, Italy from September 10 to 12, 2017:: S68–S70.

5. Blacher, E., Bashiardes, S., Shapiro, H. et al. (2019). Potential roles of gut microbiome and metabolites in modulating ALS in mice. *Nature* 572 (7770): 474–480. Nature Publishing Group.

6. Manzo, E., O'Conner, A.G., Barrows, J.M. et al. (2018). Medium-chain fatty acids, beta-hydroxybutyric acid and genetic modulation of the carnitine shuttle are protective in a drosophila model of ALS based on TDP-43. *Front. Mol. Neurosci.* 11: 182.

7. Zarei, S., Carr, K., Reiley, L. et al. (2015). A comprehensive review of amyotrophic lateral sclerosis. *Surg. Neurol. Int.* 6 (1): 171.

8. Wu, S., Yi, J., Zhang, Y.-G. et al. (2015). Leaky intestine and impaired microbiome in an amyotrophic lateral sclerosis mouse model. *Physiol Rep.* 3 (4): e12356–e12356.

9. Figueroa-Romero, C., Guo, K., Murdock, B.J. et al. (2019). Temporal evolution of the microbiome, immune system and epigenome with disease progression in ALS mice. *Dis. Model Mech.* 13 (2): dmm041947.

10. Burberry, A., Wells, M.F., Limone, F. et al. (2020). C9orf72 suppresses systemic and neural inflammation induced by gut bacteria. *Nature* 582 (7810): 89–94.

11. Rowin, J., Xia, Y., Jung, B., and Sun, J. (2017). Gut inflammation and dysbiosis in human motor neuron disease. *Physiol. Rep.* 5 (18): e13443.

12. Brenner, D., Hiergeist, A., Adis, C. et al. (2018). The fecal microbiome of ALS patients. *Neurobiol. Aging* 61: 132–137.

13. Bischoff, S.C., Barbara, G., Buurman, W. et al. (2014). Intestinal permeability–a new target for disease prevention and therapy. *BMC Gastroenterol.* 14 (1): 189–125. Bio Med Central.

14. Gassler, N. (2017). Paneth cells in intestinal physiology and pathophysiology. *World J. Gastrointest. Pathophysiol.* 8 (4): 150–160.

15. Ostaff, M.J., Stange, E.F., and Wehkamp, J. (2013). Antimicrobial peptides and gut microbiota in homeostasis and pathology. *EMBO Mol. Med.* 5 (10): 1465–1483.

16. Duncan, S.H., Barcenilla, A., Stewart, C.S. et al. (2002). Acetate utilization and butyryl coenzyme A (CoA):acetate-CoA transferase in butyrate-producing bacteria from the human large intestine. *Appl. Environ. Microbiol.* 68 (10): 5186–5190.

17. Sanna, S., van Zuydam, N.R., Mahajan, A. et al. (2019). Causal relationships among the gut microbiome, short-chain fatty acids and metabolic diseases. *Nat. Genet.* 51 (4): 600–605. Nature Publishing Group.

18. Chriett, S., Dąbek, A., Wojtala, M. et al. (2019). Prominent action of butyrate over β-hydroxybutyrate as histone deacetylase inhibitor, transcriptional modulator and anti-inflammatory molecule. *Sci. Rep.* 9 (1): 742–714. Nature Publishing Group.

19. Srinivasan, B., Kolli, A.R., Esch, M.B. et al. (2015). TEER measurement techniques for in vitro barrier model systems. *J. Lab. Autom.* 20 (2): 107–126. 3rd ed. SAGE Publications Sage CA: Los Angeles, CA.

20. Gurney, M.E., Pu, H., Chiu, A.Y. et al. (1994). Motor neuron degeneration in mice that express a human Cu,Zn superoxide dismutase mutation. *Science* 264 (5166): 1772–1775.

21. Donohoe, D.R., Garge, N., Zhang, X. et al. (2011). The microbiome and butyrate regulate energy metabolism and autophagy in the mammalian colon. *Cell Metab.* 13 (5): 517–526.

22. Salim, S. (2017). Oxidative stress and the central nervous system. *J. Pharmacol. Exp. Ther.* 360 (1): 201–205. American Society for Pharmacology and Experimental Therapeutics.

23. Davie, J.R. (2003). Inhibition of histone deacetylase activity by butyrate. *J. Nutr.* 133 (7 Suppl): 2485S–2493S.

24. Yuille, S., Reichardt, N., Panda, S. et al. (2018). Human gut bacteria as potent class I histone deacetylase inhibitors in vitro through production of butyric acid and valeric acid. Nie D, editor. *PLoS One* 13 (7): e0201073.

25. Shukla, S. and Tekwani, B.L. (2020). Histone deacetylases inhibitors in neurodegenerative diseases, neuroprotection and neuronal differentiation. *Front. Pharmacol.* 11: 537.

26. Dentel, C., Palamiuc, L., Henriques, A. et al. (2013). Degeneration of serotonergic neurons in amyotrophic lateral sclerosis: a link to spasticity. *Brain* 136 (Pt 2): 483–493.

27. Fang, E.F., Lautrup, S., Hou, Y. et al. (2017). NAD+ in aging: molecular mechanisms and translational implications. *Trends Mol. Med.* 23 (10): 899–916.

28. Dobson, G.P., Letson, H.L., Biros, E., and Morris, J. (2019). Specific pathogen-free (SPF) animal status as a variable in biomedical research: have we come full circle? *EBioMedicine* 41: 42–43.

29. Heiman-Patterson, T.D., Deitch, J.S., Blankenhorn, E.P. et al. (2005). Background and gender effects on survival in the TgN (SOD1-G93A)1Gur mouse model of ALS. *J. Neurol. Sci.* 236 (1–2): 1–7.

30. Islam, M.T. (2017). Oxidative stress and mitochondrial dysfunction-linked neurodegenerative disorders. *Neurol. Res.* 39 (1): 73–82.

31. Smith, E.F., Shaw, P.J., and De Vos, K.J. (2019). The role of mitochondria in amyotrophic lateral sclerosis. *Neurosci. Lett.* 710: 132933.

32. Calle, M.L. (2019). Statistical analysis of metagenomics data. *Genomics Inform.* 17 (1): e6. Korea Genome Organization.

33. O'Rourke, J.G., Bogdanik, L., Yáñez, A. et al. (2016). C9orf72 is required for proper macrophage and microglial function in mice. *Science* 351 (6279): 1324–1329.

34. Burberry, A., Suzuki, N., Wang, J.-Y. et al. (2016). Loss-of-function mutations in the C9ORF72 mouse ortholog cause fatal autoimmune disease. *Sci. Transl. Med.* 8 (347): 347ra93–347ra93.

35. Ugolino, J., Ji, Y.J., Conchina, K. et al. (2016). Loss of C9orf72 enhances autophagic activity via deregulated mTOR and TFEB signaling. Cox GA, editor. *PLoS Genet.* 12 (11): e1006443.

36. Jiang, J., Zhu, Q., Gendron, T.F. et al. (2016). Gain of toxicity from ALS/FTD-linked repeat expansions in C9ORF72 is alleviated by antisense oligonucleotides targeting GGGGCC-containing RNAs. *Neuron* 90 (3): 535–550.

37. Whary, M.T. and Fox, J.G. (2004). Natural and experimental helicobacter infections. *Comp. Med.* 54 (2): 128–158.

38. Aziz, Q., Doré, J., Emmanuel, A. et al. (2013). Gut microbiota and gastrointestinal health: current concepts and future directions. *Neurogastroenterol. Motil.* 25 (1): 4–15.

39. Sommer, F. and Bäckhed, F. (2013). The gut microbiota–masters of host development and physiology. *Nat. Rev. Microbiol.* 11 (4): 227–238.

40. Lloyd-Price, J., Abu-Ali, G., and Huttenhower, C. (2016). The healthy human microbiome. *Genome Med.* 8 (1): 51–11. BioMed Central.

41. Sampson, T.R., Debelius, J.W., Thron, T. et al. (2016). Gut microbiota regulate motor deficits and neuroinflammation in a model of Parkinson's disease. *Cell* 167 (6): 1469–1480.e12.

42. Herdewyn, S., Cirillo, C., Van Den Bosch, L. et al. (2014). Prevention of intestinal obstruction reveals progressive neurodegeneration in mutant TDP-43 (A315T) mice. *Mol. Neurodegener.* 9 (1): 24.

43. Nübling, G.S., Mie, E., Bauer, R.M. et al. (2014). Increased prevalence of bladder and intestinal dysfunction in amyotrophic lateral sclerosis. *Amyotroph. Lateral Scler. Frontotemporal Degener.* 15 (3–4): 174–179.

44. Forshew, D.A. and Bromberg, M.B. (2003). A survey of clinicians' practice in the symptomatic treatment of ALS. *Amyotroph. Lateral Scler. Other Motor Neuron Disord.* 4 (4): 258–263.

45. Haghikia, A., Jörg, S., Duscha, A. et al. (2015). Dietary fatty acids directly impact central nervous system autoimmunity via the small intestine. *Immunity* 43 (4): 817–829.

46. Kouchaki, E., Tamtaji, O.R., Salami, M. et al. (2017). Clinical and metabolic response to probiotic supplementation in patients with multiple sclerosis: a randomized, double-blind, placebo-controlled trial. *Clin. Nutr.* 36 (5): 1245–1249.

47. Weingarden, A., González, A., Vázquez-Baeza, Y. et al. (2015). Dynamic changes in short- and long-term bacterial composition following fecal microbiota transplantation for recurrent Clostridium difficile infection. *Microbiome* 3 (1): 10–18. BioMed Central.

48. Mandrioli, J., Amedei, A., Cammarota, G. et al. (2019). FETR-ALS study protocol: a randomized clinical trial of fecal microbiota transplantation in amyotrophic lateral sclerosis. *Front. Neurol.* 10: 1021.

49. Turnbaugh, P.J., Ley, R.E., Hamady, M. et al. (2007). The human microbiome project. *Nature* 449 (7164): 804–810. Nature Publishing Group.

50. Jeffery, I.B., Lynch, D.B., and O'Toole, P.W. (2016). Composition and temporal stability of the gut microbiota in older persons. *ISME J.* 10 (1): 170–182. Nature Publishing Group.

51. Spielman, L.J., Gibson, D.L., and Klegeris, A. (2018). Unhealthy gut, unhealthy brain: the role of the intestinal microbiota in neurodegenerative diseases. *Neurochem. Int.* 120: 149–163.

52. Cryan, J.F., O'Riordan, K.J., Cowan, C.S.M. et al. (2019). The microbiota-gut-brain axis. *Physiol. Rev.* 99 (4): 1877–2013.

53. Winkler, E.A., Sengillo, J.D., Sullivan, J.S. et al. (2013). Blood-spinal cord barrier breakdown and pericyte reductions in amyotrophic lateral sclerosis. *Acta Neuropathol.* 125 (1): 111–120.

54. Winkler, E.A., Sengillo, J.D., Sagare, A.P. et al. (2014). Blood-spinal cord barrier disruption contributes to early motor-neuron degeneration in ALS-model mice. *Proc. Natl. Acad. Sci. U. S. A.* 111 (11): E1035–E1042.

55. Henkel, J.S., Beers, D.R., Wen, S. et al. (2009). Decreased mRNA expression of tight junction proteins in lumbar spinal cords of patients with ALS. *Neurology* 72 (18): 1614–1616.

56. Nicaise, C., Mitrecic, D., Demetter, P. et al. (2009). Impaired blood-brain and blood-spinal cord barriers in mutant SOD1-linked ALS rat. *Brain Res.* 1301: 152–162.

57. Huntley, M.A., Bien-Ly, N., Daneman, R., and Watts, R.J. (2014). Dissecting gene expression at the blood-brain barrier. *Front. Neurosci.* 8 (124): 355.

58. Braniste, V., Al-Asmakh, M., Kowal, C. et al. (2014). The gut microbiota influences blood-brain barrier permeability in mice. *Sci. Transl. Med.* 6 (263): 263ra158–263ra158.

59. Meister, S., Storck, S.E., Hameister, E. et al. (2015). Expression of the ALS-causing variant hSOD1 (G93A) leads to an impaired integrity and altered regulation of claudin-5 expression in an in vitro blood-spinal cord barrier model. *J. Cereb. Blood Flow Metab.* 35 (7): 1112–1121, SAGE Publications Sage UK: London, England.

60. Catanzaro, R., Anzalone, M., Calabrese, F. et al. (2015). The gut microbiota and its correlations with the central nervous system disorders. *Panminerva Med.* 57 (3): 127–143.

61. Rooks, M.G. and Garrett, W.S. (2016). Gut microbiota, metabolites and host immunity. *Nat. Rev. Immunol.* 16 (6): 341–352. Nature Publishing Group.

62. Kato, L.M., Kawamoto, S., Maruya, M., and Fagarasan, S. (2014). The role of the adaptive immune system in regulation of gut microbiota. *Immunol. Rev.* 260 (1): 67–75. John Wiley & Sons, Ltd (10.1111).

63. McCauley, M.E. and Baloh, R.H. (2019). Inflammation in ALS/FTD pathogenesis. *Acta Neuropathol.* 137 (5): 715–730. Springer Berlin Heidelberg.

64. Zhang, R., Miller, R.G., Gascon, R. et al. (2009). Circulating endotoxin and systemic immune activation in sporadic amyotrophic lateral sclerosis (sALS). *J. Neuroimmunol.* 206 (1–2): 121–124.

65. Rentzos, M., Rombos, A., Nikolaou, C. et al. (2010). Interleukin-17 and interleukin-23 are elevated in serum and cerebrospinal fluid of patients with ALS: a reflection of Th17 cells activation? *Acta Neurol. Scand.* 122 (6): 425–429. John Wiley & Sons, Ltd (10.1111).

66. Fung, T.C., Olson, C.A., and Hsiao, E.Y. (2017). Interactions between the microbiota, immune and nervous systems in health and disease. *Nat. Neurosci.* 20 (2): 145–155. Nature Publishing Group.

67. Shamim, A., Mahmood, T., Ahsan, F. et al. (2018). Lipids: an insight into the neurodegenerative disorders. *Clin. Nutr. Exp.* 20: 1–19.

68. Kespohl, M., Vachharajani, N., Luu, M. et al. (2017). The microbial metabolite butyrate induces expression of Th1-associated factors in CD4+ T cells. *Front. Immunol.* 8: 1036.

69. Kadowaki, A., Miyake, S., Saga, R. et al. (2016). Gut environment-induced intraepithelial autoreactive CD4(+) T cells suppress central nervous system autoimmunity via LAG-3. *Nat. Commun.* 7 (1): 11639–11616. Nature Publishing Group.

70. Pellegrini, C., Antonioli, L., Colucci, R. et al. (2018). Interplay among gut microbiota, intestinal mucosal barrier and enteric neuro-immune system: a common path to neurodegenerative diseases? *Acta Neuropathol.* 136 (3): 345–361.

71. Shi, N., Li, N., Duan, X., and Niu, H. (2017). Interaction between the gut microbiome and mucosal immune system. *Mil. Med. Res.* 4 (1): 14–17.BioMed Central.

72. Erny, D., Hrabě de Angelis, A.L., Jaitin, D. et al. (2015). Host microbiota constantly control maturation and function of microglia in the CNS. *Nat. Neurosci.* 18 (7): 965–977. Nature Publishing Group.

73. Pablo, J., Banack, S.A., Cox, P.A. et al. (2009). Cyanobacterial neurotoxin BMAA in ALS and Alzheimer's disease. *Acta Neurol. Scand.* 120 (4): 216–225. John Wiley & Sons, Ltd (10.1111).

74. Bradley, W.G. and Mash, D.C. (2009). Beyond Guam: the cyanobacteria/BMAA hypothesis of the cause of ALS and other neurodegenerative diseases. *Amyotroph. Lateral Scler.* 10 (Suppl 2(sup 2)): 7–20. 5 ed. Taylor & Francis.

75. Kurland, L.T. (1988). Amyotrophic lateral sclerosis and Parkinson's disease complex on Guam linked to an environmental neurotoxin. *Trends Neurosci.* 11 (2): 51–54.

76. Grif, K., Patscheider, G., Dierich, M.P., and Allerberger, F. (2003). Incidence of fecal carriage of listeria monocytogenes in three healthy volunteers: a one-year prospective stool survey. *Eur. J. Clin. Microbiol. Infect Dis.* 22 (1): 16–20. Springer-Verlag.

77. Dehhaghi, M., Kazemi Shariat Panahi, H., and Guillemin, G.J. (2018). Microorganisms' footprint in neurodegenerative diseases. *Front. Cell Neurosci.* 12: 466.

78. Viala, J.P.M., Mochegova, S.N., Meyer-Morse, N., and Portnoy, D.A. (2008). A bacterial pore-forming toxin forms aggregates in cells that resemble those associated with neurodegenerative diseases. *Cell Microbiol.* 10 (4): 985–993. John Wiley & Sons, Ltd (10.1111).

79. Disson, O. and Lecuit, M. (2012). Targeting of the central nervous system by listeria monocytogenes. *Virulence* 3 (2): 213–221. Taylor & Francis.

80. Alonso, R., Pisa, D., Marina, A.I. et al. (2015). Evidence for fungal infection in cerebrospinal fluid and brain tissue from patients with amyotrophic lateral sclerosis. *Int. J. Biol. Sci.* 11 (5): 546–558.

81. French, P.W., Ludowyke, R., and Guillemin, G.J. (2019). Fungal neurotoxins and sporadic amyotrophic lateral sclerosis. *Neurotox. Res.* 35 (4): 969–980. Springer US.

82. Oliveira, D., Borges, A., and Simões, M. (2018). Staphylococcus aureus toxins and their molecular activity in infectious diseases. *Toxins (Basel)* 10 (6): 252. Multidisciplinary Digital Publishing Institute.

83. Wagley, S., Bokori-Brown, M., Morcrette, H. et al. (2019). Evidence of clostridium perfringens epsilon toxin associated with multiple sclerosis. *Mult. Scler.* 25 (5): 653–660.

84. Longstreth, W.T., Meschke, J.S., Davidson, S.K. et al. (2005). Hypothesis: a motor neuron toxin produced by a clostridial species residing in gut causes ALS. *Med Hypotheses* 64 (6): 1153–1156.

85. Goonetilleke, A. and Harris, J.B. (2004). Clostridial neurotoxins. *J. Neurol. Neurosurg. Psychiatr.* 75 (Suppl 3(suppl_3)): iii35–iii39.

86. Yang, N.J. and Chiu, I.M. (2017). Bacterial signaling to the nervous system through toxins and metabolites. *J. Mol. Biol.* 429 (5): 587–605.

87. Almeida, A., Mitchell, A.L., Boland, M. et al. (2019). A new genomic blueprint of the human gut microbiota. *Nature* 568 (7753): 499–504. Nature Publishing Group.

88. Vandoorne, T., De Bock, K., and Van Den Bosch, L. (2018). Energy metabolism in ALS: an underappreciated opportunity? *Acta Neuropathol.* 135 (4): 489–509. Springer Berlin Heidelberg.

89. LeBlanc, J.G., Chain, F., Martín, R. et al. (2017). Beneficial effects on host energy metabolism of short-chain fatty acids and vitamins produced by commensal and probiotic bacteria. *Microb. Cell Fact.* 16 (1): 79–10. BioMed Central.

90. Lautrup, S., Sinclair, D.A., Mattson, M.P., and Fang, E.F. (2019). NAD+ in brain aging and neurodegenerative disorders. *Cell Metab.* 30 (4): 630–655.

91. Abe, K., Itoyama, Y., Sobue, G. et al. (2014). Confirmatory double-blind, parallel-group, placebo-controlled study of efficacy and safety of edaravone (MCI-186) in amyotrophic lateral sclerosis patients. *Amyotroph. Lateral Scler. Frontotemporal Degener.* 15 (7–8): 610–617. Taylor & Francis.

92. Miller, R.G., Mitchell, J.D., and Moore, D.H. (2012). Riluzole for amyotrophic lateral sclerosis (ALS)/motor neuron disease (MND). Miller RG, editor. *Cochrane Database Syst Rev.* 3: CD001447. Chichester, UK: John Wiley & Sons, Ltd.

93. Nagase, M., Yamamoto, Y., Miyazaki, Y., and Yoshino, H. (2016). Increased oxidative stress in patients with amyotrophic lateral sclerosis and the effect of edaravone administration. *Redox Rep.* 21 (3): 104–112. Taylor & Francis.

94. Takahashi, F., Takei, K., Tsuda, K., and Palumbo, J. (2017). Post-hoc analysis of MCI186–17, the extension study to MCI186–16, the confirmatory double-blind, parallel-group, placebo-controlled study of edaravone in amyotrophic lateral sclerosis. *Amyotroph. Lateral Scler. Frontotemporal Degener.* Taylor & Francis 18 (sup1): 32–39.

95. Hogg, M.C., Halang, L., Woods, I. et al. (2018). Riluzole does not improve lifespan or motor function in three ALS mouse models. *Amyotroph. Lateral Scler. Frontotemporal Degener.* 19 (5–6): 438–445.

96. Haro, C., Rangel-Zúñiga, O.A., Alcalá-Díaz, J.F. et al. (2016). Intestinal microbiota is influenced by gender and body mass index. Sanz Y, editor. *PLoS One* 11 (5): e0154090.

CHAPTER 6

Protein Aggregation in Amyotrophic Lateral Sclerosis

Christen G. Chisholm[1,2], Justin J. Yerbury[1,2], and Luke McAlary[1,2]

[1] *Illawarra Health and Medical Research Institute, University of Wollongong, Wollongong, New South Wales, Australia*
[2] *Molecular Horizons and School of Chemistry and Molecular Biosciences, University of Wollongong, Wollongong, New South Wales, Australia*

INTRODUCTION

Misfolding of proteins and their subsequent aggregation into insoluble inclusions is a common pathological hallmark of many neurodegenerative diseases [1]. Generally, specific neurodegenerative diseases are characterized by the aggregation and deposition of specific proteins in distinct regions and cell types of the central nervous system (CNS). Amyotrophic lateral sclerosis (ALS) is a progressive neurodegenerative disease characterized by the loss of motor neurons in the brain and spinal cord causing developing paralysis of limb and bulbar function, with death due to respiratory failure within an average of three to five years from symptom onset. ALS is classified on the basis of whether there is a family history of disease (familial amyotrophic lateral sclerosis – fALS) or not (sporadic amyotrophic lateral sclerosis – sALS). Although a diverse set of genes are implicated in ALS and the associated protein aggregates contain many different co-aggregating proteins, ALS is characterized by protein aggregates primarily containing either TAR DNA-binding protein of 43 kDa (TDP-43) [2, 3], Cu/Zn superoxide dismutase (SOD1) [4], or fused in sarcoma (FUS) [5, 6]. Indeed, genetic screening has identified disease-associated mutations in many of the proteins identified in inclusions in ALS (reviewed in [7]). Collectively, this suggests that protein aggregation is not only a marker of disease but also strongly tied to the etiology and pathomechanisms of neurodegeneration.

PATHOLOGICAL PROTEIN INCLUSIONS ASSOCIATED WITH ALS

Many of the proteins encoded by fALS-associated genes can be found in the neuronal protein aggregates of sALS patients in their wild-type (WT) form (reviewed in [8]), indicating that misfolding and aggregation are not entirely dependent on mutation. For example, TDP-43 mislocalization and aggregation are observed in ~97% of all ALS cases, including all sALS cases, whereas SOD1 (2%) and FUS (1%) inclusions are associated with the remaining cases [9]. The most common genetic cause of ALS is the expansion of an intronic hexanucleotide repeat (GGGGCC) in chromosome 9 open reading frame 72 (*C9orf72*) [10, 11]. This expansion is present in 5–10% of sALS cases and 40–50% of fALS cases [12–14]. Translation of these hexanucleotide sequences produces dipeptide repeat polypeptides (DPRs), which can form pathological cytoplasmic aggregates. In the majority of ALS cases with *C9orf72* mutations, TDP-43 aggregates are also present, and some evidence suggests that the deposition of DPRs initiates TDP-43 proteinopathy [15–18].

Other WT ALS-associated proteins are also found in sALS aggregates, including OPTN [19], UBQLN2 [20], and p62 [21, 22]. The aggregation of these key proteins suggests that they may be intimately tied to the pathobiology of ALS in general. The aggregation of TDP-43 and FUS is also associated with frontotemporal lobar degeneration (FTLD) [2, 23], a disease that is thought to exist on the same spectrum as ALS due to pathological and genetic similarities [9].

Although our understanding of the fundamental physiological mechanisms underlying ALS is incomplete, the key neuropathological hallmark of the disease is the aggregation and accumulation of ubiquitinated proteinaceous inclusions in the cytoplasm of degenerating motor neurons and surrounding support cells [24]. The anatomical regions of the CNS where these inclusions form include the motor cortex, brain stem, spinal cord, frontal cortex, temporal cortex, hippocampus, and cerebellum [25]. ALS is characterized by a number of distinct pathological protein inclusions: star-like *C9orf72*-associated DPR inclusions, bunina bodies, spheroids, basophilic inclusions, and ubiquitin immunoreactive inclusions (reviewed in [24]). The type of inclusions present in a case varies depending on ALS genotype or lack thereof.

Symptomatically, ALS is a progressive disorder, and attempts have been made to examine pathology throughout the disease course. By assessing the levels and distribution of phosphorylated TDP-43 (pTDP-43) throughout the CNS, it was suggested that the progression of pTDP-43 pathology in ALS could be divided into four stages. Initially, pTDP-43 is found in the agranular neocortex, spinal motor neurons, and bulbar somatomotor neurons. Pathology then spreads sequentially through axonally connected areas throughout the CNS (reviewed in [26]). Both bulbar onset and spinal cases showed a similar pattern of TDP-43 pathology. Interestingly, there is reported to be a statistically significant correlation of pTDP-43 pathology with cell loss in several CNS regions, including beyond motor areas, as the disease progresses. These include the superior and middle temporal gyrus, cingulate gyrus, amygdala, hippocampal formation, entorhinal cortex, and occasionally Onuf's nucleus [27]. Aggregates of pTDP-43 have also been observed in the interneurons of Clarke's column and the cerebellar dentate nucleus with significant loss of dopaminergic neurons of the substantia nigra [28]. Neuronal lesions also correlate with similar lesions in grey and white matter oligodendroglial cells and astrocytes [29].

Whether these inclusions are a result or cause of toxicity remains to be conclusively demonstrated. Such diversity of inclusion characteristics (size, shape, subcellular distribution, protein constituents) indicates that different biochemical pathways govern their formation, yet the clinical phenotype of ALS is not specific to the observed pathological features. It is important within the field to answer, "What causes these inclusions?" Determining this may uncover a deeper understanding of what is at the heart of neuronal dysfunction in ALS.

Protein Homeostasis and Misfolded Protein Partitioning in ALS

To understand the implications of protein aggregation in neurodegeneration, an understanding of protein homeostasis (proteostasis) is required. *Proteostasis* is the maintenance of all proteins in the cell in the correct and functioning conformation, location, and concentration [30]. Disruption of these key characteristics can lead to pathological protein aggregation [31].

Protein folding is best understood as a thermodynamic funnel in which entropy drives an unfolded protein from a high-free-energy, disordered state to a lower-free-energy, ordered state, where these low-energy states include both native conformations and misfolded/aggregated states [32]. Mistakes during protein folding can be exacerbated by environmental conditions such as macromolecular crowding, ion concentration, oxidation, pH, and temperature [33]. These same environmental conditions are also known to promote partial protein unfolding in natively folded proteins [34], suggesting that proteins in their native conformation can transition to aggregation-prone states under the right conditions.

To protect the cell from aggregating proteins, a complex quality control network exists to maintain proteostasis, requiring coordination and control of both protein synthesis and protein degradation pathways. It is especially necessary in post-mitotic cells, such as motor neurons, where a misfolded/aggregated protein build-up cannot be divided between daughter cells through division [35, 36]. The proteostasis network comprises multiple pathways and processes involved in the generation, folding, transport, and disposal of proteins (reviewed in [31]).

A key feature of the proteostasis network is the partitioning of misfolded proteins into specific compartments within cells [37]. In this way, aggregation is not just a passive stochastic process but is actively pursued by cells during times of stress to maintain proper proteostasis. Sequestration of aggregation-prone proteins (such as TDP-43, SOD1, and FUS) into distinct compartments [38] prevents them from undergoing interactions that may lead to the formation of toxic oligomers or damage to the cell. Several compartments have been proposed, including insoluble protein deposits (IPOD), juxtanuclear quality control (JUNQ) [37], and RNA interactor specific compartments/inclusions (RISCI) [38].

IPOD inclusions are dense, almost static structures thought to be composed mainly of amyloidogenic proteins. IPOD inclusions are ubiquitinated late after their formation [37] and are suggested to be protective in the case of huntingtin protein aggregation in cultured cells [39]. In comparison, JUNQ compartments are dynamic and colocalize with ubiquitin at the earliest time point measured, suggesting that ubiquitinated proteins primarily sequester to this compartment [37, 38]. Interestingly, the partitioning of SOD1 mutants (*mSOD1*) to JUNQ has been shown to significantly impair the dynamic nature of the JUNQ compartment [40], suggesting that this may be a mechanism through which misfolded SOD1 becomes toxic. Further, there is growing evidence that misfolded mutant SOD1 can disrupt the ubiquitin proteasome system [41–43], potentially resulting in sequestration of ubiquitin from its other essential functioning such as cell signaling.

TDP-43 inclusions in patients are known to be ubiquitinated [2, 3]; however, studies into the inclusion formation of TDP-43 in cultured cells suggest that the colocalization of ubiquitin with these inclusions occurs late after their initial formation [38], similar to what is observed for IPOD inclusions [37]. Interestingly, although TDP-43 contains a prion-like domain (on the basis of sequence physicochemical properties being similar to yeast sup35 protein [44]) capable of aggregating into amyloid-like structures and associates with ubiquitin late, it does not sequester to IPOD in cultured cells [38]. Rather, TDP-43 variably localizes to SOD1-positive inclusions (JUNQ) when co-expressed, signifying that there may be competing aggregation pathways for TDP-43 in cells [38], perhaps mediated by its RNA-binding roles.

CONSEQUENCES OF PROTEIN AGGREGATION IN ALS

While the deposition of TDP-43, SOD1, and FUS into aggregates is well established, how and indeed whether these protein aggregates cause cell death remains under debate. There are a number of possible mechanisms for how protein aggregation in ALS may result in cell toxicity (see Figure 6.1). There is strong evidence linking many aggregating proteins, including SOD1, TDP-43, and FUS, to mitochondrial dysfunction and, indeed, complete mitochondrial degeneration [45–47]. The mechanism for this is yet to be elucidated, but possibilities include blocking mitochondrial transport pores, accumulating inside the intermembrane space, and/or activating the mitochondrial unfolded protein response. Protein aggregation is also known to disrupt the proteostasis network, including impairment of the key protein degradation pathways, the ubiquitin proteasome system, and autophagy (reviewed in [48]). The sequestration of other essential cellular molecules into protein aggregates would also be detrimental to cell health by inducing a loss of function in essential proteins (reviewed in [49]). Indeed, expression of amyloidogenic proteins in cultured cells is found to sequester other proteins belonging to essential biochemical pathways such as proteostasis, cytoskeletal maintenance, chromatin organization, and RNA metabolism [50], some pathways of which are found disrupted in ALS [7, 51]. Finally, evidence suggests protein aggregation in the cytoplasm inhibits nucleocytoplasmic transport, including the transport of mRNA, disrupting global RNA metabolism [52]. Considering the diversity of

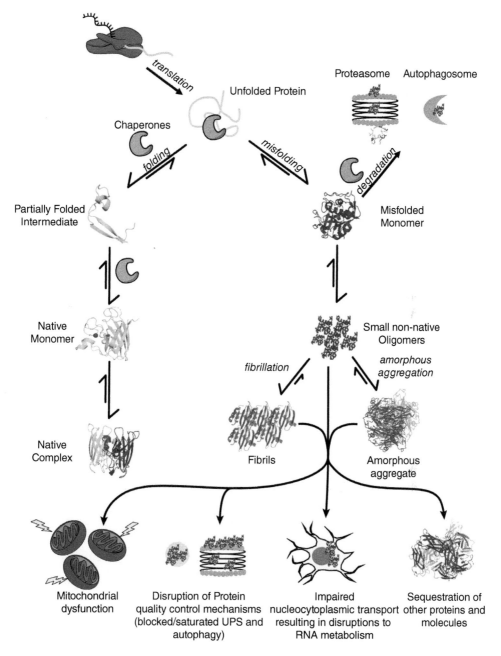

FIGURE 6.1   Schematic of protein misfolding and aggregation process and the associated cytotoxic consequences. Following synthesis, proteins fold into a partially folded intermediate with the assistance of chaperones. Due to mutations or stress, the intermediate can misfold into an incorrect conformation. Misfolded proteins can then go on to aggregate into small oligomers and fibrils when proteins misfold. Misfolded monomers and small oligomers are separately thought to be neurotoxic as well as able to contribute to the formation of larger aggregates. How these aggregates cause cytotoxicity is still debated; however, mitochondrial dysfunction, disruption of UPS and autophagy, impaired nucleocytoplasmic transport, disruptions to RNA metabolism, and sequestration of other proteins and molecules are all correlated with ALS.

downstream effects that protein aggregation has on cellular health, it remains difficult to identify specific interactions that would be viable therapeutic targets, other than the key aggregating proteins themselves [52].

THE PRIMARY AGGREGATING PROTEINS IN ALS

Although ALS can be caused by mutations in over 20 different genes, all ALS cases are characterized by protein inclusions containing SOD1, TDP-43, or FUS. This indicates that understanding the physiological and disease roles of these proteins is key to understanding what may cause ALS.

Superoxide Dismutase-1 (SOD1)

The gene encoding Cu/Zn superoxide dismutase (SOD1) was the first to be genetically linked to ALS [53]. Currently, over 160 different mutations within SOD1 are thought to be associated with ALS [54], and these mutations are considered to account for ~20% of fALS cases [7]. SOD1 is a 32 kDa homodimeric metalloenzyme that catalyzes the dismutation of oxygen free radicals to both molecular oxygen and hydrogen peroxide [55], thereby protecting cells from oxidative damage. It was first proposed that mutations in SOD1 were ALS-causative via a loss of enzymatic function [53]; however, subsequent studies in SOD1 mice refuted this [56, 57]. mSOD1 that retained partial or complete enzymatic function still induced ALS-like phenotypes [56], and knockout of *SOD1* in mice did not induce ALS-like phenotypes [57]. It is now accepted that the misfolding and aggregation of SOD1 is the primary mechanism by which SOD1 elicits motor neuron toxicity [4].

Although it is a small protein, SOD1 requires extensive post-translational modification to fold into its native conformation. This includes binding of zinc and copper ions and the formation of an intrasubunit disulfide bond, processes that are facilitated by the "copper chaperone for SOD1" [58–60]. Once these modifications have been made, SOD1 monomers can associate into the native and functional homodimer. ALS-associated mutations can affect any of the steps in the SOD1 maturation pathway, leading to misfolding [61] and subsequent aggregation [62]. More recently, advances in performing in-cell nuclear magnetic resonance (NMR) has revealed the intracellular conformation of ALS-associated mSOD1 to be primarily metal-depleted and disulfide-reduced [63], indicating that the unfolded form of mSOD1 is the primary aggregation-prone species. *In vivo* examination of several mouse models expressing different human mSOD1 variants also supports the notion that the primary aggregation competent conformation of mSOD1 is likely unfolded [64].

A curious observation is that different ALS-associated mSOD1 result in highly variable patient survival [65]. In line with this, the level of mSOD1 aggregation and inclusion formation in cultured cells is often reported to be dependent on the mutation within SOD1 [66, 67]. Discrepancies currently exist as to whether a soluble non-native oligomeric form of mSOD1 is responsible for cellular toxicity [68–70] or if the larger aggregates themselves are toxic [40, 66]. Indeed, the exact mechanism by which mSOD1 is toxic remains elusive and requires further investigation.

Transactivation Response DNA Binding Protein 43 (TDP-43)

In 2006, two separate research groups identified ubiquitinated TDP-43 as the major component in protein inclusions in FTLD and ALS [2, 3]. Up to 97% of all sALS patients and all fALS patients, with the exception of those with SOD1 or FUS mutations, show TDP-43–positive aggregates in affected tissues [71, 72]. As such, the study of TDP-43 aggregation *in vitro* and *in vivo* has implications for both fALS and sALS cases.

TDP-43 is a DNA/RNA binding protein involved in RNA metabolism [73]. Structurally, TDP-43 is composed of four domains: a ubiquitin-like N-terminal domain, tandem RNA recognition motifs (RRM), and a low-complexity C-terminal domain [73]. The C-terminal domain is considered to be prion-like on the basis of its sequence being similar to yeast prion-protein [44], and most of the ALS-associated mutations occur in this domain [54]. ALS-associated mutations in the TDP-43 C-terminal domain have been shown to increase aggregation propensity and *in vivo* toxicity [74–76].

In ALS patients, the pathological signatures of TDP-43 include cleavage into 35 and 25 kDa C-terminal fragments, hyperphosphorylation, ubiquitination, and mislocalization from the nucleus to the cytoplasm [2, 3, 71, 73]. It is plausible that the cytoplasmic accumulation and aggregation of TDP-43 results in both a loss of function and a gain of toxic function, given the integral roles of nuclear TDP-43 in mRNA regulation and transport [77, 78].

The mechanisms by which TDP-43 forms intracellular aggregates are debated. The C-terminal low-complexity domain of TDP-43 controls its ability to undergo liquid–liquid phase separation [79]. Some evidence suggests that TDP-43 partitioning into stress granules is responsible for the formation of inclusions [80, 81], whereas other evidence suggests that phase transitions independent of stress granules are responsible for pathological aggregation [82, 83]. Evidence also suggests that TDP-43 can aggregate through a ubiquitin proteasome system-associated pathway [38]. Regardless, the ability of TDP-43 to undergo phase transitions in the cell appears to be important for understanding both disease etiology and pathology.

Fused in Sarcoma (FUS)

Mutations in FUS were reported to cause ALS in 2009 [5, 6], and genomic analysis has shown that this gene accounts for 4–5% of fALS and 1% of sALS cases [7]. Like TDP-43, FUS is a DNA/RNA binding protein with a key role in RNA metabolism. Indeed, the FUS structure is somewhat similar to that of TDP-43, in that it contains an N-terminal low-complexity prion-like domain, a single RRM, and a C-terminal Arg/Gly-rich region containing a zinc-finger motif [73]. Interestingly, ALS-associated mutations in FUS are spread throughout the protein; however, the majority occur in the C-terminal nuclear localization sequence [73]. Accordingly, under healthy conditions, FUS is primarily localized to the nucleus; but in ALS-affected brains and spinal cords, FUS is found aggregated in the cytoplasm [5, 6].

Evidence strongly suggests that the toxic effects of FUS are due to its aberrant cytoplasmic localization, perhaps disrupting nucleocytoplasmic transport [84]. This finding is supported by work in *Drosophila*, where deletion of the nuclear export signal reduced the toxicity of FUS [85]. Interestingly, aggregation and subsequent neurodegeneration occur when either WT FUS and mutant TDP-43 are co-expressed, or WT TDP-43 and mutant FUS are co-expressed, suggesting that aggregation can involve an interaction between TDP-43 and FUS [85], perhaps mediated by their ability to undergo liquid phase separation.

Similar to TDP-43, FUS can also undergo phase transitions in the cell [86] and partition to stress granules [87]. *In vitro* examination of FUS has suggested that ALS mutations can exacerbate a solidification of phase-separated material [86]. Furthermore, increasing the levels of FUS localized to the cytoplasm by an ALS mutation (or a tagged protein) results in promotion of the formation of stress granules beyond that seen with WT FUS [88], suggesting that cytoplasmic mislocalization of FUS is a key determinant in its toxicity. It remains to be determined whether the localization of ALS-associated FUS mutants to stress granules results in the formation of cytoplasmic aggregates, or if aggregates can spontaneously occur due to increased cytoplasmic concentration.

PRION-LIKE PROPAGATION OF PROTEIN AGGREGATION IN ALS

There is strong evidence to suggest that prion-like propagation of protein misfolding and/or aggregation is a key mechanism in ALS. The prion paradigm stems from the transmissive properties of the Prion protein (PrP). While PrP is typically found in a native healthy conformation, the extraordinary discovery was made that the scrapie-associated misfolded pathological conformation of PrP was capable of interacting with the healthy conformation and converting it to the pathological conformation in sheep and goats [89]. The pathological conformation of PrP can spread from cell to cell and from organism to organism in an infectious manner, transmitting disease in the absence of a nucleic acid component [89]. Additionally, the neuropathology of the prion diseases is highly similar to that of neurodegenerative diseases, including the hallmark characteristic of the accumulation of key proteins into aggregates [90].

The pathology and clinical manifestation of ALS support a role for prion-like propagation. The primary observations supporting a prion-like mechanism include protein aggregation as a key hallmark of disease, spread of symptoms from a focal point of onset, and aggregation of specific proteins (SOD1, TDP-43, FUS). Interestingly, SOD1, TDP-43, and FUS are all capable of forming amyloid fibrils, a structure with properties that allow for prion-like propagation [91]. Although the idea that ALS is an amyloid disease is contentious, some evidence suggests that inclusions from ALS patients can contain amyloid-like or filamentous components [92–94].

The first evidence for prion-like propagation in ALS came when SOD1 mouse spinal cord homogenates were used to seed the amyloid aggregation of recombinant SOD1 [95]. Several cell culture studies showing the seeded aggregation and template-directed misfolding of SOD1 soon followed [96, 97] and have been further substantiated [98, 99]. *In vivo* evidence of the prion-like propagation of SOD1 has come from the injection of aggregated material from recombinant sources [100], other mice [100–103], and even human post mortem samples [104] into the nervous system of non-symptomatic or pre-symptomatic SOD1 transgenic mice. Although misfolded SOD1 is implicated in sALS, evidence supporting its prion-like transmission is less clear than in the case of SOD1-fALS.

As with SOD1, initial evidence of the prion-like properties of TDP-43 came from using recombinant protein, where *in vitro* generated TDP-43 fibrils were used to seed the aggregation of overexpressed TDP-43 in cultured cells [105]. Shortly after this, lipofection of immortalized neuronal cells with TDP-43–enriched extracts from ALS patients showed a potent seeding effect and resulted in ubiquitinated TDP-43 inclusions in recipient cells [106]. Multiple studies have now shown that cultured cells can be effectively seeded through the addition of pathological TDP-43 aggregates [107–112]. Evidence for the ability of TDP-43 aggregates to transmit disease *in vivo* has also been reported, although the initial seed was from FTLD patients [109]. It was observed that injection of TDP-43–enriched extracts from patient tissue into the nervous system of either mice expressing the human TDP-43 transgene or WT mice induced the formation of TDP-43 inclusions along connected anatomical pathways [109].

In comparison to both SOD1 and TDP-43, evidence supporting the prion-like propagation of FUS is currently lacking. Previous work has shown that the ALS-associated G156E mutation in FUS enhances its propensity to form amyloid fibrils *in vitro* and also that co-transfection of primary cultured neurons with WT FUS and/or G156E FUS would result in the deposition of the WT FUS only when mutant G156E FUS was present in cells [113]. Several experiments remain to be performed to confirm FUS as having bona fide prion-like properties, including *in vitro* assays and seeding cell lines with exogenous FUS aggregates.

Although there is strong cell culture and *in vivo* evidence supporting prion-like propagation of pathological SOD1 and TDP-43 in ALS, we still do not know the exact molecular structures of these propagating particles. Improvements in the structural biology toolkit afford new opportunities to examine these assemblies in detail and perhaps even identify specific disease-associated conformations and target them therapeutically.

CONCLUSION

Over the past decade, the evidence linking protein misfolding and aggregation to neurodegenerative disease has become substantial to the point where these diseases are now considered protein-misfolding disorders. The pathological signature of protein-misfolding diseases is the deposition of insoluble inclusions detectable in cell models, *in vivo* models, and human histological samples. While there are differences in the vulnerability of various regions of the nervous system and different proteins constitute the depositions, this common feature links these diseases and possibly provides a clue to unraveling their cause. In the case of ALS, there is growing evidence that a correlation exists between protein aggregate load and neuronal loss in the spinal cord. Although ALS can be caused by mutations in a number of genes or by unknown factors, all cases are characterized by the deposition of protein aggregates, notably TDP-43, FUS, or SOD1. Furthermore, these disease-associated proteins also interact with a number of other binding partners that are involved in a multitude of important physiological functions that may be affected by or contribute to disease pathogenesis. Evidence is also growing to implicate these misfolded proteins in the infectious spread of the disease throughout the nervous system. Elucidating the role that protein aggregation and proteostasis breakdown play in the pathobiological mechanisms of ALS may provide unique opportunities to identify biomarkers and therapeutic targets for earlier diagnosis and effective treatment for this devastating disease.

ACKNOWLEDGMENTS

CGC was supported by an Australian Government Research Training Program Scholarship from the University of Wollongong. JJY is supported by an NHMRC Career Development Fellowship (1084144) and a Dementia Teams Grant (1095215). LM is supported by funding from The Motor Neurone Disease Research Institute of Australia (Dr. Paul Brock MND NSW Research Grant).

CONFLICT OF INTEREST

The authors declare no potential conflict of interest with respect to research, authorship, and/or publication of this manuscript.

COPYRIGHT AND PERMISSION STATEMENT

REFERENCES

1. Chiti, F. and Dobson, C.M. (2017). Protein misfolding, amyloid formation, and human disease: a summary of progress over the last decade. *Annu Rev Biochem* 86: 27–68.
2. Neumann, M., Sampathu, D.M., Kwong, L.K. et al. (2006). Ubiquitinated TDP-43 in frontotemporal lobar degeneration and amyotrophic lateral sclerosis. *Science* 314 (5796): 130–133.

3. Arai, T., Hasegawa, M., Akiyama, H. et al. (2006). TDP-43 is a component of ubiquitin-positive tau-negative inclusions in frontotemporal lobar degeneration and amyotrophic lateral sclerosis. *Biochem Biophys Res Commun* 351 (3): 602–611.

4. Bruijn, L.I., Houseweart, M.K., Kato, S. et al. (1998). Aggregation and motor neuron toxicity of an ALS-linked SOD1 mutant independent from wild-type SOD1. *Science* 281 (5384): 1851–1854.

5. Kwiatkowski, T.J. Jr., Bosco, D.A., Leclerc, A.L. et al. (2009). Mutations in the FUS/TLS gene on chromosome 16 cause familial amyotrophic lateral sclerosis. *Science* 323 (5918): 1205–1208.

6. Vance, C., Rogelj, B., Hortobágyi, T. et al. (2009). Mutations in FUS, an RNA processing protein, cause familial amyotrophic lateral sclerosis type 6. *Science* 323 (5918): 1208–1211.

7. Taylor, J.P., Brown, R.H. Jr., and Cleveland, D.W. (2016). Decoding ALS: from genes to mechanism. *Nature* 539 (7628): 197–206.

8. Blokhuis, A.M., Groen, E.J.N., Koppers, M. et al. (2013). Protein aggregation in amyotrophic lateral sclerosis. *Acta Neuropathol* 125 (6): 777–794.

9. Ling, S.-C., Polymenidou, M., and Cleveland, D.W. (2013). Converging mechanisms in ALS and FTD: disrupted RNA and protein homeostasis. *Neuron* 79 (3): 416.

10. DeJesus-Hernandez, M., Mackenzie, I.R., Boeve, B.F. et al. (2011). Expanded GGGGCC hexanucleotide repeat in noncoding region of C9ORF72 causes chromosome 9p-linked FTD and ALS. *Neuron* 72 (2): 245–256.

11. Renton, A.E., Majounie, E., Waite, A. et al. (2011). A hexanucleotide repeat expansion in C9ORF72 is the cause of chromosome 9p21-linked ALS-FTD. *Neuron* 72 (2): 257–268.

12. Byrne, S., Elamin, M., Bede, P. et al. (2012). Cognitive and clinical characteristics of patients with amyotrophic lateral sclerosis carrying a C9orf72 repeat expansion: a population-based cohort study. *Lancet Neurol* 11 (3): 232–240.

13. Majounie, E., Renton, A.E., Mok, K. et al. (2012). Frequency of the C9orf72 hexanucleotide repeat expansion in patients with amyotrophic lateral sclerosis and frontotemporal dementia: a cross-sectional study. *Lancet Neurol* 11 (4): 323–330.

14. Umoh, M.E., Fournier, C., Li, Y. et al. (2016). Comparative analysis of C9orf72 and sporadic disease in an ALS clinic population. *Neurology* 87 (10): 1024–1030.

15. Solomon, D.A., Stepto, A., Au, W.H. et al. (2018). A feedback loop between dipeptide-repeat protein, TDP-43 and karyopherin-α mediates C9orf72-related neurodegeneration. *Brain* 141 (10): 2908–2924.

16. Nonaka, T., Masuda-Suzukake, M., Hosokawa, M. et al. (2018). C9ORF72 dipeptide repeat poly-GA inclusions promote: intracellular aggregation of phosphorylated TDP-43. *Hum Mol Genet*.

17. Khosravi, B., Hartmann, H., May, S. et al. Cytoplasmic poly-GA aggregates impair nuclear import of TDP-43 in C9orf72 ALS/FTLD. *Hum Mol Genet* 26 (4): 790–800.

18. Cooper-Knock, J., Hewitt, C., Highley, J.R. et al. (2012). Clinico-pathological features in amyotrophic lateral sclerosis with expansions in C9ORF72. *Brain J Neurol* 135 (Pt 3): 751–764.

19. Maruyama, H., Morino, H., Ito, H. et al. (2010). Mutations of optineurin in amyotrophic lateral sclerosis. *Nature* 465 (7295): 223–226.

20. Deng, H.-X., Chen, W., Hong, S.-T. et al. (2011). Mutations in UBQLN2 cause dominant X-linked juvenile and adult-onset ALS and ALS/dementia. *Nature* 477 (7363): 211–215.

21. Gal, J., Ström, A.-L., Kilty, R. et al. (2007). p62 accumulates and enhances aggregate formation in model systems of familial amyotrophic lateral sclerosis. *J Biol Chem* 282 (15): 11068–11077.

22. Mizuno, Y., Amari, M., Takatama, M. et al. (2006). Immunoreactivities of p 62, an ubiqutin-binding protein, in the spinal anterior horn cells of patients with amyotrophic lateral sclerosis. *J Neurol Sci* 249 (1): 13–18.

23. Neumann, M., Rademakers, R., Roeber, S. et al. (2009). A new subtype of frontotemporal lobar degeneration with FUS pathology. *Brain* 132 (Pt 11): 2922–2931.

24. Saberi, S., Stauffer, J.E., Schulte, D.J., and Ravits, J. (2015). Neuropathology of amyotrophic lateral sclerosis and its variants. *Neurol Clin* 33 (4): 855–876.

25. Al-Chalabi, A., Jones, A., Troakes, C. et al. (2012). The genetics and neuropathology of amyotrophic lateral sclerosis. *Acta Neuropathol* 124 (3): 339–352.

26. Braak, H., Brettschneider, J., Ludolph, A.C. et al. (2013). Amyotrophic lateral sclerosis--a model of corticofugal axonal spread. *Nat Rev Neurol* 9 (12): 708–714.

27. Brettschneider, J., Del Tredici, K., Toledo, J.B. et al. (2013). Stages of pTDP-43 pathology in amyotrophic lateral sclerosis. *Ann Neurol* 74 (1): 20–38.

28. Brettschneider, J., Arai, K., Del Tredici, K. et al. (2014). TDP-43 pathology and neuronal loss in amyotrophic lateral sclerosis spinal cord. *Acta Neuropathol* 128 (3): 423–437.

29. Geser, F., Brandmeir, N.J., Kwong, L.K. et al. (2008). Evidence of multisystem disorder in whole-brain map of pathological TDP-43 in amyotrophic lateral sclerosis. *Arch Neurol* 65 (5): 636–641.

30. Balch, W.E., Morimoto, R.I., Dillin, A., and Kelly, J.W. (2008). Adapting proteostasis for disease intervention. *Science* 319 (5865): 916.

31. Yerbury, J.J., Ooi, L., Dillin, A. et al. (2016). Walking the tightrope: proteostasis and neurodegenerative disease. *J Neurochem* 137 (4): 489–505.

32. Jahn, T.R. and Radford, S.E. (2005). The yin and yang of protein folding. *FEBS J* 272 (23): 5962–5970.

33. Gidalevitz, T., Prahlad, V., and Morimoto, R.I. (2011). The stress of protein misfolding: from single cells to multicellular organisms. *Cold Spring Harb Perspect Biol* 3 (6): a009704.

34. Sherman, M.Y. and Goldberg, A.L. (2001). Cellular defenses against unfolded proteins: a cell biologist thinks about neurodegenerative diseases. *Neuron* 29 (1): 15–32.

35. Nyström, T. and Liu, B. (2014). Protein quality control in time and space – links to cellular aging. *FEMS Yeast Res* 14 (1): 40–48.

36. Ogrodnik, M., Salmonowicz, H., Brown, R. et al. (2014). Dynamic JUNQ inclusion bodies are asymmetrically inherited in mammalian cell lines through the asymmetric partitioning of vimentin. *Proc Natl Acad Sci U S A* 111 (22): 8049–8054.

37. Kaganovich, D., Kopito, R., and Frydman, J. (2008). Misfolded proteins partition between two distinct quality control compartments. *Nature* 454 (7208): 1088.

38. Farrawell, N.E., Lambert-Smith, I.A., Warraich, S.T. et al. (2015). Distinct partitioning of ALS associated TDP-43, FUS and SOD1 mutants into cellular inclusions. *Sci Rep* 5: 13416.

39. Arrasate, M., Mitra, S., Schweitzer, E.S. et al. (2004). Inclusion body formation reduces levels of mutant huntingtin and the risk of neuronal death. *Nature* 431 (7010): 805.

40. Weisberg, S.J., Lyakhovetsky, R., Werdiger, A.-C. et al. (2012). Compartmentalization of superoxide dismutase 1 (SOD1G93A) aggregates determines their toxicity. *Proc Natl Acad Sci U S A* 109 (39): 15811–15816.

41. Urushitani, M., Kurisu, J., Tsukita, K., and Takahashi, R. (2002). Proteasomal inhibition by misfolded mutant superoxide dismutase 1 induces selective motor neuron death in familial amyotrophic lateral sclerosis. *J Neurochem* 83 (5): 1030–1042.

42. Basso, M., Massignan, T., Samengo, G. et al. (2006). Insoluble mutant SOD1 is partly oligoubiquitinated in amyotrophic lateral sclerosis mice. *J Biol Chem* 281 (44): 33325–33335.

43. Farrawell, N.E., Lambert-Smith, I., Mitchell, K. et al. (2018). SOD1 aggregation alters ubiquitin homeostasis in a cell model of ALS. *J Cell Sci* 131 (11): jcs209122.

44. King, O.D., Gitler, A.D., and Shorter, J. (2012). The tip of the iceberg: RNA-binding proteins with prion-like domains in neurodegenerative disease. *Brain Res* 1462: 61–80.

45. Nakaya, T. and Maragkakis, M. (2018). Amyotrophic lateral sclerosis associated FUS mutation shortens mitochondria and induces neurotoxicity. *Sci Rep* 8 (1): 15575.

46. Wang, P., Deng, J., Dong, J. et al. (2019). TDP-43 induces mitochondrial damage and activates the mitochondrial unfolded protein response. *PLoS Genet* 15 (5): e1007947.

47. Tafuri, F., Ronchi, D., Magri, F. et al. (2015). SOD1 misplacing and mitochondrial dysfunction in amyotrophic lateral sclerosis pathogenesis. *Front Cell Neurosci* 9: 336.

48. Medinas, D.B., Valenzuela, V., and Hetz, C. (2017). Proteostasis disturbance in amyotrophic lateral sclerosis. *Hum Mol Genet* 26 (R2): R91–R104.

49. Yang, H. and Hu, H.-Y. (2016). Sequestration of cellular interacting partners by protein aggregates: implication in a loss-of-function pathology. *FEBS J* 283 (20): 3705–3717.

50. Olzscha, H., Schermann, S.M., Woerner, A.C. et al. (2011). Amyloid-like aggregates sequester numerous metastable proteins with essential cellular functions. *Cell* 144 (1): 67–78.

51. Ciryam, P., Lambert-Smith, I.A., Bean, D.M. et al. (2017). Spinal motor neuron protein supersaturation patterns are associated with inclusion body formation in ALS. *Proc Natl Acad Sci U S A* 114 (20): E3935–e43.

52. Woerner, A.C., Frottin, F., Hornburg, D. et al. (2016). Cytoplasmic protein aggregates interfere with nucleocytoplasmic transport of protein and RNA. *Science* 351 (6269): 173.

53. Rosen, D. (1993). Mutations in Cu/Zn superoxide dismutase gene are associated with familial amyotrophic lateral sclerosis. *Nature* 364 (6435): 362.

54. Wroe, R., Wai-Ling Butler, A., Andersen, P.M. et al. (2008). ALSOD: the amyotrophic lateral sclerosis online database. *Amyotroph Lateral Scler* 9 (4): 249–250.

55. McCord, J.M. and Fridovich, I. (1969). Superoxide dismutase. an enzymic function for erythrocuprein (hemocuprein). *J Biol Chem* 244 (22): 6049–6055.

56. Gurney, M., Pu, H., Chiu, A. et al. (1994). Motor neuron degeneration in mice that express a human Cu, Zn superoxide dismutase mutation. *Science* 264 (5166): 1772–1775.

57. Reaume, A.G., Elliott, J.L., Hoffman, E.K. et al. (1996). Motor neurons in Cu/Zn superoxide dismutase-deficient mice develop normally but exhibit enhanced cell death after axonal injury. *Nat Genet* 13 (1): 43–47.

58. Wright, G.S.A., Antonyuk, S.V., and Samar, H.S. (2016). A faulty interaction between SOD1 and hCCS in neurodegenerative disease. *Sci Rep* 6 (1): 27691.

59. Banci, L., Barbieri, L., Bertini, I. et al. (2011). In-cell NMR in *E. coli* to monitor maturation steps of hSOD1. *PLoS One* 6 (8): e23561.

60. Banci, L., Bertini, I., Cantini, F. et al. (2012). Human superoxide dismutase 1 (hSOD1) maturation through interaction with human copper chaperone for SOD1 (hCCS). *Proc Natl Acad Sci U S A* 109 (34): 13555–13560.

61. Lindberg, M.J., Normark, J., Holmgren, A., and Oliveberg, M. (2004). Folding of human superoxide dismutase: disulfide reduction prevents dimerization and produces marginally stable monomers. *Proc Natl Acad Sci U S A* 101 (45): 15893–15898.

62. Chattopadhyay, M., Durazo, A., Sohn, S.H. et al. (2008). Initiation and elongation in fibrillation of ALS-linked superoxide dismutase. *Proc Natl Acad Sci* 105 (48): 18663–18668.

63. Luchinat, E., Barbieri, L., Rubino, J.T. et al. (2014). In-cell NMR reveals potential precursor of toxic species from SOD1 fALS mutants. *Nat Commun* 5: 5502.

64. Lang, L., Zetterström, P., Brännström, T. et al. (2015). SOD1 aggregation in ALS mice shows simplistic test tube behavior. *Proc Natl Acad Sci U S A* 112 (32): 9878–9883.

65. Wang, Q., Johnson, J.L., Agar, N.Y.R., and Agar, J.N. (2008). Protein aggregation and protein instability govern familial amyotrophic lateral sclerosis patient survival. *PLoS Biol* 6 (7): e170.

66. McAlary, L., Andrew Aquilina, J., and Yerbury, J.J. (2016). Susceptibility of mutant SOD1 to form a destabilized monomer predicts cellular aggregation and toxicity but not in vitro aggregation propensity. *Front Neurosci* 10: 499.

67. Turner, B.J., Atkin, J.D., Farg, M.A. et al. (2005). Impaired extracellular secretion of mutant superoxide dismutase 1 associates with neurotoxicity in familial amyotrophic lateral sclerosis. *J Neurosci* 25 (1): 108–117.

68. Zhu, C., Beck, M.V., Griffith, J.D. et al. (2018). Large SOD1 aggregates, unlike trimeric SOD1, do not impact cell viability in a model of amyotrophic lateral sclerosis. *Proc Natl Acad Sci U S A* 115 (18): 4661–4665.

69. Sangwan, S., Zhao, A., Adams, K.L. et al. (2017). Atomic structure of a toxic, oligomeric segment of SOD1 linked to amyotrophic lateral sclerosis (ALS). *Proc Natl Acad Sci U S A* 114 (33): 8770–8775.

70. Gill, C., Phelan, J.P., Hatzipetros, T. et al. (2019). SOD1-positive aggregate accumulation in the CNS predicts slower disease progression and increased longevity in a mutant SOD1 mouse model of ALS. *Sci Rep* 9 (1): 6724.

71. Mackenzie, I.R.A., Bigio, E.H., Ince, P.G. et al. (2007). Pathological TDP-43 distinguishes sporadic amyotrophic lateral sclerosis from amyotrophic lateral sclerosis with SOD1 mutations. *Ann Neurol* 61 (5): 427–434.

72. Prasad, A., Bharathi, V., Sivalingam, V. et al. (2019). Molecular mechanisms of TDP-43 misfolding and pathology in amyotrophic lateral sclerosis. *Front Mol Neurosci* 12: 25.

73. Lagier-Tourenne, C., Polymenidou, M., and Cleveland, D.W. (2010). TDP-43 and FUS/TLS: emerging roles in RNA processing and neurodegeneration. *Hum Mol Genet* 19 (R1): R46–R64.

74. Berning, B.A. and Walker, A.K. (2019). The pathobiology of TDP-43 C-terminal fragments in ALS and FTLD. *Front Neurosci* 13: 335.

75. Santamaria, N., Alhothali, M., Alfonso, M.H. et al. (2017). Intrinsic disorder in proteins involved in amyotrophic lateral sclerosis. *Cell Mol Life Sci* 74 (7): 1297–1318.

76. Johnson, B.S., Snead, D., Lee, J.J. et al. (2009). TDP-43 is intrinsically aggregation-prone, and amyotrophic lateral sclerosis-linked mutations accelerate aggregation and increase toxicity. *J Biol Chem* 284 (30): 20329–20339.

77. Vanden Broeck, L., Callaerts, P., and Dermaut, B. (2014). TDP-43-mediated neurodegeneration: towards a loss-of-function hypothesis? *Trends Mol Med* 20 (2): 66–71.

78. Ederle, H. and Dormann, D. (2017). TDP-43 and FUS en route from the nucleus to the cytoplasm. *FEBS Lett* 591 (11): 1489–1507.

79. Conicella, A.E., Zerze, G.H., Mittal, J., and Fawzi, N.L. (2016). ALS mutations disrupt phase separation mediated by α-helical structure in the TDP-43 low-complexity C-terminal domain. *Structure* 24 (9): 1537–1549.

80. Zhang, P., Fan, B., Yang, P. et al. (2019). Chronic optogenetic induction of stress granules is cytotoxic and reveals the evolution of ALS-FTD pathology. *elife* 8: e39578.

81. Mackenzie, I.R., Nicholson, A.M., Sarkar, M. et al. (2017). TIA1 mutations in amyotrophic lateral sclerosis and frontotemporal dementia promote phase separation and alter stress granule dynamics. *Neuron* 95 (4): 808–816. e9.

82. Mann, J.R., Gleixner, A.M., Mauna, J.C. et al. (2019). RNA binding antagonizes neurotoxic phase transitions of TDP-43. *Neuron* 102 (2): 321–338. e8.

83. Gasset-Rosa, F., Lu, S., Yu, H. et al. (2019). Cytoplasmic TDP-43 de-mixing independent of stress granules drives inhibition of nuclear import, loss of nuclear TDP-43, and cell death. *Neuron* 102 (2): 339–357. e7.

84. Dormann, D., Rodde, R., Edbauer, D. et al. (2010). ALS-associated fused in sarcoma (FUS) mutations disrupt transportin-mediated nuclear import. *EMBO J* 29 (16): 2841–2857.

85. Lanson, N.A. Jr., Maltare, A., King, H. et al. (2011). A drosophila model of FUS-related neurodegeneration reveals genetic interaction between FUS and TDP-43. *Hum Mol Genet* 20 (13): 2510–2523.

86. Patel, A., Lee, H.O., Jawerth, L. et al. (2015). A liquid-to-solid phase transition of the ALS protein FUS accelerated by disease mutation. *Cell* 162 (5): 1066–1077.

87. Andersson, M.K., Ståhlberg, A., Arvidsson, Y. et al. (2008). The multifunctional FUS, EWS and TAF15 proto-oncoproteins show cell type-specific expression patterns and involvement in cell spreading and stress response. *BMC Cell Biol* 9: 37.

88. Marrone, L., Poser, I., Casci, I. et al. (2018). Isogenic FUS-eGFP iPSC reporter lines enable quantification of FUS stress granule pathology that Is rescued by drugs inducing autophagy. *Stem Cell Reports* 10 (2): 375–389.

89. Prusiner, S.B. (1982). Novel proteinaceous infectious particles cause scrapie. *Science* 216 (4542): 136–144.

90. Prusiner, S.B. (2001). Neurodegenerative diseases and prions. *N Engl J Med* 344 (20): 1516–1526.

91. Marchante, R., Beal, D.M., Koloteva-Levine, N. et al. (2017). The physical dimensions of amyloid aggregates control their infective potential as prion particles. *elife* 6.

92. Kato, S., Takikawa, M., Nakashima, K. et al. (2000). New consensus research on neuropathological aspects of familial amyotrophic lateral sclerosis with superoxide dismutase 1 (SOD1) gene mutations: inclusions containing SOD1 in neurons and astrocytes. *Amyotroph Lateral Scler Other Motor Neuron Disord* 1 (3): 163–184.

93. Bigio, E.H., Wu, J.Y., Deng, H.-X. et al. (2013). Inclusions in frontotemporal lobar degeneration with TDP-43 proteinopathy (FTLD-TDP) and amyotrophic lateral sclerosis (ALS), but not FTLD with FUS proteinopathy (FTLD-FUS), have properties of amyloid. *Acta Neuropathol* 125 (3): 463–465.

94. Mori, F., Tanji, K., Zhang, H.-X. et al. (2008). Maturation process of TDP-43-positive neuronal cytoplasmic inclusions in amyotrophic lateral sclerosis with and without dementia. *Acta Neuropathol* 116 (2): 193–203.

95. Chia, R., Tattum, M.H., Jones, S. et al. (2010). Superoxide dismutase 1 and tg SOD1 mouse spinal cord seed fibrils, suggesting a propagative cell death mechanism in amyotrophic lateral sclerosis. *PLoS One* 5 (5): e10627.

96. Münch, C., O'Brien, J., and Bertolotti, A. (2011). Prion-like propagation of mutant superoxide dismutase-1 misfolding in neuronal cells. *Proc Natl Acad Sci U S A* 108 (9): 3548–3553.

97. Grad, L.I., Guest, W.C., Yanai, A. et al. (2011). Intermolecular transmission of superoxide dismutase 1 misfolding in living cells. *Proc Natl Acad Sci U S A* 108 (39): 16398–16403.

98. Pokrishevsky, E., Hong, R.H., Mackenzie, I.R., and Cashman, N.R. (2017). Spinal cord homogenates from SOD1 familial amyotrophic lateral sclerosis induce SOD1 aggregation in living cells. *PLoS One* 12 (9): e0184384.

99. Zeineddine, R., Pundavela, J.F., Corcoran, L. et al. (2015). SOD1 protein aggregates stimulate macropinocytosis in neurons to facilitate their propagation. *Mol Neurodegener* 10: 57.

100. Ayers, J.I., Diamond, J., Sari, A. et al. (2016). Distinct conformers of transmissible misfolded SOD1 distinguish human SOD1-FALS from other forms of familial and sporadic ALS. *Acta Neuropathol* 132 (6): 827–840.

101. Ayers, J.I., Fromholt, S., Koch, M. et al. (2014). Experimental transmissibility of mutant SOD1 motor neuron disease. *Acta Neuropathol* 128 (6): 791–803.

102. Ayers, J.I., Fromholt, S.E., O'Neal, V.M. et al. (2016). Prion-like propagation of mutant SOD1 misfolding and motor neuron disease spread along neuroanatomical pathways. *Acta Neuropathol* 131 (1): 103–114.

103. Bidhendi, E.E., Bergh, J., Zetterström, P. et al. (2016). Two superoxide dismutase prion strains transmit amyotrophic lateral sclerosis-like disease. *J Clin Invest* 126 (6): 2249–2253.

104. Ekhtiari Bidhendi, E., Bergh, J., Zetterström, P. et al. (2018). Mutant superoxide dismutase aggregates from human spinal cord transmit amyotrophic lateral sclerosis. *Acta Neuropathol* 136 (6): 939–953.

105. Furukawa, Y., Kaneko, K., Watanabe, S. et al. (2011). A seeding reaction recapitulates intracellular formation of sarkosyl-insoluble transactivation response element (TAR) DNA-binding protein-43 inclusions. *J Biol Chem* 286 (21): 18664–18672.

106. Nonaka, T., Suzukake, M., Arai, T. et al. (2013). Insoluble TDP-43 prepared from diseased brains has prion-like properties. *Alzheimers Dement* 9 (4): 720.

107. Shimonaka, S., Nonaka, T., Suzuki, G. et al. (2016). Templated aggregation of TAR DNA-binding protein of 43 kDa (TDP-43) by seeding with TDP-43 peptide fibrils. *J Biol Chem* 291 (17): 8896–8907.

108. Laferrière, F., Maniecka, Z., Pérez-Berlanga, M. et al. (2019). TDP-43 extracted from frontotemporal lobar degeneration subject brains displays distinct aggregate assemblies and neurotoxic effects reflecting disease progression rates. *Nat Neurosci* 22 (1): 65–77.

109. Porta, S., Xu, Y., Restrepo, C.R. et al. (2018). Patient-derived frontotemporal lobar degeneration brain extracts induce formation and spreading of TDP-43 pathology in vivo. *Nat Commun* 9 (1): 4220.

110. Zeineddine, R., Whiten, D.R., Farrawell, N.E. et al. (2017). Flow cytometric measurement of the cellular propagation of TDP-43 aggregation. *Prion* 11 (3): 195–204.

111. Smethurst, P., Newcombe, J., Troakes, C. et al. (2016). in vitro prion-like behaviour of TDP-43 in ALS. *Neurobiol Dis* 96: 236–247.

112. Feiler, M.S., Strobel, B., Freischmidt, A. et al. (2015). TDP-43 is intercellularly transmitted across axon terminals. *J Cell Biol* 211 (4): 897–911.

113. Nomura, T., Watanabe, S., Kaneko, K. et al. (2014). Intranuclear aggregation of mutant FUS/TLS as a molecular pathomechanism of amyotrophic lateral sclerosis. *J Biol Chem* 289 (2): 1192–1202.

CHAPTER 7

Evidence for a Growing Involvement of Glia in Amyotrophic Lateral Sclerosis

Rowan A. W. Radford[1], Andres Vidal-Itriago[1], Natalie M. Scherer[1], Albert Lee[1], Manuel Graeber[2], Roger S. Chung[1], and Marco Morsch[1]

[1] Motor Neuron Disease Research Centre, Faculty of Medicine and Health Sciences, Macquarie University, Sydney, New South Wales, Australia
[2] Brain Tumor Research Laboratories, Brain and Mind Centre, The University of Sydney, Sydney, New South Wales, Australia

INTRODUCTION

NON-NEURONAL CELLS PLAY IMPORTANT ROLES IN NEURODEGENERATION INCLUDING IN ALS

Glial Cells and Their Established Functions

Glia are the non-neuronal cells that occupy the parenchyma of the central nervous system (CNS). They are essential for homeostasis and include astrocytes, oligodendrocytes, and microglia. Astrocytes are a diverse population of cells that provide structural and metabolic support in many forms, such as neurotransmitter recycling, innate immunity of the CNS, maintenance of ion-homeostasis, and the extracellular CNS environment [1, 2]. Oligodendrocyte-lineage cells are the most abundant in the CNS and crucial to myelination and ion regulation [3, 4]. Finally, microglia tile the CNS in discrete niches, continuously surveying the environment and operating as resident macrophage precursor and primary innate immune cells that respond to injury, invading pathogens, and degenerative changes of the CNS [5, 6].

Neurodegeneration and the Role of Glial Cells

Neurodegenerative diseases are primarily characterized by the progressive dysfunction of neurons. Glial dysfunction and primary glial degeneration can contribute to this neuronal breakdown, and this is particularly well known in leukodystrophies, where glial-specific genes and processes are affected and lead to neurodegeneration [7]. Similarly, numerous studies have demonstrated that non-neuronal processes are major contributors to neuronal dysfunction in amyotrophic lateral sclerosis (ALS) and other neurodegenerative diseases (reviewed, for example, in [8–10]). It remains to be clarified to what extent the glial response is driven by a "healthy" reaction or whether glial cells are affected themselves by the disease process underlying ALS.

Glia in ALS

ALS is a heterogeneous and devastating progressive neurodegenerative syndrome affecting the neurons controlling skeletal muscle motor control [11]. Attesting to the heterogeneity of ALS, the clinical phenotype can significantly vary among patients [12]. So far, over 30 genes have been identified, including highly penetrant mutations and sequence variants that confer different levels of risk of developing ALS [13, 14]. Cytoplasmic inclusions in motor neurons and glia are a characteristic hallmark of ALS, and at least three distinct subtypes are found upon neuropathological assessment [15]. These three proteins are TAR DNA binding protein 43 (TDP-43), superoxide dismutase-1 (SOD1), and fused in sarcoma (FUS). Mutations in these genes can lead to the development of ALS, and pathological inclusions can be detected in basically all ALS cases, including sporadic forms. Altogether, these distinctive manifestations suggest the existence of different pathomechanisms that can lead to motor neuron dysfunction and loss. Interestingly, TDP-43, SOD1, and FUS are not restricted to motor neurons (or even neurons) but are expressed ubiquitously, including by glial cells. A graphical summary of the glial-related changes in TDP-43, SOD1, and FUS pathology is depicted in Figure 7.1. In addition, several other ALS-related genes have been previously shown to influence glial function [16].

While direct motor neuron involvement in ALS is indisputable, there is a large body of evidence in support of glia also actively impacting ALS pathogenesis and progression [17, 18]. In this chapter, we summarize the extensive evidence that glia directly contribute to ALS via disruption of normal tissue homeostasis and mechanisms that can directly result in ALS pathology and motor neuron loss. Overall, there can be no doubt about the importance of non-neuronal cells such as glial cells in regulating mechanisms that are involved in motor neuron survival, ALS pathogenesis, and progression. Moreover, the homeostatic imbalance between neurons and glia may be a significant factor that contributes to the wide-ranging disease heterogeneity (onset, duration, and severity) observed in familial and sporadic ALS patients. We highlight the current limitations of the concept that links glia activation to accelerated disease progression and emphasize the importance of differentiating glial responses according to the disease state.

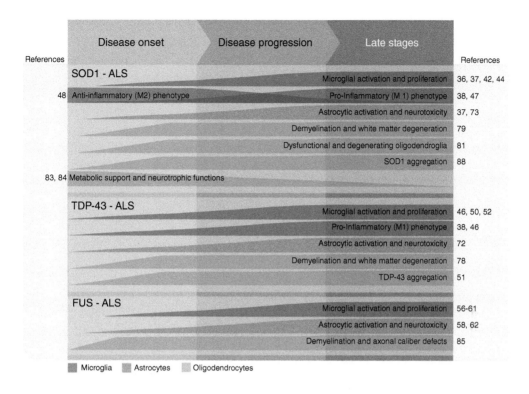

	Disease onset	Disease progression	Late stages	
References				**References**
	SOD1 - ALS			
			Microglial activation and proliferation	36, 37, 42, 44
48	Anti-inflammatory (M2) phenotype		Pro-Inflammatory (M 1) phenotype	38, 47
			Astrocytic activation and neurotoxicity	37, 73
			Demyelination and white matter degeneration	79
			Dysfunctional and degenerating oligodendroglia	81
			SOD1 aggregation	88
83, 84	Metabolic support and neurotrophic functions			
	TDP-43 - ALS			
			Microglial activation and proliferation	46, 50, 52
			Pro-Inflammatory (M1) phenotype	38, 46
			Astrocytic activation and neurotoxicity	72
			Demyelination and white matter degeneration	78
			TDP-43 aggregation	51
	FUS - ALS			
			Microglial activation and proliferation	56-61
			Astrocytic activation and neurotoxicity	58, 62
			Demyelination and axonal caliber defects	85

■ Microglia   ■ Astrocytes   ☐ Oligodendrocytes

FIGURE 7.1   Schematic of the time course of how glial cells have been reported to affect TDP-43, SOD1, and FUS pathology.

Glial Dysfunction Is a Common Hallmark of ALS Patients

Upon *post mortem* neuropathological examination, the classical neuropathological hallmark of ALS is the loss of motor neurons in the anterior horn of the spinal cord as well as brainstem motor nuclei and giant pyramidal neurons of the motor cortex (Betz cells). Neuronal loss is accompanied by glial activation, degeneration of the corticospinal tracts and spinal anterior nerve roots, and the presence of ubiquitinated cytoplasmic inclusions in remaining neurons and glia [19, 20]. Glial activation is typically simplified to changes in the morphology and proliferation of astrocytes and microglia [21]. Astrocytic activation has been reported in the brain and spinal cord of ALS patients, and neurotoxic astrocytes have been observed in ALS *post mortem* tissue in areas corresponding to neurodegeneration [22, 23]. Additionally, microglial activation and expression of phagocytic markers such as CD68 have been shown to correlate with neuronal loss, axonal degeneration, and TDP-43 pathology *post mortem* in patient tissue [24–26]. Recent advances in neuroimaging of patients have allowed direct visualization of glial dysfunction and activation. Positron emission tomography (PET) and single positron emission computed tomography (SPECT) or magnetic resonance imaging (MRI) in patients, targeting predominately activated microglia (ligands against Translocator protein 18 kDa (TSPO)) or astrocytic metabolites, have shown activation in anatomical areas corresponding to neurodegeneration throughout various symptomatic stages of ALS while being absent in non-disease controls [27–30].

In vivo neuroimaging and *post mortem* neuropathological studies of ALS cohorts are invaluable in directly observing the pathogenic process and verifying a connection between glial activation and ALS. However, these approaches are limited, if not static, and lack the versatility of experimental manipulation. Glial activation can change over time and is now considered protective or toxic depending upon the scenario [31, 32]. Therefore, cell and animal models of ALS are of fundamental importance for elucidating the role of glia and especially glial activation in ALS pathogenesis.

GLIAL ACTIVATION IN ALS MODELS

Major Pathological Forms of ALS

While dozens of genes have been identified as playing a role in ALS, there are historically three pathological forms that have been studied in greater detail. SOD1 inclusion pathology is seen in ~2% of ALS cases, and SOD1 mutations are found in 1–2% of sporadic and 12–20% of familial cases [15, 16]. In contrast, ~97% of ALS patients show cytoplasmic accumulation of the hallmark protein TDP-43. Mutations in the *FUS* gene account for approximately 4% of familial and 1% of sporadic ALS cases [33]. FUS protein inclusions are found in ~1% of ALS [16, 34].

Microglia-Related ALS Pathology

The innate and adaptive immune system is the first defense line for a mammalian host to combat pathogens and infection. Microglia, the resident macrophages of the CNS, are part of this response system, and their "activation" has been linked to disease states for over 100 years (reviewed in [35]). They play a key role in the response to various pathological processes [6, 36] and, along with astrocytes, have been strongly linked to the progressive phase of pathogenesis in ALS [37]. However, microglial activation is a very dynamic and heterogeneous process that can be protective or cytotoxic, and there is evidence of both functions in ALS microglia [31, 38]. Targeting microglia and the inflammatory cascade in ALS might therefore be therapeutically relevant to modify the onset or progression of neurodegeneration.

Microglia in SOD1-ALS Pathology

A wealth of studies have linked microglia activation to ALS, originally in human cases and later in SOD1 pathology, describing a speculative switch from a neuroprotective phenotype to a harmful "proinflammatory" microglia response [38, 39]. Chimeric rodent models, where wild-type (WT) cells and mutant SOD1-expressing cells ($SOD1^{G85R}$, $SOD1^{G37R}$, $SOD1^{G93A}$) were co-expressed together in a controlled fashion, were particularly informative and strongly suggested that surrounding glial cells affect the survival of motor neurons and influence disease onset and progression (reviewed by [40, 41]).

Early studies reported an increase in microglial reactivity found in *post mortem* tissue of all but one sporadic ALS-patients [24, 39] and SOD1^{G93A} mice [42]. Replacing SOD1^{G93A}-expressing microglia with WT microglia through a bone marrow transplantation extended the survival by ~30 days and led to a 40% longer disease duration in SOD1^{G93A} mice, with no significant change in the time point of disease onset, implying a contribution of mSOD1-expressing microglia in ALS disease progression [43]. Furthermore, it has been shown that repressing human SOD1 in microglia significantly improved the mean survival of mutant SOD1^{G37R} mice by 99 days with minor effects on early disease phases [44]. Finally, pharmacologically depleting microglia and reducing monocytes using a CSF1R antagonist reduced motor neuron cell death, slowed disease progression, and increased the maximal lifespan by 12% in the SOD1^{G93A} model [45]. These results suggest that microglia can play a modulating role during the different phases of disease as reflected by their wide spectrum of phenotypes (neuroprotective vs. neurotoxic) [40, 46, 47].

Microglia isolated from SOD1^{G93A} mice during late disease stages presented a decreased level of anti-inflammatory markers compared to microglia isolated during the early stages at 11 weeks of age [48]. Interestingly, the anti-inflammatory markers were similar between 11-week old mice and age-matched WT counterparts. Motor neurons in co-culture with end-stage microglia showed a significant decrease in neurite number and survival rate when compared to co-cultures with early-stage or WT microglia [48]. Those results support the idea of a microglia transformation during disease progression from a neuroprotective phenotype at early stages toward a reactive, neuro-damaging one at later disease stages [45, 48, 49].

Microglia in TDP-43-ALS Pathology

As stated above, only ~3% of patients carry mutations in SOD1 and are characterized by the pathological presence of cytoplasmic SOD1 inclusions in motor neurons. In contrast, ~97% of ALS patients show cytoplasmic accumulation of the hallmark protein TDP-43. Therefore, SOD1-ALS can be considered as a more "pure" form of ALS, while many other genes (including TDP-43) are associated with ALS as well as other neurodegenerative diseases, including frontotemporal dementia (FTD) [16].

In a mutant mouse model of TDP-43 pathology, motor deficits correlated with an increase in the activation and number of microglia [50]. *Post mortem* analysis of TDP-43–positive ALS patients, as well as imaging studies, have further linked microglia to TDP-43 pathology [25, 27, 51]. Two animal studies have recently demonstrated that microglia can clear TDP-43 from stressed/dying motor neurons [52, 53], suggesting a different role for microglia compared to the SOD1 experimental model (where microglia have been described mainly as neurotoxic). Notably, inhibition (functional elimination) of microglia resulted in cytoplasmic and abnormal axonal localization of TDP-43 [53]. Microglia in older mice displayed a reduced ability to clear TDP-43 [52], correlating with a more severe phenotype in older transgenic TDP-43 mice. These data provide a complementary explanation of how microglia may contribute to neuroprotection and regulate TDP-43 pathology. They further challenge the current thinking about the role of microglia in ALS and provide a new direction for considering two longstanding questions in the field: (i) in what way does microglia activation contribute to neurodegeneration in ALS? and (ii) what is the fate of TDP-43 that accumulates in dying motor neurons [54]? Phagocytosis of dead motor neurons containing TDP-43 inclusions by macrophages/microglia can also be seen in *post mortem* ALS tissue, giving credence to microglia/macrophages being a vector and/or regulating TDP-43 pathology [55].

Microglia in FUS-ALS Pathology

Mutations in the *FUS* gene account for approximately 4% of familial ALS cases and are found in 1% of sporadic ALS cases [33]. FUS protein inclusions are detectable in ~1% of ALS cases [16, 34]. However, studies assessing the role of microglial cells in FUS-ALS are scarce. Several studies have reported extensive microgliosis in the brain and spinal cord of FUS-ALS patients and animal models [56–61]. On the other hand, one study assessing mouse FUS-R521C spinal cords found no detectable levels of WTFUS or MTFUS in microglia (despite its ubiquitous expression and detection in astrocytes and oligodendrocytes), suggesting that microgliosis might be reactive, i.e. a consequence of neuronal death and/or astrocytic activation [62].

One *in vitro* study has shown that primary microglia from rats adopted a proinflammatory phenotype with increased production of IL-6, iNOS, and TNFα when treated with a conditioned medium of astrocytes over-expressing WT FUS [58]. Other studies, describing mutant FUS-related disruption of synaptic homeostasis, might suggest a microglial involvement unrelated to inflammation. Transgenic mice expressing low levels of R521G mutant FUS showed significant loss of dendritic arbors, mature spines, and major impairments of synaptic homeostasis [63]. It is well known that microglia play a key role in pruning, remodeling, and eliminating synapses during embryonic development, experience-related brain rewiring, and nerve injury [64–66]. Importantly, microglia-mediated synaptic loss has also been observed in common neurodegenerative disorders such as Alzheimer's and Parkinson's disease [67, 68]. However, whether microglia are involved in the elimination of synapses in this model of FUS-ALS remains unknown. Thus, further studies assessing the role of microglia in FUS related ALS are needed, not only to investigate the contribution of FUS and microglia within a proinflammatory environment but also to study potential new functions that may be completely unrelated to inflammation.

Astrocyte-Related ALS Pathology

Astrocytic dysfunction is implicated in ALS pathogenesis via multiple pathways. Ubiquitous RNA knockdown of endogenous TDP-43 notably reduced astrocytic TDP-43 expression compared to TDP-43 in motor neurons and related to a more severe phenotype and progression compared to knockdown of only neuronal TDP-43 in mouse models [69–71]. On the other hand, driving expression of mutant TDP-43 in astrocytes has been shown to induce progressive loss of motor neurons and an ALS phenotype in transgenic rats [72]. These data implicate altered astrocytic TDP-43 expression in the pathogenesis of ALS. Astrocytic dysfunction is also prevalent in humanized models, suggesting that it is not limited to rodents. Astrocytes isolated *post mortem* from SOD1 negative ALS cases show neurotoxicity toward cultured motor neurons [73, 74]. Similarly, induced pluripotent stem cells (iPSCs) derived from sporadic and familial ALS cases with *C9orf72* (chromosome 9 open reading frame 72) and *SOD1* mutations and differentiated into an astrocyte-like phenotype also displayed neurotoxicity toward co-cultured motor neurons [75]. Human glial progenitors derived from iPSCs have been shown to differentiate and functionally replace endogenous murine astrocytes when xenografted into the rodent spinal cord. It is of note, therefore, that rodents xenografted with glial progenitors from SOD1 and sALS (sporadic ALS) patients exhibited behavioral motor deficits and reduced numbers of motor neurons, with the remaining motor neurons displaying cytoskeletal and ubiquitylation dysfunction [76, 77]. Furthermore, markers of neurotoxic astrocytes have been reported in ALS *post mortem* tissue [23]. Taken together, these data highlight that astrocytes can be a driver of neurotoxicity in various ALS models.

Oligodendrocyte-Related ALS Pathology and Glial Inclusion Formation

Compared to microglia and astrocytes, the role of oligodendrocytes in ALS pathology has been less extensively studied. However, there is accumulating evidence for a requirement of TDP-43 for oligodendrocyte survival and myelination. Whether oligodendrocyte impairment is a consequence or a cause of motor neuron loss is an important question that remains to be answered.

Oligodendrocytes dysfunction leads to demyelination and degeneration in the grey matter of patients and demyelination of the corticospinal tracts [78, 79]. Thinning of the pyramidal tracts in ALS patients is particularly evident in the corticospinal portion and detectable *antemortem* using MRI. Whether this precedes axonal/neuronal loss from the motor cortex or is merely a consequence of neuronal loss remains to be seen. A conditional knockout of *TARDBP* in mature oligodendrocytes leads to increased mortality and a progressive motor phenotype induced by necroptotic degeneration of mature oligodendrocytes resulting in decreased myelination and motor neuron dysfunction, despite no obvious motor neuron degeneration [80]. This indicates that TDP-43 is vital for proper myelination by oligodendrocytes and normal motor neuron function *in vivo* and that pathological deposition of TDP-43 in multiple cell types can contribute to ALS.

Philips et al. investigated the role of oligodendrocytes in ALS after observing degenerative changes in ALS patients [81]. They showed that oligodendrocytes degenerated before motor neuron loss occurred. Furthermore, the overall number of oligodendrocytes remained constant throughout disease progression. This was attributed to oligodendrocyte precursor cell proliferation, with the striking fact that newly differentiated cells seemed to be dysfunctional in their key roles in forming the myelin sheet and providing metabolic support. Similar results were also observed by Kang et al., who reported a loss of grey matter oligodendrocytes in the spinal cord of SOD1^{G93A} mice before disease symptom onset [79]. They reported that the selective depletion of mutant human SOD1^{G37R} from oligodendrocytes resulted in delayed disease onset and prolonged survival in mice. These results suggest that ALS linked genes are capable of weakening motor neuron function by impairing oligodendrocytes.

The nervous system consumes a disproportionate amount of the overall produced energy [82]. A lack of energy metabolites such as glucose or lactate impairs the overall function and survival of neurons. Oligodendrocytes play a key role in providing metabolic support to the axon by releasing lactate exclusively through monocarboxylate transporter 1 (MCT1). It has been shown *in vivo* and *in vitro* that a reduction of MCT1 levels impairs neuronal function, resulting in damage and loss [83]. A decreased expression of MCT1 in oligodendrocytes found in SOD1^{G93A} mice and ALS patients suggests that mutant SOD1 affects oligodendrocytes by changing their MCT1 expression, resulting in decreased neurotrophic support for motor neurons. Further evidence indicating that metabolic support of axons by oligodendrocytes plays an important role at disease onset comes from an *in vitro* co-culture study. Ferraiuolo et al. obtained human-induced pluripotent stem cell-derived (iPSC-derived) oligodendrocytes from sporadic and familial SOD1-ALS cases and showed that these cells had a reduced ability to produce and release lactate resulting in decreased motor neuron survival [84].

Increased FUS inclusions in oligodendrocytes were also observed in a mouse model expressing FUS lacking a nuclear localization sequence NLS (FUS$^{\Delta NLS}$) [85]. Interestingly, rescuing the mutation specifically in motor neurons prevented motor neuron degeneration but only delayed motor function impairments. The authors also reported a downregulation in the expression of genes related to myelination and an increase in the number of oligodendrocytes in the spinal cord, even after reversal of the FUS mutation in motor neurons. These changes were accompanied by myelination defects such as a smaller caliber of motor axons that may explain motor function impairment even when there was no significant motor neuron death. Taken together, these findings suggest that oligodendrocytes may play an important role in FUS-ALS pathology, regardless of the effects of the genetic defect on motor neurons and other glial cells. Additional studies are required.

GLIAL INCLUSION FORMATION IN ALS

Oligodendrocytes

Oligodendrocytes contain TDP-43 inclusions in ALS, especially in the motor cortex, where they are the most common cell-type to harbor inclusions [86]. However, TDP-43 inclusion formation is not a feature of all oligodendroglia in all brain regions and seems to be specific to myelinating oligodendrocytes of large motor tracts, demonstrating that these cells are susceptible to developing TDP-43 inclusions [87]. The formation of oligodendrocyte TDP-43 inclusions has been proposed to potentially precede neuronal TDP-43 inclusion formation in the spinal cord, based on an ALS neuropathological staging scheme [51]. This fits with observations in SOD1^{G93A} mutant mice where mutant SOD1 was detected in processes of oligodendrocytes even before SOD1 aggregation in motor neurons and astrocytes was detected [88]. Other SOD1 animal studies have shown that oligodendrocytes and their precursors influence the onset of motor dysfunction [79, 81, 89]. Additionally, a study using chimeric mice indicated that nonpathogenic cytosolic proteins such as SOD1 could be intercellularly transported between neurons and oligodendrocytes in the spinal cord [90]. Whether this phenomenon extends to TDP-43, and the mechanism for this intercellular transport between oligodendrocytes and neurons, needs to be identified; however, it may prove to be relevant to both the development of oligodendrial pathology and the spread of pathological stimuli between cells.

A study using *post mortem* tissue from familial and sporadic ALS patients carrying different FUS mutations has reported the presence of FUS immunoreactive (FUSir) inclusions in the cytoplasm of oligodendrocytes, while none were found in astrocytes or microglia [91]. Interestingly, the abundance of the FUS cytoplasmic inclusions was different depending on the age of onset of the disease. The late-onset group, age of onset between 44 and 62 years, showed abundant FUSir inclusions in oligodendrocytes and adjacent neurons. In contrast, FUS inclusions were infrequent in those patients with an early onset of the disease, between 18 and 22 years.

Astrocytes

SOD1 patients display prominent astrocytic inclusions in patient *post mortem* tissue and also in certain rodent SOD1 models. In particular, the role of astrocytes in glutamate clearance has been widely recognized, and loss of the astrocytic EAAT2/GLT1 transporter is associated with ALS pathology in rodent models and patients [92, 93]. In fact, one of the two clinically approved drugs for the treatment of ALS is riluzole, a pharmacological agent that is considered to reduce glutamate excitotoxicity. Recent studies also highlighted the critical role of astrocytes in providing neurotrophic as well as detrimental factors that can determine the fate of a motor neuron [94].

THE ROLE OF GLIAL CELLS IN SOD1 PATHOLOGY MIGHT BE DIFFERENT FROM OTHER FORMS OF ALS

The discovery of the gene encoding for SOD1 has greatly contributed to our understanding of the involvement of glial cells during disease progression. The SOD1 mouse model is arguably the best-characterized ALS animal model to date, and elegant studies using genetic and chimeric tools have unequivocally demonstrated that glial cells influence and are essential for the progression of SOD1 pathology.

The finding that microglia are linked to disease progression has led to several clinical trials that target glial cells (mainly the suppression thereof) to treat ALS patients. However, these have not been effective or tolerated in patients, and confounding factors (such as study design and cohort size) may have potentially contributed to the failure of translating the research results into successful treatments for patients. While this is disappointing, it is important to consider that disease mechanisms might not be the same for all forms of ALS. SOD1-ALS in particular appears to represent a "pure" form of ALS, whereas TDP-43-ALS embodies a somewhat "entangled" form with TDP-43 pathology evident in ALS as well as in frontotemporal lobar degeneration (FTLD). It is therefore important to evaluate the contribution of glial cells in non-SOD1 models of ALS, and the first animal studies are beginning to emerge [52, 53].

Most genes known to cause ALS-FTD are not restricted to motor neurons; they are often ubiquitously expressed and have been shown to be essential in pathways required for normal microglial function such as inflammatory responses and phagocytosis [16]. *C9orf72* is essential for proper myeloid and microglial homeostasis in mice with loss of function, leading to accumulation of lysosomes and a proinflammatory phenotype [95, 96]. *C9orf72* expansions have been shown to exhibit epigenetic hypermethylation of the promoter, leading to transcriptional silencing of *C9orf72*. Meanwhile, ALS-*C9orf72* patient tissue showed increased RNA expression of immune and inflammatory pathways, with microglia showing large accumulation of lysosomes, suggesting that a similar mechanism may be contributing to the phenotype in *C9orf72* carriers [96, 97]. Additionally, known ALS-FTD genes such as optineurin (*OPTN*), sequestosome 1 (*SQSTM1*), TANK binding kinase 1 (*TBK1*), and valosin containing protein (*VCP*) are vital for phagocytosis, intercellular waste clearance, and regulating inflammation by modulating nuclear factor kappa B (NF-κB) signaling [98–104]. NF-κB is one of the crucial regulators of glial inflammatory responses; its induction is seen in *post mortem* tissue along with SOD1 and TDP-43 models, where it has been shown to also coincide with motor neurotoxicity induced by astrocytes and microglia [22, 49, 105].

The recent identification of microglia-specific genes such as triggering receptors expressed on myeloid cells (*TREM2*), colony stimulating factor 1 receptor (*CSF1R*), and *TYRO* protein tyrosine kinase-binding protein (*TYROBP*) further highlights the complex molecular mechanisms underlying glial activation. Their precise pro- or anti-inflammatory contributions are critically dependent on the timing and magnitude of their activation. In particular, TREM2-mediated signaling and dysregulation of this pathway have been demonstrated to play a critical role in several neurodegenerative and other neurological diseases (for review, see [106]).

CONCLUSION

There is compelling evidence that glia play an important role in ALS and other neurodegenerative diseases. Glial cells both respond to pathological changes in neurons and can be affected themselves, depending on disease mechanism. Some of the key data presented in this chapter regarding how glial cells affect TDP-43, SOD1, and FUS pathology are summarized in Figure 7.1. While there is clear support for the effects of gain as well as loss of function in glial cells, their exact role during disease progression and how they may influence the course of disease will undoubtedly remain a key topic in the field for years to come.

Another important question is whether the suppression of inflammation in ALS (and other neurodegenerative diseases) will be an effective strategy to delay or halt disease progression, or whether it will fail as in the case of Alzheimer's disease. There has been confusion surrounding the term *neuroinflammation*, which is currently applied uncritically [107] by many authors to both classical inflammation, as in multiple sclerosis, and gliosis in numerous other conditions ranging from depression to autism. Careful characterization of neuron–glial communication pathways for different ALS subtypes is more likely to hold the key to a better understanding of disease mechanisms. An answer to the question of whether glial activation constitutes a response to neurodegeneration – i.e. whether glial cells are healthy and reactive, or whether activated glia are undergoing degeneration themselves and display a specific glial ALS phenotype – is therefore of major importance.

One ongoing question is how comparable experimental animal pathology is to human disease conditions. A classic example is that the antibiotic minocycline delayed disease progression in transgenic mice but exacerbated symptoms in Phase III clinical trials in ALS patients [108, 109]. However, it is important to consider that animal models may present different overt phenotypes, while the underlying mechanisms may still be identical [110]. Two inducible transgenic TDP-43 mouse models that have been recently established [111, 112] are of particular interest in this context as they may permit a detailed characterization of the disease mechanisms that underpin the hallmark TDP-43 pathology in ALS and the role of glia during that process. Other animal models will also continue to make seminal contributions to our understanding of the dynamic nature of neuron–glia interactions in the CNS [53, 113–116] and help to identify novel disease modifiers that are directly relevant for patients and can't be easily monitored in patients or rodent models. Furthermore, the development of iPSCs has become a powerful model to address the pathological divergence between familial and sporadic ALS patients and the role of glial cells [117, 118]. iPSCs are an especially critical tool for the stratification of disease phenotypes and to facilitate targeted treatment and drug discovery. As is true for other conditions like cancer, personalized approaches together with multi-drug regimens are likely to be the future treatment paradigm for ALS patients.

Our understanding of the functional importance of microglia during ALS pathogenesis has grown significantly in recent years. This includes their morphological changes (beyond the amoeboid-ramified classification) as well as the activation of ligands (pro- or anti-inflammatory) and their receptors. For example, recent advances in the characterization of microglia have shed new light on genetic influences of their function and the control of their functions by motor neurons, with important implications for neuron degeneration and disease [96, 119]. However, much is to be learned about the microglial activation cascade and their contribution to disease (prevention and/or exacerbation). The simplistic idea that microglia induce motor neuron death in

ALS (specifically non-SOD1-ALS) and possibly other neurodegenerative diseases through enhanced "inflammatory" activation is certainly outdated. Microglia can be active in an immunologically neutral state, and harvesting the potential of these neurotropic properties is of significant interest in future multi-factorial treatment paradigms.

Taken together, a better understanding of neuron–glia interactions will have important implications for the pathological mechanisms in ALS and other neurodegenerative diseases. Defining the molecular fingerprint of glial cells and influencing their role in neurodegeneration will help to design and develop novel strategies that can interfere with the rapid progression that affects people suffering from ALS.

ACKNOWLEDGMENTS

This work was supported by the Motor Neuron Disease Research Institute of Australia (GIA 1838, BLP 1901), the Australian Research Council (DP150104472), the National Health and Medical Research Council of Australia (Dementia Teams Grant 1 095 215), the Snow Foundation Fellowship (MM), and donations made toward MND research at Macquarie University. We also wish to thank the zebrafish facility staff (past and present) for assistance in zebrafish care.

CONFLICT OF INTEREST

The authors declare no potential conflict of interest with respect to research, authorship, and/or publication of this manuscript.

COPYRIGHT AND PERMISSION STATEMENT

REFERENCES

1. Sofroniew, M.V. and Vinters, H.V. (2010). Astrocytes: biology and pathology. *Acta Neuropathologica* 119 (1): 7–35.
2. Khakh, B.S. and Sofroniew, M.V. (2015). Diversity of astrocyte functions and phenotypes in neural circuits. *Nature Neuroscience* 18 (7): 942–952.
3. Bradl, M. and Lassmann, H. (2010). Oligodendrocytes: biology and pathology. *Acta Neuropathologica* 119 (1): 37–53.
4. Valério-Gomes, B., Guimarães, D.M., Szczupak, D., and Lent, R. (2018). The absolute number of oligodendrocytes in the adult mouse brain. *Frontiers in Neuroanatomy* 12 (90).

5. Tremblay, M.-È., Stevens, B., Sierra, A. et al. (2011). The role of microglia in the healthy brain. *The Journal of Neuroscience* 31 (45): 16064–16069.

6. Graeber, M. and Streit, W. (2010). Microglia: biology and pathology. *Acta Neuropathologica* 119 (1): 89–105.

7. Verkhratsky, A., Sofroniew, M.V., Messing, A. et al. (2012). Neurological diseases as primary gliopathies: a reassessment of neurocentrism. *ASN Neuro* 4 (3): AN20120010.

8. Filipi, T., Hermanova, Z., Tureckova, J. et al. (2020). Glial cells—the strategic targets in amyotrophic lateral sclerosis treatment. *Journal of Clinical Medicine* 9 (1): 261.

9. Peters, O.M., Ghasemi, M., and Brown, R.H. Jr. (2015). Emerging mechanisms of molecular pathology in ALS. *The Journal of Clinical Investigation* 125 (5): 1767–1779.

10. Yamanaka, K. and Komine, O. (2018). The multi-dimensional roles of astrocytes in ALS. *Neuroscience Research* 126: 31–38.

11. Kiernan, M.C., Vucic, S., Cheah, B.C. et al. (2011). Amyotrophic lateral sclerosis. *Lancet* 377 (9769): 942–955.

12. Al-Chalabi, A., Hardiman, O., Kiernan, M.C. et al. (2016). Amyotrophic lateral sclerosis: moving towards a new classification system. *Lancet Neurology* 15 (11): 1182–1194.

13. Boylan, K. (2015). Familial ALS. *Neurologic Clinics* 33 (4): 807–830.

14. Chia, R., Chiò, A., and Traynor, B.J. (2018). Novel genes associated with amyotrophic lateral sclerosis: diagnostic and clinical implications. *Lancet Neurology* 17 (1): 94–102.

15. Al-Chalabi, A., Jones, A., Troakes, C. et al. (2012). The genetics and neuropathology of amyotrophic lateral sclerosis. *Acta Neuropathologica* 124 (3): 339–352.

16. Radford, R.A.W., Morsch, M., Rayner, S.L. et al. (2015). The established and emerging roles of astrocytes and microglia in amyotrophic lateral sclerosis and frontotemporal dementia. *Frontiers in Cellular Neuroscience* 9: 414.

17. Robberecht, W. and Philips, T. (2013). The changing scene of amyotrophic lateral sclerosis. *Nature Reviews. Neuroscience* 14 (4): 248–264.

18. Ilieva, H., Polymenidou, M., and Cleveland, D.W. (2009). Non–cell autonomous toxicity in neurodegenerative disorders: ALS and beyond. *The Journal of Cell Biology* 187 (6): 761–772.

19. Brooks, B.R., Miller, R.G., Swash, M., and Munsat, T.L. (2000). El escorial revisited: revised criteria for the diagnosis of amyotrophic lateral sclerosis. *Amyotrophic Lateral Sclerosis and Other Motor Neuron Disorders* 1 (5): 293–299.

20. Saberi, S., Stauffer, J.E., Schulte, D.J., and Ravits, J. (2015). Neuropathology of amyotrophic lateral sclerosis and its variants. *Neurologic Clinics* 33 (4): 855–876.

21. Burda, J.E. and Sofroniew, M.V. (2014). Reactive gliosis and the multicellular response to CNS damage and disease. *Neuron* 81 (2): 229–248.

22. Schiffer, D., Cordera, S., Cavalla, P., and Migheli, A. (1996). Reactive astrogliosis of the spinal cord in amyotrophic lateral sclerosis. *Journal of the Neurological Sciences* 139: 27–33.

23. Liddelow, S.A., Guttenplan, K.A., Clarke, L.E. et al. (2017). Neurotoxic reactive astrocytes are induced by activated microglia. *Nature* 541 (7638): 481–487.

24. Kawamata, T., Akiyama, H., Yamada, T., and McGeer, P.L. (1992). Immunologic reactions in amyotrophic lateral sclerosis brain and spinal cord tissue. *The American Journal of Pathology* 140 (3): 691–707.

25. Brettschneider, J., Libon, D., Toledo, J. et al. (2012). Microglial activation and TDP-43 pathology correlate with executive dysfunction in amyotrophic lateral sclerosis. *Acta Neuropathologica* 123 (3): 395–407.

26. Brettschneider, J., Toledo, J.B., Van Deerlin, V.M. et al. (2012). Microglial activation correlates with disease progression and upper motor neuron clinical symptoms in amyotrophic lateral sclerosis. *PLoS One* 7 (6): e39216.

27. Turner, M.R., Cagnin, A., Turkheimer, F.E. et al. (2004). Evidence of widespread cerebral microglial activation in amyotrophic lateral sclerosis: an [11C](R)-PK11195 positron emission tomography study. *Neurobiology of Disease* 15 (3): 601–609.

28. Corcia, P., Tauber, C., Vercoullie, J. et al. (2013). Molecular imaging of microglial activation in amyotrophic lateral sclerosis. *PLoS One* 7 (12): e52941.

29. Zürcher, N.R., Loggia, M.L., Lawson, R. et al. (2015). Increased in vivo glial activation in patients with amyotrophic lateral sclerosis: assessed with [(11)C]-PBR28. *NeuroImage. Clinical* 7: 409–414.

30. Chiò, A., Pagani, M., Agosta, F. et al. (2014). Neuroimaging in amyotrophic lateral sclerosis: insights into structural and functional changes. *Lancet Neurology* 13 (12): 1228–1240.

31. Prinz, M. and Priller, J. (2014). Microglia and brain macrophages in the molecular age: from origin to neuropsychiatric disease. *Nature Reviews. Neuroscience* 15 (5): 300–312.

32. Liddelow, S.A. and Barres, B.A. (2017). Reactive astrocytes: production, function, and therapeutic potential. *Immunity* 46 (6): 957–967.

33. Renton, A.E., Chio, A., and Traynor, B.J. (2014). State of play in amyotrophic lateral sclerosis genetics. *Nature Neuroscience* 17 (1): 17–23.

34. Mackenzie, I.R.A., Rademakers, R., and Neumann, M. (2010). TDP-43 and FUS in amyotrophic lateral sclerosis and frontotemporal dementia. *Lancet Neurology* 9 (10): 995–1007.

35. Rock, R.B., Gekker, G., Hu, S. et al. (2004). Role of microglia in central nervous system infections. *Clinical Microbiology Reviews* 17 (4): 942–964.

36. Hall, E.D., Oostveen, J.A., and Gurney, M.E. (1998). Relationship of microglial and astrocytic activation to disease onset and progression in a transgenic model of familial ALS. *Glia* 23 (3): 249–256.

37. Philips, T. and Robberecht, W. (2011). Neuroinflammation in amyotrophic lateral sclerosis: role of glial activation in motor neuron disease. *Lancet Neurology* 10 (3): 253–263.

38. Geloso, M.C., Corvino, V., Marchese, E. et al. (2017). The dual role of microglia in ALS: mechanisms and therapeutic approaches. *Frontiers in Aging Neuroscience* 9: 242.

39. Troost, D., van den Oord, J.J., and JMBVD, J. (1990). Immunohistochemical characterization of the inflammatory infiltrate in amyotrophic lateral sclerosis. *Neuropathology and Applied Neurobiology* 16 (5): 401–410.

40. Philips, T. and Rothstein, J.D. (2014). Glial cells in amyotrophic lateral sclerosis. *Experimental Neurology* 262: 111–120.

41. Clement, A.M., Nguyen, M.D., Roberts, E.A. et al. (2003). Wild-type nonneuronal cells extend survival of SOD1 mutant motor neurons in ALS mice. *Science* 302 (5642): 113–117.

42. Alexianu, M.E., Kozovska, M., and Appel, S.H. (2001). Immune reactivity in a mouse model of familial ALS correlates with disease progression. *Neurology* 57 (7): 1282–1289.

43. Beers, D.R., Henkel, J.S., Xiao, Q. et al. (2006). Wild-type microglia extend survival in PU.1 knockout mice with familial amyotrophic lateral sclerosis. *Proceedings of the National Academy of Sciences* 103 (43): 16021–16026.

44. Boillée, S., Yamanaka, K., Lobsiger, C.S. et al. (2006). Onset and progression in inherited ALS determined by motor neurons and microglia. *Science* 312 (5778): 1389–1392.

45. Martínez-Muriana, A., Mancuso, R., Francos-Quijorna, I. et al. (2016). CSF1R blockade slows the progression of amyotrophic lateral sclerosis by reducing microgliosis and invasion of macrophages into peripheral nerves. *Scientific Reports* 6 (1): 25663.

46. Tang, Y. and Le, W. (2016). Differential roles of M1 and M2 microglia in neurodegenerative diseases. *Molecular Neurobiology* 53 (2): 1181–1194.

47. Henkel, J.S., Beers, D.R., Zhao, W., and Appel, S.H. (2009). Microglia in ALS: the good, the bad, and the resting. *Journal of Neuroimmune Pharmacology* 4 (4): 389–398.

48. Liao, B., Zhao, W., Beers, D.R. et al. (2012). Transformation from a neuroprotective to a neurotoxic microglial phenotype in a mouse model of ALS. *Experimental Neurology* 237 (1): 147–152.

49. Frakes Ashley, E., Ferraiuolo, L., Haidet-Phillips Amanda, M. et al. (2014). Microglia induce motor neuron death via the classical NF-κB pathway in amyotrophic lateral sclerosis. *Neuron* 81 (5): 1009–1023.

50. Lee, J.D., Levin, S.C., Willis, E.F. et al. (2018). Complement components are upregulated and correlate with disease progression in the TDP-43 (Q331K) mouse model of amyotrophic lateral sclerosis. *Journal of Neuroinflammation* 15 (1): 171.

51. Brettschneider, J., Arai, K., Del Tredici, K. et al. (2014). TDP-43 pathology and neuronal loss in amyotrophic lateral sclerosis spinal cord. *Acta Neuropathologica* 128 (3): 423–437.

52. Spiller, K.J., Restrepo, C.R., Khan, T. et al. (2018). Microglia-mediated recovery from ALS-relevant motor neuron degeneration in a mouse model of TDP-43 proteinopathy. *Nature Neuroscience* 21 (3): 329–340.

53. Svahn, A.J., Don, E.K., Badrock, A.P. et al. (2018). Nucleo-cytoplasmic transport of TDP-43 studied in real time: impaired microglia function leads to axonal spreading of TDP-43 in degenerating motor neurons. *Acta Neuropathologica* 136 (3): 445–459.

54. Polymenidou, M. and Cleveland, D.W. (2011). The seeds of neurodegeneration: prion-like spreading in ALS. *Cell* 147 (3): 498–508.

55. Pamphlett, R. and Kum, J.S. (2008). TDP-43 inclusions do not protect motor neurons from sporadic ALS. *Acta Neuropathologica* 116 (2): 221–222.

56. López-Erauskin, J., Tadokoro, T., Baughn, M.W. et al. (2018). ALS/FTD-linked mutation in FUS suppresses intra-axonal protein synthesis and drives disease without nuclear loss-of-function of FUS. *Neuron* 100 (4): 816–830. e7.

57. Ling, S.-C., Dastidar, S.G., Tokunaga, S. et al. (2019). Overriding FUS autoregulation in mice triggers gain-of-toxic dysfunctions in RNA metabolism and autophagy-lysosome axis. *eLife* 8: e40811.

58. Ajmone-Cat, M.A., Onori, A., Toselli, C. et al. (2019). Increased FUS levels in astrocytes leads to astrocyte and microglia activation and neuronal death. *Scientific Reports* 9 (1): 4572.

59. Sharma, A., Lyashchenko, A.K., Lu, L. et al. (2016). ALS-associated mutant FUS induces selective motor neuron degeneration through toxic gain of function. *Nature Communications* 7 (1): 10465.

60. Mitchell, J.C., McGoldrick, P., Vance, C. et al. (2013). Overexpression of human wild-type FUS causes progressive motor neuron degeneration in an age- and dose-dependent fashion. *Acta Neuropathologica* 125 (2): 273–288.

61. Rossaert, E., Pollari, E., Jaspers, T. et al. (2019). Restoration of histone acetylation ameliorates disease and metabolic abnormalities in a FUS mouse model. *Acta Neuropathologica Communications* 7 (1): 107.

62. Qiu, H., Lee, S., Shang, Y. et al. (2014). ALS-associated mutation FUS-R521C causes DNA damage and RNA splicing defects. *The Journal of Clinical Investigation* 124 (3): 981–999.

63. Sephton, C.F., Tang, A.A., Kulkarni, A. et al. (2014). Activity-dependent FUS dysregulation disrupts synaptic homeostasis. *Proceedings of the National Academy of Sciences* 111 (44): E4769–E4778.

64. Paolicelli, R.C., Bolasco, G., Pagani, F. et al. (2011). Synaptic pruning by microglia is necessary for normal brain development. *Science* 333 (6048): 1456–1458.

65. Tremblay, M.-È., Lowery, R.L., and Majewska, A.K. (2010). Microglial interactions with synapses are modulated by visual experience. *PLoS Biology* 8 (11): e1000527.

66. Moran, L.B. and Graeber, M.B. (2004). The facial nerve axotomy model. *Brain Research Reviews* 44 (2): 154–178.

67. Rajendran, L. and Paolicelli, R.C. (2018). Microglia-mediated synapse loss in alzheimer's disease. *The Journal of Neuroscience* 38 (12): 2911–2919.

68. Aono, H., Choudhury, M.E., Higaki, H. et al. (2017). Microglia may compensate for dopaminergic neuron loss in experimental parkinsonism through selective elimination of glutamatergic synapses from the subthalamic nucleus. *Glia* 65 (11): 1833–1847.

69. Wu, L.-S., Cheng, W.-C., and Shen, C.K.J. (2012). Targeted depletion of TDP-43 expression in the spinal cord motor neurons leads to the development of amyotrophic lateral sclerosis-like phenotypes in mice. *The Journal of Biological Chemistry* 287 (33): 27335–27344.

70. Iguchi, Y., Katsuno, M., Niwa, J.-i. et al. (2013). Loss of TDP-43 causes age-dependent progressive motor neuron degeneration. *Brain* 136 (5): 1371–1382.

71. Yang, C., Wang, H., Qiao, T. et al. (2014). Partial loss of TDP-43 function causes phenotypes of amyotrophic lateral sclerosis. *Proceedings of the National Academy of Sciences* 111 (12): E1121–E1129.

72. Tong, J., Huang, C., Bi, F. et al. (2013). Expression of ALS-linked TDP-43 mutant in astrocytes causes non-cell-autonomous motor neuron death in rats. *The EMBO Journal* 32 (13): 1917–1926.

73. Haidet-Phillips, A.M., Hester, M.E., Miranda, C.J. et al. (2011). Astrocytes from familial and sporadic ALS patients are toxic to motor neurons. *Nature Biotechnology* 29 (9): 824–828.

74. Re Diane, B., Le Verche, V., Yu, C. et al. (2014). Necroptosis drives motor neuron death in models of both sporadic and familial ALS. *Neuron* 81 (5): 1001–1008.

75. Meyer, K., Ferraiuolo, L., Miranda, C.J. et al. (2014). Direct conversion of patient fibroblasts demonstrates non-cell autonomous toxicity of astrocytes to motor neurons in familial and sporadic ALS. *Proceedings of the National Academy of Sciences* 111 (2): 829–832.

76. Chen, H., Qian, K., Chen, W. et al. (2015). Human-derived neural progenitors functionally replace astrocytes in adult mice. *The Journal of Clinical Investigation* 125 (3): 1033–1042.

77. Qian, K., Huang, H., Peterson, A. et al. (2017). Sporadic ALS astrocytes induce neuronal degeneration in vivo. *Stem Cell Reports* 8 (4): 843–855.

78. Rohan, Z., Matej, R., Rusina, R., and Kovacs, G.G. (2014). Oligodendroglial response in the spinal cord in TDP-43 proteinopathy with motor neuron involvement. *Neurodegenerative diseases* 14 (3): 117–124.

79. Kang, S.H., Li, Y., Fukaya, M. et al. (2013). Degeneration and impaired regeneration of gray matter oligodendrocytes in amyotrophic lateral sclerosis. *Nature Neuroscience* 16 (5): 571–579.

80. Wang, J., Ho, W.Y., Lim, K. et al. (2018). Cell-autonomous requirement of TDP-43, an ALS/FTD signature protein, for oligodendrocyte survival and myelination. *Proceedings of the National Academy of Sciences* 115 (46): E10941.

81. Philips, T., Bento-Abreu, A., Nonneman, A. et al. (2013). Oligodendrocyte dysfunction in the pathogenesis of amyotrophic lateral sclerosis. *Brain* 136 (2): 471–482.

82. Mink, J.W., Blumenschine, R.J., and Adams, D.B. (1981). Ratio of central nervous system to body metabolism in vertebrates: its constancy and functional basis. *American Journal of Physiology—Regulatory, Integrative and Comparative Physiology* 241 (3): R203–R212.

83. Lee, Y., Morrison, B.M., Li, Y. et al. (2012). Oligodendroglia metabolically support axons and contribute to neurodegeneration. *Nature* 487 (7408): 443–448.

84. Ferraiuolo, L., Meyer, K., Sherwood, T.W. et al. (2016). Oligodendrocytes contribute to motor neuron death in ALS via SOD1-dependent mechanism. *Proceedings of the National Academy of Sciences* 113 (42): E6496–E6505.

85. Scekic-Zahirovic, J., Oussini, H.E., Mersmann, S. et al. (2017). Motor neuron intrinsic and extrinsic mechanisms contribute to the pathogenesis of FUS-associated amyotrophic lateral sclerosis. *Acta Neuropathologica* 133 (6): 887–906.

86. Fatima, M., Tan, R., Halliday, G.M., and Kril, J.J. (2015). Spread of pathology in amyotrophic lateral sclerosis: assessment of phosphorylated TDP-43 along axonal pathways. *Acta Neuropathologica Communications* 3: 47.

87. Brettschneider, J., Del Tredici, K., Toledo, J.B. et al. (2013). Stages of pTDP-43 pathology in amyotrophic lateral sclerosis. *Annals of Neurology* 74 (1): 20–38.

88. Stieber, A., Gonatas, J.O., and Gonatas, N.K. (2000). Aggregates of mutant protein appear progressively in dendrites, in periaxonal processes of oligodendrocytes, and in neuronal and astrocytic perikarya of mice expressing the SOD1G93A mutation of familial amyotrophic lateral sclerosis. *Journal of the Neurological Sciences* 177 (2): 114–123.

89. Yamanaka, K., Boillee, S., Roberts, E.A. et al. (2008). Mutant SOD1 in cell types other than motor neurons and oligodendrocytes accelerates onset of disease in ALS mice. *Proceedings of the National Academy of Sciences of the United States of America* 105 (21): 7594–7599.

90. Thomas, E.V., Fenton, W.A., McGrath, J., and Horwich, A.L. (2017). Transfer of pathogenic and nonpathogenic cytosolic proteins between spinal cord motor neurons in vivo in chimeric mice. *Proceedings of the National Academy of Sciences of the United States of America* 114 (15): E3139–E3148.

91. Mackenzie, I.R.A., Ansorge, O., Strong, M. et al. (2011). Pathological heterogeneity in amyotrophic lateral sclerosis with FUS mutations: two distinct patterns correlating with disease severity and mutation. *Acta Neuropathologica* 122 (1): 87–98.

92. Rothstein, J.D., Van Kammen, M., Levey, A.I. et al. (1995). Selective loss of glial glutamate transporter GLT-1 in amyotrophic lateral sclerosis. *Annals of Neurology* 38 (1): 73–84.

93. Lin, C.-L.G., Bristol, L.A., Jin, L. et al. (1998). Aberrant RNA processing in a neurodegenerative disease: the cause for absent EAAT2, a glutamate transporter, in amyotrophic lateral sclerosis. *Neuron* 20 (3): 589–602.

94. Mariana, P., Benjamin, A.H., Kelby, M.K., and Marcelo, R.V. (2017). Role and therapeutic potential of astrocytes in amyotrophic lateral sclerosis. *Current Pharmaceutical Design* 23 (33): 5010–5021.

95. Burberry, A., Suzuki, N., Wang, J.-Y. et al. (2016). Loss-of-function mutations in the C9ORF72 mouse ortholog cause fatal autoimmune disease. *Science Translational Medicine* 8 (347): 347ra93–ra93.

96. O'Rourke, J.G., Bogdanik, L., Yáñez, A. et al. (2016). C9orf72 is required for proper macrophage and microglial function in mice. *Science* 351 (6279): 1324–1329.

97. Liu, E.Y., Russ, J., Wu, K. et al. (2014). C9orf72 hypermethylation protects against repeat expansion-associated pathology in ALS/FTD. *Acta Neuropathologica* 128 (4): 525–541.

98. Seto, S., Tsujimura, K., Horii, T., and Koide, Y. (2013). Autophagy adaptor protein p 62/SQSTM1 and autophagy-related gene Atg5 mediate autophagosome formation in response to *mycobacterium tuberculosis* infection in dendritic cells. *PLoS One* 8 (12): e86017.

99. Pilli, M., Arko-Mensah, J., Ponpuak, M. et al. (2012). TBK-1 promotes autophagy-mediated antimicrobial defense by controlling autophagosome maturation. *Immunity* 37 (2): 223–234.

100. Tresse, E., Salomons, F.A., Vesa, J. et al. (2010). VCP/p 97 is essential for maturation of ubiquitin-containing autophagosomes and this function is impaired by mutations that cause IBMPFD. *Autophagy* 6 (2): 217–227.

101. Duran, A., Linares, J.F., Galvez, A.S. et al. (2008). The signaling adaptor p62 Is an important NF-κB mediator in tumorigenesis. *Cancer Cell* 13 (4): 343–354.

102. Zhu, G., Wu, C.-J., Zhao, Y., and Ashwell, J.D. (2007). Optineurin negatively regulates TNFα-induced NF-κB activation by competing with NEMO for ubiquitinated RIP. *Current Biology* 17 (16): 1438–1443.

103. Asai, T., Tomita, Y., Nakatsuka, S.-i. et al. (2002). VCP (p97) regulates NFKB signaling pathway, which is important for metastasis of osteosarcoma cell line. *Japanese Journal of Cancer Research* 93 (3): 296–304.

104. Pomerantz, J.L. and Baltimore, D. (1999). NF-kappaB activation by a signaling complex containing TRAF2, TANK and TBK1, a novel IKK-related kinase. *The EMBO Journal* 18 (23): 6694–6704.

105. Migheli, A., Piva, R., Atzori, C.A. et al. (1997). c-Jun, JNK/SAPK kinase and transcription factor NF-[kappa]B are selectively activated in astrocytes, but not motor neurons, in amyotrophic lateral sclerosis. *Journal of Neuropathology and Experimental Neurology* 56 (12): 1314–1322.

106. Konishi, H. and Kiyama, H. (2018). Microglial TREM2/DAP12 signaling: a double-edged sword in neural diseases. *Frontiers in Cellular Neuroscience* 12 (206).

107. Graeber, M.B. (2014). Neuroinflammation: no rose by any other name. *Brain Pathology* 24 (6): 620–622.

108. Gordon, P.H., Moore, D.H., Miller, R.G. et al. (2007). Efficacy of minocycline in patients with amyotrophic lateral sclerosis: a phase III randomised trial. *Lancet Neurology* 6 (12): 1045–1053.

109. Kriz, J., Nguyen, M.D., and Julien, J.-P. (2002). Minocycline slows sisease progression in a mouse model of amyotrophic lateral sclerosis. *Neurobiology of Disease* 10 (3): 268–278.

110. Ittner, L.M., Halliday, G.M., Kril, J.J. et al. (2015). FTD and ALS[mdash]translating mouse studies into clinical trials. *Nature Reviews. Neurology* 11 (6): 360–366.

111. Walker, A.K., Spiller, K.J., Ge, G. et al. (2015). Functional recovery in new mouse models of ALS/FTLD after clearance of pathological cytoplasmic TDP-43. *Acta Neuropathologica* 130 (5): 643–660.

112. Ke, Y.D., van Hummel, A., Stevens, C.H. et al. (2015). Short-term suppression of A315T mutant human TDP-43 expression improves functional deficits in a novel inducible transgenic mouse model of FTLD-TDP and ALS. *Acta Neuropathologica* 130 (5): 661–678.

113. Krug, L., Chatterjee, N., Borges-Monroy, R. et al. (2017). Retrotransposon activation contributes to neurodegeneration in a drosophila TDP-43 model of ALS. *PLoS Genetics* 13 (3): e1006635.

114. Van Damme, P., Robberecht, W., and Van Den Bosch, L. (2017). Modelling amyotrophic lateral sclerosis: progress and possibilities. *Disease Models & Mechanisms* 10 (5): 537–549.

115. Formella, I., Svahn, A.J., Radford, R.A.W. et al. (2018). Real-time visualization of oxidative stress-mediated neurodegeneration of individual spinal motor neurons in vivo. *Redox Biology* 19: 226–234.

116. Morsch, M., Radford, R., Lee, A. et al. (2015). in vivo characterization of microglial engulfment of dying neurons in the zebrafish spinal cord. *Frontiers in Cellular Neuroscience* 9: 321.

117. Lee, S. and Huang, E.J. (2017). Modeling ALS and FTD with iPSC-derived neurons. *Brain Research* 1656: 88–97.

118. Halpern, M., Brennand, K.J., and Gregory, J. (2019). Examining the relationship between astrocyte dysfunction and neurodegeneration in ALS using hiPSCs. *Neurobiology of Disease* 132: 104562.

119. Ayata, P., Badimon, A., Strasburger, H.J. et al. (2018). Epigenetic regulation of brain region-specific microglia clearance activity. *Nature Neuroscience* 21 (8): 1049–1060.

CHAPTER 8

Animal Models of ALS – Current and Future Perspectives

Robert A. Déziel[1], Amber L. Marriott[1], Denis G. Kay[2], and Daphne A. Gill[1,3]

[1] CNS Contract Research Corp, Charlottetown, Prince Edward Island, Canada
[2] Alpha Cognition Inc., Charlottetown, Prince Edward Island, Canada
[3] Department of Biomedical Sciences, University of Prince Edward Island, Charlottetown, Prince Edward Island, Canada

INTRODUCTION

In the 150 years since Charcot first described the grouping of signs and symptoms that would eventually be called amyotrophic lateral sclerosis (ALS) [1], there has been significant progress in the understanding of this disease. Yet our current knowledge regarding ALS is still lacking due in part to our incomplete modeling of this disease. This failure to properly model ALS is a consequence of a number of factors, not least the lack of a clear understanding of where and how the disease begins in the nervous system.

In this chapter, we will first describe the basic clinical manifestations of this disease, treatment options for those afflicted, and potential genetic and environmental causes. From there, we will discuss current cell and animal models of the disease as well as our recommendations for potential future models to best represent the complex etiology and pathogenesis of ALS.

THE CLINICAL MANIFESTATIONS OF ALS

The development of ALS symptoms is insidious, and once the diagnosis has been established, a patient's estimated remaining lifespan is typically two to three years, with a median survival rate of less than 10% five years post diagnosis [2]. Classic

Spectrums of Amyotrophic Lateral Sclerosis: Heterogeneity, Pathogenesis and Therapeutic Directions,
First Edition. Edited by Christopher A. Shaw and Jessica R. Morrice.
© 2021 John Wiley & Sons Ltd. Published 2021 by John Wiley & Sons Ltd.

initial signs of ALS include muscle atrophy and weakness, cranial nerve dysfunction, and, less frequently, respiratory distress. There is no definitive clinical biomarker available, and a definitive diagnosis relies on electrophysiological assessment in conjunction with a neurologist familiar with the disease [3].

ALS initially presents in the clinic in one of the following manners, discussed in descending order of relative frequency in patients.

Limb Onset

In more common cases, patients enter the clinic with initial concerns of unilateral muscle weakness in the absence of pain in the upper limbs, complaints of clumsiness, or loss of fine motor movements in the hand [3]. Less frequently, patients present with lower limb dysfunction, including gait disturbances and foot drop, which cannot be explained by other potential diagnoses.

Bulbar Onset

On occasion, patients first present with bulbar aspects of disease, including glossal atrophy, dysphagia, dysarthria, and other symptoms associated with the decline of proper use of specific cranial nerves [4]. Confirmation of these symptoms with a diagnosis of ALS can be achieved by performing a cranial nerve exam, electromyography, or magnetic resonance imaging (MRI). Many of these assessments are performed to rule out other diseases that can mimic some of these symptoms, including myasthenia gravis, oculopharyngeal muscular dystrophy, and others [5].

Respiratory Onset

Infrequently, patients first present at the clinic with respiratory symptoms, although this occurs in less than 5% of initial diagnoses [6, 7]. In these cases, patients typically present with shortness of breath during rest or after some form of activity. Surprisingly, even though the onset of respiratory dysfunction typically occurs in the later stages of the disease, those who first present with respiratory symptoms have similar survival times as those presenting with bulbar symptoms [7]. Why this is the case is yet unknown. However, individuals first presenting with either bulbar or respiratory symptoms typically have a worse prognosis than those presenting with muscle weakness [8].

ALS's typical progression can be classified in stages, beginning with the onset of the patient's first symptom (stage 1). From there, the disease continues in the following order over the course of the next two to three years [9]:

- Stage 2A: Diagnosis
- Stage 2B: Involvement of a second region
- Stage 3: Involvement of a third region
- Stage 4A: Need for gastrostomy
- Stage 4B: Need for respiratory support

Although less prominent than muscle weakness or bulbar symptoms, approximately half of patients with ALS also develop some form of cognitive impairment within 18 months of diagnosis [10]. This cognitive decline is thought to be due to the atrophy of the frontal and temporal lobes from damage incurred through the pathological aggregation of transactivation response DNA binding protein 43 kDa (TDP-43) in these areas [11].

Patients who present with ALS are typically males in their early 60s, with a slightly higher prevalence among Caucasian populations in the United States [12]. The severity and timeline of symptoms appear to worsen the older the patient is at the time of diagnosis [13, 14].

The hypothesized causes of the disease are many-fold and involve both genetic and environmental origins, which will be discussed further in this chapter. Despite the extensive investigation of ALS pathogenesis, it is still unclear exactly where the disease begins. Theories include the "dying-forward" of cells in the motor cortex, wherein cells in the cortex cause motor neurons in the anterior horn to die. Another theory includes the "dying-back" of neurons proximal to the neuromuscular junction, wherein distal portions of peripheral neurons degrade first [15]. It is also possible for both of these to occur simultaneously due to a yet-unknown cause. More research is required to answer these questions with any certainty.

CURRENT AND EXPERIMENTAL PHARMACOLOGICAL INTERVENTIONS

At present, there are few effective pharmacological treatments for ALS. Most available interventions are used to alleviate symptoms and increase quality of life but have little effect on continued muscle atrophy or long-term survival. To date, only two Food and Drug Administration (FDA) approved medications have been demonstrated to increase survival time and improve motor signs and symptoms inherent in the disease: riluzole and edaravone.

Riluzole

Riluzole (trade name: Rilutek®) has been in use for the treatment of ALS since 1995 after the completion of a Phase III clinical trial indicating its effectiveness [16]. It has been shown that the drug not only increases survival time by approximately three months but also improves limb function in ALS patients [17], although it appears to have no effect on overall muscle strength. This drug has been hypothesized to work through a number of different pathways, the best-characterized of which is the reduction of glutamate excitoxicity supposedly present in ALS through the blockage of N-Methyl-d-aspartate (NMDA) and α-amino-3-hydroxy-5-methyl-4-isoxazolepropionic acid (AMPA) channels. Other potential mechanisms of action have also been proposed, including the selective blockage of voltage-gated calcium channels, sodium ion channels, the modification of GABAergic systems, or a synergistic combination of all of these effects, reducing neuronal damage and death [18].

Paradoxically, the purported benefits of riluzole may not transfer effectively to animal models. A recent publication by Hogg et al. found that the drug did not increase lifespan or improve muscle function in three separate rodent models of ALS, indicating that our current rodent models are insufficiently recapitulating the pathophysiology of this disease [19].

Edaravone

Developed initially in Japan as a treatment for stroke [20], edaravone (trade name: Radicut®) has been approved by the FDA for the treatment of ALS as of 2017 [21]. A recent clinical trial has demonstrated that treatment with edaravone significantly increases patient lifespan as well as their amyotrophic lateral sclerosis functional rating scale (ALSFRS-R) compared to placebo [22]. This drug has been hypothesized to work by scavenging free radicals, thereby reducing oxidative stress, which has shown to protect both neurons and their nearby supporting cells [23].

Future Directions for Pharmacological Interventions

A number of other experimental treatments have been attempted, but unfortunately, most of them have failed to demonstrate efficacy in Phase II and III clinical trials [24]. Only one recent discovery, masitinib (a tyrosine-kinase inhibitor) in conjunction with riluzole, has been demonstrated to be effective in treating ALS by slowing the rate of functional decline by 27% as compared to placebo [25], and it may eventually be found in clinics as a third FDA-approved option for ALS patients.

Currently, there is a limited repertoire of effective treatments for ALS. More research into the basic biology of this disease is needed, along with the development of new animal models that better represent the pathogenesis of ALS.

CAUSATIVE FACTORS IN THE DEVELOPMENT OF ALS

Genetic Factors

While the cause of ALS is unknown, scientific evidence shows both sporadic and familial origins. It is estimated that 90% of cases are considered sporadic and 10% familial [6]. Several gene mutations have been found to cause familial ALS and are also associated with the development of a small number of sporadic ALS cases. Over 25 genes are now associated with ALS [26]. Of these, four genes are predominantly associated with familial ALS: superoxide dismutase 1 (*SOD1*), chromosome 9 open reading frame 72 (*C9orf72*), the RNA and DNA binding proteins TAR DNA-binding protein 43 (*TARDBP*), and fused in sarcoma (*FUS*).

SOD1 mutations are associated with 12–20% autosomal dominant familial ALS cases and about 1–2% of sporadic cases [27, 28]. In 1993, an international consortium identified *SOD1* as a gene responsible for autosomal dominant familial ALS cases. The *SOD1* gene is responsible for making the superoxide dismutase enzyme, which binds to molecules of copper and zinc to break down superoxide radicals. These molecules are byproducts of normal cell processes and must be broken down to avoid cell damage. Mutations of the *SOD1* gene prevent the breakdown of toxic substances, leading to their build-up in nerve cells and eventually causing cell death [28].

Mutations in the first intron of *C9orf72* are the most common genetic cause of ALS, resulting in 25–40% of familial ALS and a small percentage of sporadic cases. Haeusler et al. [29] identified a molecular mechanism by which structural polymorphisms of the *C9orf72* hexanucleotide repeat expansion (HRE) lead to ALS. The HRE forms DNA and RNA G-quadruplexes with distinct structures and promotes RNA/DNA hybrids (R-loops). This structural polymorphism causes a repeat length-dependent accumulation of transcripts aborted in the HRE region. These transcribed repeats bind to ribonucleoproteins in a conformation-dependent manner. Specifically, nucleolin binds to the HRE G-quadruplex, and patients' cells show evidence of nucleolar stress. The authors concluded that the *C9orf72* HRE structural polymorphism at both the DNA and RNA levels initiates molecular cascades, leading to ALS pathologies.

Deposition of ubiquitin inclusion in motor neurons is one of the leading pathogenic mechanisms of ALS. Okamoto et al. [30] first noted the appearance of ubiquitin-positive tau-negative neuronal cytoplasmic inclusions and dystrophic neurites in ALS patients. TDP-43 is the main component of intracellular ubiquitin inclusion bodies in these pathological deposits. Primarily distributed in the nucleus of neurons, TDP-43 participates in nuclear RNA transcription, alternative splicing, and mRNA stability regulation [31, 32]. Pathological TDP-43–mediated neuronal death is typically caused by neurotoxicity consequent to the loss of TDP-43 function [33]. At least seven ALS-associated genes (including *C9orf72*) are linked to TDP-43 proteinopathy [34]. Mutations of the *TARDBP* gene encoding TDP-43 have been identified in a minority of both sporadic and familial ALS cases [35–38], with the vast majority of sporadic ALS cases (>90%) found to be associated with TDP-43 pathology [38].

The mutant *SOD1* mouse model and other ALS mouse models, such as Wobbler mice (due to mutant *Vps54* gene), show upregulation, mislocalization, and accumulation of TDP-43 in the brain [39, 40]. In human studies, not all TDP-43 inclusion bodies have been ubiquitinated, especially in the early stages of ALS, which suggests that ubiquitination is an advanced metabolic phenomenon in ALS disease [41]. Thus, the attendant disruption of normal RNA metabolism resulting from the high prevalence of TDP-43 mislocalization, both loss of nuclear localization and accumulation of pathological cytoplasmic aggregates, likely plays a significant role in the pathogenesis of ALS.

Like TDP-43, mutations in *FUS* are associated with only a few percent of familial ALS cases [42] where cytoplasmic mislocalization has been ascribed to disruption of nuclear import with the consequent recruitment of FUS into stress granules [43]. Also, like TDP-43, widespread cytoplasmic localization of aggregated FUS has been documented in sporadic ALS (where it is often found co-localized with TDP-43) [42]. More recently, widespread cytoplasmic mislocalization of unaggregated FUS has been documented in sporadic ALS post mortem tissue, and a putative mechanism has been described for its mislocalization [44]. Thus nucleocytoplasmic transport defects are a common feature of several key proteins in ALS [45].

In summary, both TDP-43 and FUS are mislocalized to the cytoplasm in the vast majority of sporadic ALS cases. Together with the disturbance of RNA metabolism resulting from mutations in *C9orf72*, the consequences of these mislocalized proteins underscore the importance of compromised RNA metabolism in the pathogenesis of ALS.

Environmental and Epigenetic Factors

While genetic predisposition is an unquestionable player in ALS pathogenesis, it is now well understood that non-genetic/environmental factors provide an additional layer to the complex tapestry of this multifactorial disease. Exactly what these additional non-genetic factors may be, and why and how they contribute to ALS pathophysiology, however, remains elusive. Given the variety of ALS subtypes and the propensity for ALS to manifest in later life, it is not surprising that this confusion exists, nor that such a broad range of putative environmental triggers have been connected to the disorder.

Non-genetic factors that have been investigated in association with ALS range from lifestyle (e.g. smoking, exercise, body mass) to exposures (e.g. chemicals, heavy metals, pesticides/herbicides, electric shock, electromagnetic fields), injury (e.g. head trauma, nerve damage), inflammatory processes (e.g. viruses, fungi, neuroinflammation), treatments (e.g. statins, antibacterial drugs), and diet (e.g. foods containing β-methylamino-L-alanine [BMAA] found in cyanobacteria-contaminated seafood, β-sitosterol-β-D-glucoside [BSSG] found in plants). There is currently significant disagreement regarding the actual impact of any given factor on ALS development, again reflecting the complexity of this progressive disorder (e.g. for review, see [46–49]).

Linking genetics and environment, epigenetic modifications have also been suggested as important factors in ALS pathogenesis. Although currently in very early stages, research into post-translational histone modifications, DNA methylation, and microRNA activity has revealed intriguing mechanistic aberrations with potential relevance to ALS [50].

Gut and Microbial Factors

Most recently, research has uncovered a possible connection between the gut microbiome and ALS development, a connection that is made even more intriguing by its unique ability to tie in many of the factors that have been individually implicated in earlier investigations.

Changes in gut microbiota are now understood to be an ongoing process, with initial colonization beginning at vaginal birth [51]. From this time onward, the composition of intestinal microbiota may be influenced by a variety of factors, both internal and external. Functions of the gut microbiota include essential processes related to metabolism and immunity [52]. Physiological oversight of intestinal processes (e.g. peristalsis, secretions, permeability, etc.) relies on a network of neural, hormonal, and immunological signaling, with intricate bidirectional connections between gut and brain. It is this complex connectivity that is believed to be the route through which gut microbiota can influence brain function [53].

Initial animal research implicating the gut microbiome in ALS pathology by Wu et al. [54] reported changes in gut microbiome profiles between SOD1^{G93A} mice compared to wild type (WT), with administration of butyrate (a short-chain fatty acid produced in the gut by bacterial metabolic activity) in drinking water prolonging lifespan and decreasing aggregation of the G93A-SOD1 mutated protein [55]. Further support for dysregulated gut microbiome in ALS pathology has been reported by Blacher and colleagues [56], who further demonstrate the impact of the environment on the microbiome in SOD1^{G93A} mice, noting that animals from different labs show different microbiome profiles. A more detailed investigation of gut bacteria in these mice resulted in the identification of a particular species, *Akkermansia muciniphila* (which produces the metabolite nicotinamide), as protective against pathogenesis in SOD1^{G93A} mouse models. In humans, microbial dysbiosis in ALS has also been reported [56–59], although not universally [60]. These types of investigations are still in very early stages, and further research is required.

The concept of gut-brain interactions as an initiating factor for central nervous system (CNS) disorders is not unique to ALS. Parkinson's disease (PD), a neurodegenerative movement disorder that involves the destruction of dopamine-producing neuronal cells in the substantia nigra, has been shown to be associated with gastrointestinal dysfunction [61]. In fact, evidence is mounting that changes in gut microbiota are not simply a part of the PD pathology but may actually be an initiating factor [62]. Another neurodegenerative disorder that has been increasingly linked with dysregulation of gut microbiota is Alzheimer's disease (AD) [63], particularly with respect to a high-fat diet [64]. A variety of connections to the gut microbiome have been described, including associations between microbial metabolites and cognitive decline [65], along with microbial dysbiosis from antibiotic use [66]. Similarly, autism spectrum disorder (*ASD*), characterized by early-life onset of deficits in language and social communication, has long been associated with intestinal dysfunction and inflammation [67]. Connections between ASD pathogenesis and specific microbial metabolites have been reported in humans [68], with evidence mounting for therapeutic interventions targeting gastrointestinal activity (for review, see [69]). Schizophrenia, a neurological disorder that has a high co-morbidity with ASD, has also been recently linked with shifts in microbial composition profiles in both animal models and humans [70, 71], while dysregulation of gut microbiota in multiple sclerosis, a disorder characterized by degrading nervous system communication through loss of the myelin sheath on neuronal axons, has been recognized for over a decade [72, 73].

Given the association between the gut microbiome and immune function, it is unsurprising that all of the disorders mentioned are known to have significant inflammatory components, not least of which is ALS [74]. Only recently has the mediatory role of the gut microbiome in the intricate interplay between immunological, endocrine, and neural function been appreciated [75]. It is now understood that through maintenance and regulation of the immune system, the gut microbiome can subsequently impact the blood-brain barrier and produce short-chain fatty acids that subsequently activate CNS microglia [76–78]. Interestingly, gene composition can have an influence on gut microbiota as well [79], adding even greater complexity to the gene–environment interaction story in disorders such as ALS.

ANIMAL MODELS OF ALS

Research into motor neuron diseases like ALS is conducted by a variety of methods including genetic analyses, imaging studies, work within the clinical population, *post mortem* analyses of patients, and preclinical research using animal models. In addition to more obvious clinical applications such as testing novel treatments or medications, animal models can also be used to study the underlying neurobiological mechanisms that contribute to many complex human disorders.

Evaluation of the strengths and weaknesses of any animal model generally entails assessment of validity, often broken down into face, construct, and predictive validity. While ideally a model may possess all forms of validity, this is often not attainable or required. The usefulness and applicability of any individual model change over time as our understanding of the disorder changes and as our requirements of the models change. For example, while predictive validity would be required for a model designed for the purpose of exploring effective therapeutants, construct validity would be more important if the purpose of the model was to provide a better understanding of the etiology of the disorder [80].

Guided by insight into the genetic and molecular basis of ALS, researchers have created a variety of models to investigate the complex process of motor neuron degeneration. Such model systems include both *in vitro* models and *in vivo* models in species ranging from invertebrates and non-mammalian vertebrates to rodent models [81]. More recently, human patient-derived stem cells have also been investigated as a potential tool in ALS research [82].

In vivo models of ALS include a large variety of species. Models in invertebrates such as *Drosophila* and *Caenorhabditis elegans* can be used for straightforward genetic screening. In addition to being used for genetic screening, zebrafish, with their nervous system that is anatomically and functionally similar to that of a human (albeit in a simplified form), offer a number of advantages for modeling specific aspects of motor neuron disease. Additionally, zebrafish are a well-established model for research in toxicology and developmental biology and have become a common species for modeling this aspect of ALS [83, 84]. Rodent models are able to mimic human disease more closely, thus displaying greater face validity and being better suited for investigating more complex pathogenic mechanisms and testing potential therapeutants.

One-hit Models of ALS

Given the number of genes now associated with ALS [26], it is no surprise that many attempts to model the disease have focused on genetically-based models [85, 86].

Recent advances in gene-editing technology like CRISPR/Cas9 have provided the opportunity to study pathogenic mutation in a variety of genetic backgrounds, creating animal models implicating genes identified in the human clinical population. Genetically based models are not without problems. Overexpression of mutant genes is often needed in order to produce end-stage-relevant phenotypes in a time frame that is suitable to the lifespan of a mouse [87]. Indeed, the aspect of age is often overlooked in animal models of many diseases, and ALS is no exception, with significant variety seen in the age of appearance and course of progression of the disease phenotype even within models that implicate the same gene [88]. For example, the SOD1-A4V mutation does not result in pathogenesis in mice until late in life (85 weeks of age, comparable to 60+ years in humans) [89] but causes highly aggressive disease progression within the human clinical population with an average disease progression of only 1.2 years [90]. Crossing SOD1-A4V mice with mice overexpressing WT SOD1 results in a double transgenic mouse that develops the disease beginning at 35 weeks of age (comparable to a human in their mid-30s) [89, 91]. Due to familial ALS patients having only one copy for each of the normal and mutant SOD1 genes, it is no surprise to find differences in pathology and age of onset between the clinical population and animal models, and even between the various SOD1 mouse models themselves due to various levels of expression, with the pathology of mice with lower overexpression of mutant SOD1 thus more closely resembling that of the human clinical population (see [90] for review). While no single model can fully reflect the spectrum of phenotypes observed in the clinical population, the use of inbred strains can be problematic in itself: the lack of genetic diversity does not accurately reflect the variation of responses that will be seen in the human clinical population, thereby limiting the translation ability of the models and thus their utility [87]. Despite the believed genetic link, the clinical presentation of ALS is highly variable in terms of the age at onset and disease progression, suggesting the important role of disease-modifying factors and turning the focus toward more environmentally mediated models.

Perhaps it is not surprising that most animal models of ALS have focused on genetic links, given the current debate over the impact of environmental factors. However, some models have the benefit that they are based on environmental factors known to cause or contribute to disease in the human clinical population. One example of such a model that also displays a clinically relevant disease progression is BSSG exposure in mice. Mice fed pellets containing BSSG for 10–15 weeks exhibited progressive motor neuron loss in the spinal cord that continues to worsen after the exposure to BSSG ended. The mice also showed decreases in glutamate transporter and tyrosine hydroxylase immunolabeling in the brain, as well as increased amounts of glial fibrillary acid protein reactivity and caspase-3 [92].

Multi-hit Models of ALS

As our understanding of motor-neuron disease advances, so does our ability to create better animal models. A more recent trend in animal modeling is that of two-hit or multi-hit models, which combine multiple factors or insults to produce a disease that more accurately resembles the human condition in both relative age of onset and presentation. These multi-hit models have been the focus of research into a variety of diseases and disorders including schizophrenia [93], autism [94], depression [95], PD [96], and others. Sometimes these models combine a genetic predisposition with an environmental insult, but multi-hit models can also include multiple environmental influences, often at different life stages.

Recent work in a zebrafish model has highlighted the potential for a multi-hit design in modeling ALS. A combination of SOD1-G93R zebrafish of ALS genetic background and embryonic exposure to cyanobacterial neurotoxin BMAA leads to early neurodevelopmental defects and adult preclinical motor dysfunction [97, 98]. Increased incidence of ALS has been linked with exposure to BMAA in human populations [99, 100], and chronic oral dosing with BMAA leads to motor system dysfunction in animals [101, 102], indicating that this two-hit model not only shows potential for good face validity but is produced in a potentially etiologically relevant manner.

Limited work investigating gene x environment interactions in ALS have also been conducted using rodent models. Work by Su et al. [103] shows that exposure to statins (a class of medications widely prescribed to promote cardiovascular health) accelerates disease development and decreases survival in SOD1-G93A mice. Likewise, recent work with the same SOD1-G93A mouse has shown that chronic low-dose exposure to methylmercury (MeHg) accelerates the time course of SOD1-G93A-induced motor dysfunction, producing motor dysfunction weeks before it was observed in unexposed SOD1 mice [104]. Exposure to MeHg is common in populations where seafood constitutes a large portion of the diet, or in areas where contamination may be elevated, and has been associated with ALS-like symptoms [105]. However, this link has been questioned and requires further study [106]. Work by Lee and Shaw [107] found that daily oral exposure to steryl glucoside beginning at 10 weeks of age enhanced the spinal motor neuron death and pathology observed in the SOD1-G37R mouse and induced motor axon abnormalities. Research by Wilson et al. [108] using cycad flour (in which the potential causal neurotoxin is the same steryl glucoside molecule used by Tabata [92]) in Apolipoprotein E (apo E) knockout mice found that while cycad-fed WT mice developed the expected progressive behavioral deficits, including amyotrophic lateral sclerosis and parkinsonism-dementia complex (ALS-PDC)-like pathological outcomes, cycad-fed apo E knockout mice were not significantly affected. Results such as these indicate a role for genetic susceptibility factors in toxin-induced neurodegeneration.

Although current work with multi-hit models of ALS is minimal, these examples highlight the potential of this line of research. Given the current belief that the development of ALS is a multistep process arising due to a combination of genetic predisposition and environmental influence [109], this approach should continue to be a potential avenue for further investigation. Comparing phenotypic outcomes between purely genetic models and multi-hit gene x environment models provide a measure of how toxicants may influence neurological disease pathways. This also provides information on toxicities that are not involved in the disease course and identifies those that may be exacerbated by genetic predisposition [109]. Current genetically based models of ALS (in various species) could be used as a "sensitized" background with which to test various environmental influences, including exposure to toxicants, thus creating a multi-hit model. The combination of a sensitized background and exposure to environmental insults may also allow for greater control over the disease progression timeline, potentially producing a more etiologically relevant model as well as providing the opportunity for a variety of disease intervention time points. The ability to study early neuromuscular deficits (prior to diagnosable disease onset) remains crucial for finding pathways that lead to neurodegeneration, allowing for early intervention in the clinical population rather than just the identification of already progressed disease state.

FUTURE MODEL DEVELOPMENT

Animal models are vital for ALS research. To date, however, the focus of most available models has been on genetic features. As our knowledge regarding the variety and complexity of contributing factors grows, it is increasingly important to begin incorporating the information that has been gathered into the development of models that more accurately reflect pathogenesis in humans.

Throughout this chapter, a number of recurrent and important issues have been identified. Models that provide better construct validity are required, not simply reflecting one facet of ALS's complex pathogenesis but combining carefully considered genetic and environmental factors, with animal age at model induction included as an important parameter. Given the prevalence of microbial dysbiosis in such a wide variety of neurological diseases, including ALS, models induced in animals that already have a genetic predisposition to ALS and subsequently incorporate ingested neurotoxins in the induction process should be pursued more aggressively. In addition to behavioral testing, epigenetic evaluation of these gene x neurotoxin animal models along with their offspring would allow for further elucidation of etiologic possibilities. To improve model utility for evaluating putative ALS treatments, a sufficient disease progression that both mimics what is seen in the clinic and allows for testing interventions within the timeframe of disease development is needed. Finally, although not overtly discussed in this chapter, a move toward standardization of testing paradigms (both behavior and histopathology) would greatly improve efforts to increase reproducibility and better allow translation of model outcome measures to the clinic.

ACKNOWLEDGMENTS

The authors gratefully acknowledge Colleen Johns, Alpha Cognition Inc., for her contribution in the preparation of this manuscript.

CONFLICT OF INTEREST

The authors declare no potential conflict of interest with respect to research, authorship, and/or publication of this manuscript.

COPYRIGHT AND PERMISSION STATEMENT

To the best of our knowledge, the materials included in this chapter do not violate copyright laws. All original sources have been appropriately acknowledged and/or referenced. Where relevant, appropriate permissions have been obtained from the original copyright holder(s).

REFERENCES

1. Charcot, J. and Joffory, A. (1969). Deux cas d'atrophie musculaire progressive avec lesions de la substance grise et des faisceaux antero-lateraux de la moelle epiniere. *Arch Pathol Norm Pathol* 2: 744–754.
2. Marin, B., Couratier, P., Arcuti, S. et al. (2016). Stratification of ALS patients' survival: a population-based study. *J Neurol* 263 (1): 100–111.
3. Eisen, A. (2009). Amyotrophic lateral sclerosis: a 40-year personal perspective. *J Clin Neurosci* 16 (4): 505–512.
4. Yunusova, Y., Plowman, E.K., Green, J.R. et al. (2019). Clinical measures of bulbar dysfunction in ALS. *Front Neurol* 10 (106): 1–11.
5. Ghasemi, M. (2016). Amyotrophic lateral sclerosis mimic syndromes. *Iran J Neurol* 15 (2): 85–91.
6. Kiernan, M.C., Vucic, S., Cheah, B.C. et al. (2011). Amyotrophic lateral sclerosis. *Lancet* 377 (9769): 942–955.
7. Shoesmith, C.L., Findlater, K., Rowe, A., and Strong, M.J. (2007). Prognosis of amyotrophic lateral sclerosis with respiratory onset. *J Neurol Neurosurg Psychiatry* 78 (6): 629–631.
8. Chiò, A., Logroscino, G., Hardiman, O. et al. (2009). Prognostic factors in ALS: a critical review. *Amyotroph Lateral Scler* 10 (5–6): 310–323.
9. Roche, J.C., Rojas-Garcia, R., Scott, K.M. et al. (2012). A proposed staging system for amyotrophic lateral sclerosis. *Brain* 135 (3): 847–852.
10. Murphy, J., Factor-Litvak, P., Goetz, R. et al. (2016). Cognitive-behavioral screening reveals prevalent impairment in a large multicenter ALS cohort. *Neurology* 86 (9): 813–820.
11. Prudlo, J., König, J., Schuster, C. et al. (2016). TDP-43 pathology and cognition in ALS. *Neurology* 87 (10): 1019–1023.
12. Cronin, S., Hardiman, O., and Traynor, B.J. (2007). Ethnic variation in the incidence of ALS: a systematic review. *Neurology* 68 (13): 1002–1007.

13. Atsuta, N., Watanabe, H., Ito, M. et al. (2009). Age at onset influences on wide-ranged clinical features of sporadic amyotrophic lateral sclerosis. *J Neurol Sci* 276 (1–2): 163–169.

14. Zoccolella, S., Beghi, E., Palagano, G. et al. (2008). Analysis of survival and prognostic factors in amyotrophic lateral sclerosis: a population based study. *J Neurol Neurosurg Psychiatry* 79 (1): 33–37.

15. Dadon-Nachum, M., Melamed, E., and Offen, D. (2011). The "dying-back" phenomenon of motor neurons in ALS. *J Mol Neurosci* 43 (3): 470–477.

16. Bensimon, G., Lacomblez, L., and Meininger, V. (1994). A controlled trial of riluzole in amyotrophic lateral sclerosis. ALS/Riluzole Study Group. *N Engl J Med* 330 (9): 585–591.

17. Miller, R.G., Mitchell, J.D., Lyon, M., and Moore, D.H. (2007). Riluzole for amyotrophic lateral sclerosis (ALS)/motor neuron disease (MND). *Cochrane Database Syst Rev* 2: CD001447.

18. Cheah, B.C., Vucic, S., Krishnan, A.V., and Kiernan, M.C. (2010). Riluzole, neuroprotection and amyotrophic lateral sclerosis. *Curr Med Chem* 17 (18): 1942–1959.

19. Hogg, M.C., Halang, L., Woods, I. et al. (2018). Riluzole does not improve lifespan or motor function in three ALS mouse models. *Amyotroph Lateral Scler Frontotemporal Degener* 19 (5–6): 438–445.

20. Abe, K., Yuki, S., and Kogure, K. (1988). Strong attenuation of ischemic and postischemic brain edema in rats by a novel free radical scavenger. *Stroke* 19 (4): 480–485.

21. Rothstein, J.D. (2017). Edaravone: a new drug approved for ALS. *Cell* 171 (4): 725.

22. Okada, M., Yamashita, S., Ueyama, H. et al. (2018). Long-term effects of edaravone on survival of patients with amyotrophic lateral sclerosis. *eNeurologicalSci* 11: 11–14.

23. Takei, K., Watanabe, K., Yuki, S. et al. (2017). Edaravone and its clinical development for amyotrophic lateral sclerosis. *Amyotroph Lateral Scler Frontotemporal Degener* 18 (sup1): 5–10.

24. Petrov, D., Mansfield, C., Moussy, A., and Hermine, O. (2017). ALS clinical trials review: 20 years of failure. Are we any closer to registering a new treatment? *Front Aging Neurosci* 9 (68): 1–11.

25. Mora, J.S., Genge, A., Chio, A. et al. (2020). Masitinib as an add-on therapy to riluzole in patients with amyotrophic lateral sclerosis: a randomized clinical trial. *Amyotroph Lateral Scler Frontotemporal Degener* 21 (1–2): 5–14.

26. Chia, R., Chiò, A., and Traynor, B.J. (2018). Novel genes associated with amyotrophic lateral sclerosis: diagnostic and clinical implications. *Lancet Neurol* 17 (1): 94–102.

27. Chiò, A., Traynor, B.J., Lombardo, F. et al. (2008). Prevalence of SOD1 mutations in the Italian ALS population. *Neurology* 70 (7): 533–537.

28. Rosen, D.R., Siddique, T., Patterson, D. et al. (1993). Mutations in Cu/Zn superoxide dismutase gene are associated with familial amyotrophic lateral sclerosis. *Nature* 362 (6415): 59–62.

29. Haeusler, A.R., Donnelly, C.J., Periz, G. et al. (2014). C9orf72 nucleotide repeat structures initiate molecular cascades of disease. *Nature* 507 (7491): 195–200.

30. Okamoto, K., Hirai, S., Yamazaki, T. et al. (1991). New ubiquitin-positive intraneuronal inclusions in the extra-motor cortices in patients with amyotrophic lateral sclerosis. *Neurosci Lett* 129 (2): 233–236.

31. Arai, T., Hasegawa, M., Akiyama, H. et al. (2006). TDP-43 is a component of ubiquitin-positive tau-negative inclusions in frontotemporal lobar degeneration and amyotrophic lateral sclerosis. *Biochem Biophys Res Commun* 351 (3): 602–611.

32. Neumann, M., Sampathu, D.M., Kwong, L.K. et al. (2006). Ubiquitinated TDP-43 in frontotemporal lobar degeneration and amyotrophic lateral sclerosis. *Science* 314 (5796): 130–133.

33. Gendrona, T.F., Rademakersa, R., and Petrucelli, L. (2013). TARDBP mutation analysis in TDP-43 proteinopathies and deciphering the toxicity of mutant TDP-43. *J Alzheimers Dis* 33 (Suppl 1): S35–S45.

34. Weskamp, K. and Barmada, S.J. (2018). TDP43 and RNA instability in amyotrophic lateral sclerosis. *Brain Res* 1693 (Pt A): 67–74.

35. Gitcho, M.A., Baloh, R.H., Chakraverty, S. et al. (2008). TDP-43 A315T mutation in familial motor neuron disease. *Ann Neurol* 63 (4): 535–538.

36. Kabashi, E., Valdmanis, P.N., Dion, P. et al. (2008). TARDBP mutations in individuals with sporadic and familial amyotrophic lateral sclerosis. *Nat Genet* 40 (5): 572–574.

37. Sreedharan, J., Blair, I.P., Tripathi, V.B. et al. (2008). TDP-43 mutations in familial and sporadic amyotrophic lateral sclerosis. *Science* 319 (5870): 1668–1672.

38. Neumann, M. (2009). Molecular neuropathology of TDP-43 proteinopathies. *Int J Mol Sci* 10 (1): 232–246.

39. Shan, X., Vocadlo, D., and Krieger, C. (2009). Mislocalization of TDP-43 in the G93A mutant SOD1 transgenic mouse model of ALS. *Neurosci Lett* 458 (2): 70–74.

40. Dennis, J.S. and Citron, B.A. (2009). Wobbler mice modeling motor neuron disease display elevated transactive response DNA binding protein. *Neuroscience* 158 (2): 745–750.

41. Herhaus, L. and Dikic, I. (2015). Expanding the ubiquitin code through post-translational modification. *EMBO Rep* 16 (9): 1071–1083.

42. Deng, H.-X., Zhai, H., Bigio, E.H. et al. (2010). FUS-immunoreactive inclusions are a common feature in sporadic and non-SOD1 familial amyotrophic lateral sclerosis. *Ann Neurol* 67 (6): 739–748.

43. Dormann, D., Rodde, R., Edbauer, D. et al. (2010). ALS-associated fused in sarcoma (FUS) mutations disrupt transportin-mediated nuclear import. *EMBO J* 29 (16): 2841–2857.

44. Tyzack, G.E., Luisier, R., Taha, D.M. et al. (2019). Widespread FUS mislocalization is a molecular hallmark of amyotrophic lateral sclerosis. *Brain* 142 (9): 2572–2580.

45. Boeynaems, S., Bogaert, E., Van Damme, P., and Van Den Bosch, L. (2016). Inside out: the role of nucleocytoplasmic transport in ALS and FTLD. *Acta Neuropathol* 132 (2): 159–173.

46. Filippini, T., Fiore, M., Tesauro, M. et al. (2020). Clinical and lifestyle factors and risk of amyotrophic lateral sclerosis: a population-based case-control study. *Int J Environ Res Public Health* 17 (3): 1–17.

47. Gunnarsson, L.G. and Bodin, L. (2019). Occupational exposures and neurodegenerative diseases—a systematic literature review and meta-analyses. *Int J Environ Res Public Health* 16 (337): 1–17.

48. Ingre, C., Roos, P.M., Piehl, F. et al. (2015). Risk factors for amyotrophic lateral sclerosis. *Clin Epidemiol* 7: 181–193.

49. Nowicka, N., Juranek, J., Juranek, J.K., and Wojtkiewicz, J. (2019). Risk factors and emerging therapies in amyotrophic lateral sclerosis. *Int J Mol Sci* 20 (11): 1–19.

50. Bennett, S.A., Tanaz, R., Cobos, S.N., and Torrente, M.P. (2019). Epigenetics in amyotrophic lateral sclerosis: a role for histone post-translational modifications in neurodegenerative disease. *Transl Res* 204: 19–30.

51. Jiménez, E., Delgado, S., Maldonado, A. et al. (2008). Staphylococcus epidermidis: a differential trait of the fecal microbiota of breast-fed infants. *BMC Microbiol* 8 (143): 1–11.

52. Bull, M.J. and Plummer, N.T. (2014). Part 1: the human gut microbiome in health and disease. *Integr Med* 13 (6): 17–22.

53. Collins, S.M., Surette, M., and Bercik, P. (2012). The interplay between the intestinal microbiota and the immune system. *Nat Rev Microbiol* 10 (11): 735–742.

54. Wu, S., Yi, J., Zhang, Y.G. et al. (2015). Leaky intestine and impaired microbiome in an amyotrophic lateral sclerosis mouse model. *Physiol Rep* 3 (4): 1–10.

55. Zhang, Y.G., Wu, S., Yi, J. et al. (2017). Target intestinal microbiota to alleviate disease progression in amyotrophic lateral sclerosis. *Clin Ther* 39 (2): 322–336.

56. Blacher, E., Bashiardes, S., Shapiro, H. et al. (2019). Potential roles of gut microbiome and metabolites in modulating ALS in mice. *Nature* 572 (7770): 474–480.

57. Rowin, J., Xia, Y., Jung, B., and Sun, J. (2017). Gut inflammation and dysbiosis in human motor neuron disease. *Physiol Rep* 5 (18): 1–6.

58. Fang, X., Wang, X., Yang, S. et al. (2016). Evaluation of the microbial diversity in amyotrophic lateral sclerosis using high-throughput sequencing. *Front Microbiol* 7 (1479): 1–7.

59. Li, C., Cui, L., Yang, Y. et al. (2019). Gut microbiota differs between parkinson's disease patients and healthy controls in northeast China. *Front Mol Neurosci* 12 (171): 1–13.

60. Fournier, C.N., Houser, M., Tansey, M.G. et al. (2020). The gut microbiome and neuroinflammation in amyotrophic lateral sclerosis? Emerging clinical evidence. *Neurobiol Dis* 135 (104300).

61. Sampson, T.R., Debelius, J.W., Thron, T. et al. (2016). Gut microbiota regulate motor deficits and neuroinflammation in a model of parkinson's disease. *Cell* 167 (6): 1469–1480.

62. Pfeiffer, R.F. (2018). Gastrointestinal dysfunction in parkinson's disease. *Curr Treat Options Neurol* 20 (54): 1–12.

63. Bostanciklioğlu, M. (2019). The role of gut microbiota in pathogenesis of alzheimer's disease. *J Appl Microbiol* 127 (4): 954–967.

64. Thériault, P., ElAli, A., and Rivest, S. (2016). High fat diet exacerbates alzheimer's disease-related pathology in APPswe/PS1 mice. *Oncotarget* 7 (42): 67808–67827.

65. Xu, R. and Wang, Q.Q. (2016). Towards understanding brain-gut-microbiome connections in alzheimer's disease. *BMC Syst Biol* 10 ((Suppl 3(63))): 277–285.

66. Angelucci, F., Cechova, K., Amlerova, J., and Hort, J. (2019). Antibiotics, gut microbiota, and alzheimer's disease. *J Neuroinflamation* 16 (108): 1–10.

67. Mangiola, F., Ianiro, G., Franceschi, F. et al. (2016). Gut microbiota in autism and mood disorders. *World J Gastroenterol* 22 (1): 361–368.

68. Kang, D., Ilhan, Z.E., Isern, N.G. et al. (2018). Differences in fecal microbial metabolites and microbiota of children with autism spectrum disorders. *Anaerobe* 49: 121–131.

69. Pulikkan, J., Mazumder, A., and Grace, T. (2019). Role of the gut microbiome in autism spectrum disorders. *Adv Exp Med Biol* 1118: 253–269.

70. Fond, G.B., Lagier, J.C., Honore, S. et al. (2020). Microbiota-orientated treatments for major depression and schizophrenia guillaume. *Nutrients* 12 (4): 1–15.

71. Zheng, P., Zeng, B., Liu, M. et al. (2019). The gut microbiome from patients with schizophrenia modulates the glutamate-glutamine-GABA cycle and schizophrenia-relevant behaviors in mice. *Sci Adv* 5 (2): 1–12.

72. Kirby, T. and Ochoa-Repáraz, J. (2018). The gut microbiome in multiple sclerosis: a potential therapeutic avenue. *Med Sci* 6 (3): 1–20.

73. Chu, F., Shi, M., Lang, Y. et al. (2018). Gut microbiota in multiple sclerosis and experimental autoimmune encephalomyelitis: current applications and future perspectives. *Mediat Inflamm* 8168717: 1–17.

74. Kjældgaard, A.L., Pilely, K., Olsen, K.S. et al. (2018). Amyotrophic lateral sclerosis: the complement and inflammatory hypothesis. *Mol Immunol* 102: 14–25.

75. Spielman, L.J., Gibson, D.L., and Klegeris, A. (2018). Unhealthy gut, unhealthy brain: the role of the intestinal microbiota in neurodegenerative diseases. *Neurochem Int* 120: 149–163.

76. Parker, A., Fonseca, S., and Carding, S.R. (2020). Gut microbes and metabolites as modulators of blood-brain barrier integrity and brain health. *Gut Microbes* 11 (2): 135–157.

77. Sampson, T.R. and Mazmanian, S.K. (2015). Control of brain development, function, and behavior by the microbiome. *Cell Host Microbe* 17 (5): 565–576.

78. Sharon, G., Sampson, T.R., Geschwind, D.H., and Mazmanian, S.K. (2016). The central nervous system and the gut microbiome. *Cell* 167 (4): 915–932.

79. Dicksved, J., Halfvarson, J., Rosenquist, M. et al. (2008). Molecular analysis of the gut microbiota of identical twins with crohn's disease. *ISME J* 2 (7): 716–727.

80. Morrice, J.R., Gregory-Evans, C.Y., and Shaw, C.A. (2018). Animal models of amyotrophic lateral sclerosis: a comparison of model validity. *Neural Regen Res* 13 (12): 2050–2054.

81. Van Damme, P., Robberecht, W., and Van Den Bosch, L. (2017). Modelling amyotrophic lateral sclerosis: progress and possibilities. *Dis Model Mech* 10 (5): 537–549.

82. Matus, S., Medinas, D.B., and Hetz, C. (2014). Common ground: stem cell approaches find shared pathways underlying ALS. *Cell Stem Cell* 14 (6): 697–699.

83. Sakowski, S.A., Lunn, J.S., Busta, A.S. et al. (2012). Neuromuscular effects of G93A-SOD1 expression in zebrafish. *Mol Neurodegener* 7 (1): 1.

84. Morrice, J.R., Gregory-Evans, C.Y., and Shaw, C.A. (2018). Modeling environmentally-induced motor neuron degeneration in zebrafish. *Sci Rep* 8 (1): 1–11.

85. Saberi, S., Stauffer, J.E., Schulte, D.J., and Ravits, J. (2015). Neuropathology of amyotrophic lateral sclerosis and its variants. *Neurol Clin* 33 (4): 855–876.

86. Philips, T. and Rothstein, J.D. (2015). Rodent models of amyotrophic lateral sclerosis. *Curr Protoc Pharmacol* 69: 5.67.1–5. 67.21.

87. Lutz, C. (2018). Mouse models of ALS: past, present and future. *Brain Res* 1693: 1–10.

88. Joyce, P.I., Fratta, P., Fisher, E.M.C., and Acevedo-Arozena, A. (2011). SOD1 and TDP-43 animal models of amyotrophic lateral sclerosis: recent advances in understanding disease toward the development of clinical treatments. *Mamm Genome* 22 (7–8): 420–448.

89. Flurkey, K., Currer, J.M., and Harrison, D.E. (2007). Mouse models in aging research. In: *The Mouse in Biomedical Research*, 2e, vol. 3 (eds. J. Fox, S. Barthold, M. Davisson, et al.), 637–672. Burlington, MA: American College Laboratory Animal Medicine (Elsevier).

90. Siddique, T. and Deng, H.-X. (1996). Genetics of amyotrophic lateral sclerosis. *Hum Mol Genet* 5 (1): 1465–1470.

91. Deng, H., Shi, Y., Furukawa, Y. et al. (2006). Conversion to the amyotrophic lateral sclerosis phenotype is associated with intermolecular linked insoluble appregates of SOD1 in mitochondria. *Proc Natl Acad Sci* 103 (18): 7142–7147.

92. Tabata, R., Wilson, J., Ly, P. et al. (2008). Chronic exposure to dietary sterol glucosides is neurotoxic to motor neurons and induces an ALS-PDC phenotype. *Neuromolecular Med* 10 (1): 24–39.

93. Monte, A.S., Mello, B.S.F., Borella, V.C.M. et al. (2017). Two-hit model of schizophrenia induced by neonatal immune activation and peripubertal stress in rats: study of sex differences and brain oxidative alterations. *Behav Brain Res* 331 (May): 30–37.

94. van Tilborg, E., Achterberg, E.J.M., van Kammen, C.M. et al. (2018). Combined fetal inflammation and postnatal hypoxia causes myelin deficits and autism-like behavior in a rat model of diffuse white matter injury. *Glia* 66 (1): 78–93.

95. D'Souza, D. and Sadananda, M. (2019). Stressor during early adolescence in hyperreactive female wistar kyoto rats induces a 'double hit' manifested by variation in neurobehaviors and brain monoamines. *Neuroscience* 414: 200–209.

96. Buhusi, M., Olsen, K., Yang, B.Z., and Buhusi, C.V. (2016). Stress-induced executive dysfunction in GDNF-deficient mice, a mouse model of parkinsonism. *Front Behav Neurosci* 10 (June): 1–10.

97. Powers, S., Kwok, S., Lovejoy, E. et al. (2017). Embryonic exposure to the environmental neurotoxin BMAA negatively impacts early neuronal development and progression of neurodegeneration in the Sod1-G93R zebrafish model of amyotrophic lateral sclerosis. *Toxicol Sci* 157 (1): 129–140.

98. Sher, R.B. (2017). The interaction of genetics and environmental toxicants in amyotrophic lateral sclerosis: results from animal models. *Neural Regen Res* 12 (6): 902–905.

99. Cox, P.A., Davis, D.A., Mash, D.C. et al. (1823). Dietary exposure to an environmental toxin triggers neurofibrillary tangles and amyloid deposits in the brain. *Proc R Soc B Biol Sci* 2016 (283): 1–10.

100. Banack, S.A., Johnson, H.E., Cheng, R., and Cox, P.A. (2007). Production of the neurotoxin BMAA by a marine cyanobacterium. *Mar Drugs* 5 (4): 180–196.

101. Spencer, P.S., Hugon, J., Ludolph, A. et al. (1987). Discovery and partial characterization of primate motor-system toxins. *CIBA Found Symp* 126: 221–238.

102. Karamyan, V.T. and Speth, R.C. (2008). Animal models of BMAA neurotoxicity: a critical review. *Life Sci* 82 (5–6): 233–246.

103. Su, X.W., Nandar, W., Neely, E.B. et al. (2018). Statins accelerate disease progression and shorten survival in SOD1-G93A mice. *Muscle Nerve* 54 (2): 284–291.

104. Bailey, J.M., Colón-Rodríguez, A., and Atchison, W.D. (2017). Evaluating a gene-environment interaction in amyotrophic lateral sclerosis: methylmercury exposure and mutated SOD1. *Curr Environ Heal reports* 4 (2): 200–207.

105. Andrew, A.S., Chen, C.Y., Caller, T.A. et al. (2018). Toenail mercury levels are associated with amyotrophic lateral sclerosis (ALS) risk. *Muscle Nerve* 58 (1): 36–41.

106. Parkin Kullmann, J.A. and Pamphlett, R. (2018). A comparison of mercury exposure from seafood consumption and dental amalgam fillings in people with and without amyotrophic lateral sclerosis (ALS): an international online case-control study. *Int J Environ Res Public Health* 15 (2874): 1–14.

107. Lee, G. and Shaw, C.A. (2011). Early exposure to environmental toxin contributes to neuronal vulnerability and axonal pathology in a model of familial ALS. *Nat Preceedings* 80: 1–33.

108. Wilson, J.M.B., Petrik, M.S., Moghadasian, M.H., and Shaw, C.A. (2005). Examining the interaction of apo E and neurotoxicity on a murine model of ALS-PDC. *Can J Physiol Pharmacol* 83 (2): 131–141.

109. Al-Chalabi, A., Calvo, A., Chio, A. et al. (2014). Analysis of amyotrophic lateral sclerosis as a multistep process: a population-based modelling study. *Lancet Neurol* 13 (11): 1108–1113.

CHAPTER 9

Clinical Trials in ALS – Current Challenges and Strategies for Future Directions

Kristiana Salmon and Angela Genge

Montreal Neurological Institute and Hospital, Montréal, Québec, Canada

INTRODUCTION

Drug development is often viewed as a linear series of events, beginning with a laboratory discovery that is then transitioned to a sequential clinical trial program in patients. While the concept of "bench-to-bedside" is familiar in academia and industry, researchers and clinicians alike often overlook the complexities of the clinical development process, which resembles a rollercoaster, complete with serendipitous twists and unforeseen falls.

Even in the most well-characterized human diseases, bringing a potential therapy from the preclinical stage to market approval is rife with challenges. When considering a disease that is rare and with incomplete understanding of pathogenesis, such as amyotrophic lateral sclerosis (ALS), the process looks like not only a wild rollercoaster ride but one that is on an unfinished track, with pieces missing or barely held in place. Without the support of a strong, foundational understanding of the pathogenesis of the disease, successfully developing effective therapies becomes an even greater hurdle to overcome. It follows to look to cell and animal models of ALS to answer questions about disease mechanisms and inform the clinical development of potential therapies. However, models can be limited in their representativeness of the human disease, as well as their practicality in laboratory research. Researchers are therefore developing

Spectrums of Amyotrophic Lateral Sclerosis: Heterogeneity, Pathogenesis and Therapeutic Directions,
First Edition. Edited by Christopher A. Shaw and Jessica R. Morrice.
© 2021 John Wiley & Sons Ltd. Published 2021 by John Wiley & Sons Ltd.

newer laboratory models of ALS for preclinical drug development that enable both the validation of targets and the ability to screen compounds rapidly [1].

To date, only two drugs have been approved in Canada and the United States to treat ALS: riluzole (Rilutek) was the first in 1995, followed by more than 20 years of failed clinical trials until edaravone (Radicava) was first approved in 2017. Neither riluzole nor edaravone is a complete success in treating ALS; both drugs demonstrated only modest effects on survival and function in their respective trials, fueling the need for continued research in the search for more effective treatments [2, 3].

This chapter will provide an overview of some of the significant challenges in ALS that complicate designing and performing randomized controlled trials, followed by a discussion of potential solutions based on emerging practices in the field and our own experiences.

CHALLENGES IN ALS CLINICAL TRIALS

Randomized controlled trials are considered the gold standard of clinical research as they control for confounding variables to provide the strongest level of evidence for efficacy [4]. However, they are expensive, time-consuming, and challenging – particularly for rare diseases, due to their small patient populations. Rare neurological diseases are also poorly understood, with few or no established biomarkers or outcome measures upon which to base trial designs. In the 25 years since riluzole was approved, the ALS community has faced more than 40 failed therapeutic programs, a staggering number that is accompanied by high financial investment, site burden, and loss of hope for patients [5].

DISEASE HETEROGENEITY

ALS is considered a heterogeneous disease, given the difference in clinical presentation between individuals with the disease [6].

While contributions to heterogeneity from non-cell autonomous pathology have been well described, they are not well understood at this time, and the molecular pathology of the different neuronal cell types identified to play a role in ALS is proving to be increasingly complex [7]. Molecular abnormalities include, but are not limited to, intracellular protein aggregates; cytoskeletal abnormalities; mitochondrial dysfunction; defects in DNA and RNA processing, transport, and function; central nervous system (CNS) inflammation; nucleocytoplasmic transport; and disrupted oxidative homeostasis.

In addition to the heterogeneity occurring at the molecular level, the clinical manifestations of ALS are also diverse. Not only is the initial presentation different from patient to patient, but the rate of functional decline varies significantly. Historically, there has been a lack of patient stratification based on disease characteristics in trials, with the resulting heterogeneity within the trial population potentially contributing to trial failure [8]. While it may be assumed that heterogeneity is exclusive to sporadic forms of the disease, we cannot necessarily turn to familial forms to offer a more concrete, homogeneous population of patients in which to conduct clinical trials. For example, clinical features, rate of functional decline, and survival are highly variable among patients with various *SOD1* gene mutations [9].

In addition to confounding the results of un-stratified trials, disease heterogeneity can also limit attempts to generalize a positive trial to the ALS patient population at large. A study demonstrated that 59.8% of patients with ALS were ineligible for clinical trials due to eligibility criteria, including meeting criteria for a specific El Escorial category, respiratory function, and disease duration [10]. This puts into question the need for more carefully conceived eligibility criteria and a more balanced approach to limiting heterogeneity to achieve internal validity (how well a study is designed and conducted) and maximizing generalizability to achieve external validity (how applicable study results are to a real-world setting).

LACK OF ESTABLISHED BIOMARKERS

One of the most significant challenges in the field of ALS is the lack of biomarkers. In the clinical setting, biomarkers are critical not only for diagnosis of disease but also to evaluate response to an intervention and select patients who are most likely to respond to an intervention. While drug development in multiple sclerosis has greatly benefitted from using imaging as a biomarker, allowing objective and quantitative measurement of efficacy and target engagement, most trials in ALS have not had a suitable biomarker available for these purposes. In ALS, the major challenge remains that there are currently no established biomarkers indicative of disease state, projected progression, or response to treatment.

LIMITATIONS OF CONVENTIONAL OUTCOME MEASURES

Outcome measures provide the best snapshot of the functional status of a patient at a given time point. As discussed later, outcome measures in Phase II trials may not always be an appropriate justification for "go/no-go" decisions for further development. Many of the currently available outcome measures for ALS have limitations; if the field continues to only look at the generally accepted consensus measures, novel breakthroughs could be missed.

ALSFRS-R

The Amyotrophic Lateral Sclerosis Functional Rating Scale Revised (ALSFRS-R) effectively measures the functional status of the patient and can capture clinically meaningful changes over time. However, it is a subjective assessment and can be subject to rater variability and inconsistent patient reporting [11, 12]. While large numbers of ALSFRS-R score trajectories can form a linear model, individual trajectories are not linear and vary greatly [8]. On an individual basis, the timeline of a single patient's ALSFRS-R score may go through periods of rapid decline as well as plateaus [13]. Depending on the duration of a clinical trial, these fluctuations in score can have a significant impact when the ALSFRS-R is used as an outcome measure, even though it is considered the gold standard for assessing function in clinical research. Furthermore, prior to emerging predictive models, it has been used to estimate disease progression at enrollment based on the change in ALSFRS-R score from reported symptom onset. Its nonlinear nature and the effect of dropouts further reduces its reliability as an outcome measure [12].

FVC/SVC

Forced vital capacity (FVC) and slow vital capacity (SVC) are lung function tests that can be used to predict survival and are closely correlated with other disease characteristics [14, 15]. However, FVC and SVC are not highly correlated with the respiratory subscores of the ALSFRS-R [16]. Additionally, patients presenting with bulbar involvement can have great difficulty in performing these assessments due to weakened facial muscles, resulting in an inability to make a proper seal around a mouthpiece used in testing [17]. This can lead to lower, unrepresentative respiratory function results in bulbar-onset or bulbar-affected patients. Patients with historical respiratory complications, such as obstructive conditions or respiratory-onset ALS, can also have altered or unrepresentative results. Finally, the use and timing of respiratory intervention, such as lung volume recruitment and non-invasive ventilation, vary from clinic to clinic [18]. These interventions may affect the ability to obtain accurate or reliable FVC or SVC measurements. In a multicenter, international clinical trial spanning several months, this variability in clinical practice and decision-making with regard to respiratory support can inadvertently affect respiratory outcome data if not accounted for in the study protocol.

HHD

Hand-held dynamometry (HHD) measures muscle strength and is closely correlated with ALSFRS-R and SVC [19]. It produces less variable results than manual muscle testing (MMT); however, it requires qualified and certified raters, ideally with prior experience, to produce reliable results. The size and strength of the evaluator as well as prior training and experience can significantly affect the quality of data resulting from the use of this outcome measure.

Survival vs. Function

The ultimate goal for disease-modifying therapies for ALS is to extend survival; however, survival is affected by both innate and external factors. Therefore, the use of survival as a primary endpoint impacts trial feasibility as it requires very lengthy trials with large sample sizes, leading to subsequent burdens on patients and trial sites [20, 21]. While functional improvements are also desirable in a trial, the statistical analysis is often affected by dropouts and deaths of trial participants. Therefore, neither survival nor function provides a complete picture of efficacy when assessed individually. An investigational product might have a disproportionate effect on function and survival, which could lead to failure of meeting the primary endpoint if the "incorrect" outcome is selected. On the other hand, using function and survival as co-primary endpoints establishes the need to achieve a positive result for both.

PHASE II TRIAL "PARADOX"

Several of the challenges discussed so far impact clinical trial design at every phase of development; however, these challenges are of particular importance for Phase II trials. Progress in the field of ALS has been impeded by multiple failures in Phase III trials, despite promising results in the preceding Phase II trial. Prominent examples of therapies that failed in Phase III include lithium, talampanel, ceftriaxone, and dexpramipexole [22–25]. Numerous reviews have been written on this subject, with disparate results between Phase II and Phase III being attributed to limited understanding of the underlying disease biology and targets of the intervention, lack of biomarkers indicative of biological activity of the intervention, insufficient disease modeling to identify suitable candidates for participation in trials, inadequate sample sizes, and disease heterogeneity [26–28].

While guidance from the US Food and Drug Administration (FDA) with regard to traditional, sequential trial design is clear that Phase II trials should guide Phase III trial design, they should not replace the latter. Yet in recent years, we have seen Phase II trials in ALS become increasingly complex, with multiple secondary and exploratory outcomes, as sponsors attempt to capture an early efficacy signal that can be further explored in a Phase III trial. The unfortunate consequence of this approach is having to manage long, demanding Phase II programs, with pressure from the sponsor on the sites to complete recruitment to trials that suffer from patient retention.

Over-interpretation of Phase II results can lead to the delay of a potentially promising therapeutic from advancing to later stages of clinical development. The development programs of tirasemtiv and reldesemtiv (Cytokinetics), both muscle-targeting therapies, illustrate this outcome well. Although the Phase II BENEFIT-ALS trial of tirasemtiv failed to meet its primary efficacy endpoint of mean change from baseline in the ALSFRS-R score, use of SVC as a secondary outcome demonstrated a slowing in the decline of respiratory function in the tirasemtiv arm compared with the placebo arm [29]. The subsequent Phase III trial, VITALITY-ALS, implemented SVC as the primary outcome, an unprecedented first for a clinical trial in ALS, given that historically ALSFRS-R had primarily been used as the primary outcome [30]. Despite the hope that the encouraging SVC data from BENEFIT-ALS would translate into positive results when SVC was used as a primary outcome, VITALITY-ALS also failed to meet the primary outcome due to poor tolerability of the drug. Cytokinetics persevered, and reldesemtiv, the next-generation molecule of tirasemtiv, was designed to reduce penetration of the blood-brain barrier, thereby reducing the risk for CNS adverse effects as observed in VITALITY-ALS. While the Phase II trial of reldesemtiv, FORTITUDE-ALS, also failed to achieve statistical significance on its primary end-point, dose-response analysis of pooled results demonstrated less of a decline in function in patients on reldesemtiv as compared to placebo [31]. Additionally, the undesirable safety profile seen in the tirasemtiv studies that resulted in the high dropout rate was not observed in FORTITUDE-ALS. The development of reldesemtiv is ongoing at this time, and it remains to be seen how the results from FORTITUDE-ALS will influence future trial designs in this clinical program.

This Phase II trial "paradox" is often driven by a lack of funding. Many sponsors want to have a clear indication of efficacy from a Phase II trial to present to their investors prior to asking them to invest in a subsequent Phase III trial. This can lead to sponsors trying to tease out more information from a Phase II trial than is reasonable, often compromising on trial design to do so. It should be emphasized that the primary goal of Phase II trials remains evaluating safety and tolerability; it is important to achieve this goal, without over-interpreting secondary efficacy endpoint data to inform Phase III design.

PATIENT RECRUITMENT AND RETENTION

Patient recruitment to clinical trials of novel therapies, and their retention, is a recurring challenge across a wide variety of diseases and disciplines [32]. There are multiple barriers to effective recruitment, including, but not limited to, financial restraints, logistical concerns, lack of resources, inadequate recruitment strategies, and restrictive eligibility criteria. Unfortunately, there is limited guidance available on interventions to improve recruitment [33].

ASSUMPTIONS FOR LEAD-IN PHASES

Lead-in phases have previously been employed in clinical trials evaluating meman-tine, minocycline, and TCH346 for ALS [34–36]. A *lead-in phase* is a period of time between screening and randomization where the patient is assessed at predefined intervals. After the lead-in phase is complete, the patient is randomized to a treatment arm for the remainder of the trial. Lead-in phases provide an opportunity to reduce sample size and can provide a baseline rate of functional decline for each patient. However, this requires that an assumption be made that functional decline is linear, and as previously discussed, this is not the case in a heterogeneous disease such as ALS. While some current development programs have already included or are looking to include a lead-in phase as a method to reduce disease heterogeneity, the risk related to the required statistical assumptions may be disadvantageous [37]. Lead-in phases may be a useful tool in Phase I trials, to obtain natural history data to be used to shape later phases, such as how the trial population of ALS patients progresses in their diseases. However, their use in late-stage ALS trials can also spark an ethical debate, considering that patients who are living with a disease associated with constant losses must spend a significant portion of time on no treatment at all.

NAVIGATING REGULATORY NUANCES

The FDA and the European Medicines Agency (EMA) have released guidance documents for the conduct of clinical trials in ALS [38, 39]. Both documents are aligned on multiple key points, including discouraging (FDA) or prohibiting (EMA) use of historical controls as an acceptable placebo group and encouraging the use of time-to-event endpoints in the analysis, randomization methods to keep treatment arms balanced, and endpoints that evaluate both function and survival.

However, the guidance documents also differ on several key points, which can make trial design challenging for sponsors hoping to satisfy both agencies when applying for approval to conduct the trial and eventually when applying for market approval. Firstly, while the FDA recommends using the current consensus diagnosis criteria as eligibility criteria, the EMA outlines the use of the El Escorial criteria for diagnosis. Secondly, the FDA clearly states that clinical trials in ALS can evaluate scientifically justified subpopulations – for example, a trial of a disease-modifying therapy for ALS patients with a specific mutation causing their ALS; the EMA guidance is unclear on this matter. Finally, a significant point of disparity between the two documents is with regard to both trial duration and survival as an endpoint. The EMA guidance states that confirmatory clinical trials evaluating disease-modifying therapies should be 12–18 months in duration, whereas the FDA guidance recommends that 12 months is preferable for approval. Furthermore, while the EMA guidance stipulates evaluating endpoints of both function and survival, it also states that survival must be demonstrated and that extended follow-up to an efficacy trial may be needed to demonstrate this. In contrast, the FDA does not require that survival be demonstrated.

These discrepancies could result in delayed drug approvals in the future, as exemplified by the recent withdrawal of the edaravone application for approval in Europe [40]. In this case, comments on the review of the submission specifically stated that there was no demonstration of survival and that the trial, at 24 weeks, was too short.

FUTURE DIRECTIONS

While numerous challenges to conducting clinical trials in ALS have resulted in multiple failures over the years, a lot of groundwork has already been laid for addressing these challenges, as discussed below.

ADVANCES IN DISEASE UNDERSTANDING AND ASSESSMENT

As we come closer to having a better understanding of the underlying disease pathology, preclinical work is also taking advantage of better models of human ALS, including the use of induced pluripotent stem cells [41]. While the use of animal models will likely be needed as a gold standard of preclinical work, at least for the foreseeable future, use of multiple and varied models of human ALS should be employed to validate both drug targets and biomarkers so that we have as much information as possible to inform trial design. The use of multiple and varied models may also accommodate a lack of viable sporadic animal models.

Disease Heterogeneity

There has been much advancement recently in appreciating disease heterogeneity and its effect on clinical trials. Predictive models and randomization stratification methods are beginning to be employed regularly [10, 42–44]. The use of these models in randomized controlled trials for ALS is pending a definitive outcome; however, they hold strong potential to reduce heterogeneity amongst the included trial participants. Further to this, some trials currently in progress are using the rate of disease progression to enrich the patient population or stratify during randomization. As discussed above, there are some limitations to the use of lead-in phases to determine the rate of disease progression and the outcome measures frequently used for this purpose (e.g. ALSFRS-R). However, when set up carefully, the use of the rate of disease progression to stratify during randomization holds significant promise for reducing the confounding effect of disease heterogeneity in the assessment of efficacy in ALS trials. As such, a balanced and careful statistical consideration is needed when considering the use of a lead-in phase in an ALS trial.

Emerging Biomarkers

Some drug development programs have strategically used biomarker analysis to inform the design of future trials in ALS. An initial Phase II trial of NP001, an immune regulator of inflammation, failed to meet its primary endpoint; however, post hoc analysis demonstrated that patients with elevated wide range C-reactive protein (wr-CRP) levels at baseline, indicating higher baseline inflammation, appeared to respond better to treatment [45]. While these results were not statistically significant, they did guide the design of a subsequent trial in an enriched population with elevated wr-CRP levels at screening. While the subsequent trial also ultimately failed, this program was one of the first to demonstrate the use of a potential biomarker to assist in selecting patients who may respond better to treatment [46].

Several candidate biomarkers are emerging as potential pharmacodynamic markers, upon further validation, in future ALS clinical trials. Neurofilament light chain (NfL), detected in either cerebrospinal fluid (CSF) and/or blood, could potentially be used as an objective measure of disease progression [47]. While only found in reliable levels in the CSF, phosphorylated neurofilament heavy chain (pNfH) has been found to be negatively correlated with the ALSFRS-R, also making it a potential tool for evaluating disease progression [48]. Chitinases have been found to correlate with pNfH; however, further validation studies are required and ongoing [49]. Additionally, p57^{ECD} is also undergoing further investigation for its use as a marker of neurodegeneration [50]. Finally, TDP-43, which is a significant pathological marker for sporadic ALS, may be useful if the right detection methods, such as an assay that could detect altered TDP-43 in CSF or a PET tracer, can be developed [51].

The majority of ALS biomarker studies to date have focused on individual targets. As technology and our understanding evolve, it is likely that a multi-modal biomarker panel will provide a more sensitive measurement for clinical relevance in trials in the future.

Novel Outcome Measures

Some novel outcome measures are being evaluated for ALS, such as electrical impedance myography (EIM) and motor unit number index (MUNIX); however, neither is validated at this time [52, 53]. Despite not yet being validated, both are currently being used actively in various clinical trials as exploratory measures. This promotes the continuous search and development of novel outcome measures that could eventually contribute to evaluating clinically meaningful results in ALS.

As discussed earlier, the use of survival as a primary endpoint can impact the feasibility of a trial and should be combined with another endpoint or outcome measure. The Combined Assessment of Function and Survival (CAFS) allows both survival and function to be analyzed in a single endpoint. CAFS ranks each participant according to their outcome [54]. In other words, the worst rank is assigned to the participant who passes away first. The best rank is assigned to the participant who survives with the least amount of functional decline during the period of the trial. This produces an outcome that is relative to all of the other trial participants. The use of CAFS as a primary outcome in dexpramipexole trials has led to it becoming increasingly popular in ALS trials [22, 55]. While CAFS can provide a balanced analysis when used as a primary endpoint, it is still crucial to select clinically meaningful outcomes as secondary endpoints so that other potential signals are not lost.

Finally, it is becoming increasingly apparent that outcome measures used as primary and secondary efficacy endpoints in Phase III trials should not be standalone but ideally should be supported by biomarkers when possible.

NEW APPROACHES TO TRIAL DESIGN

Cautious Phase II Design

When performing Phase II trials in ALS, there needs to be a better balance between validating targets and testing quickly. In light of the multiple failures in Phase III, despite promising Phase II data, it has been postulated that conducting multiple, small Phase II trials might be a potential solution to avoiding investment in large Phase III failures [37].

Adaptive Trial Design

Adaptive trial designs are becoming increasingly popular in drug development, and the FDA already has guidance in place on this topic [56]. As per the FDA, an *adaptive trial design* is one that allows for prospectively planned modifications to one or more aspects of the design based on accumulating data from subjects in the trial. These can include modifications to patient eligibility criteria, endpoints, number of interim analyses, treatment regimen, sample size, and stratification [57]. The goal of using an adaptive design is to address clinical questions in a shorter time frame and with fewer participants than in sequential, linear drug development programs. There are multiple types of adaptive designs, and some of the most common are summarized in Table 9.1.

Adaptive trial designs have already been used in previous ALS trials, such as those that evaluated Coenzyme Q10, combination therapies (minocycline-creatine and celecoxib-creatine), ceftriaxone, and dexpramipexole [60–63]. It is likely that adaptive trial design will become a more consistent trend in ALS. Both gene therapies and in-depth biomarker analysis lend themselves to adaptive designs, whereby patients have the opportunity to be allocated to the treatment group that is most likely to benefit them.

In addition, popularized by Merck's development program of Keytruda in cancer therapy, expanding out of Phase I cohorts based on biomarker data and early efficacy signals could be employed more in the field of neurology [66]. Rapidly enrolling expansion cohorts and transitioning from Phase I through to later phases within the same trial could eventually replace the need for separate, step-wise trials for each phase. This approach, somewhat of a blend between seamless and expansion cohort designs, is being used in the ongoing VALOR-ALS trial of Tofersen, an antisense oligo-nucleotide therapy (Biogen) for *SOD1*-mutated ALS [64].

Platform Trials

Traditionally, clinical trials evaluate a single therapy under one protocol [67]. In contrast, a *platform* trial, popularized in oncology, evaluates multiple therapies under one master protocol, similar to building a stadium that can accommodate multiple sporting events as opposed to tearing down and rebuilding the stadium after each game (Figure 9.1). A platform trial allows testing of multiple therapies in a manner

TABLE 9.1   Common adaptive trial designs.

Design	Concept	Examples in ALS
Response adaptive	Modifications can be made to the randomization schedule or ratios based on participant response to the intervention.	
Group sequential	The trial can be stopped prematurely for safety, futility, or efficacy concerns, based on interim analysis results. A common example is the "3 + 3" design used in Phase 1 oncology trials.	• Minocycline-creatine combination [60] • Celecoxib-creatine combination [60]
Sample size re-estimation	Sample size can be increased or decreased to achieve target power based on interim analysis results.	
Seamless	The objectives of multiple phases are combined into one trial, and data from all participants are included in the analysis. For example, a Phase II and a Phase III design may be combined into a single trial (Phase II/III).	• Coenzyme Q10 [61] • Dexpramipexole [62] • Ceftriaxone [63] • VALOR-ALS [64]
Biomarker adaptive	Modifications can be made to the trial design based on participant response to biomarkers.	• NP001 [46]
Expansion cohort	Commonly used in Phase 1 trials. Additional participants are added after the maximum tolerated dose (MTD) has been determined to obtain more data on the estimated MTD, as well as the drug activity. Expansion cohort design has been combined with seamless design, with the most notable case being the development of Merck's Keytruda [65].	• VALOR-ALS [64]

Sources: Bhattacharyya and Rai [57], Pallmann et al. [58], and Mahajan and Gupta [59].

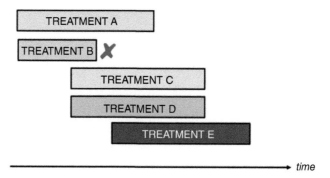

FIGURE 9.1   Platform trials allow the evaluation of multiple therapies under one clinical trial protocol and setup. Therapies under evaluation do not necessarily all commence at the same time, at the outset of the trial. Similarly, therapies can be dropped from the platform if interim analyses demonstrates either a safety concern or futility. *Source*: Based on Schultz et al. [67].

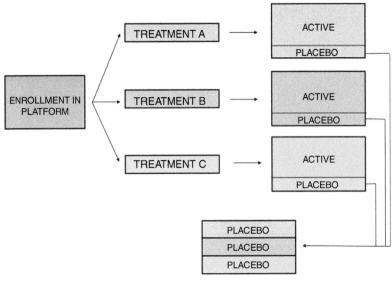

FIGURE 9.2   Platform trials reduce the number of participants assigned to the placebo group in each treatment arm. Each therapy under evaluation has its own placebo group, and all placebo groups from all treatment arms are pooled and used as the comparator for the entire trial. *Source*: Based on Schultz et al. [67].

that reduces both time to results and overall trial cost. New therapies can be added at any time, and any that meet criteria for futility can be dropped.

This marriage of a master protocol design and adaptive design reduces the placebo group size by pooling placebo groups across treatment arms (Figure 9.2).

Multiple platform trials for ALS are slated to launch in 2020, including The Sean M. Healy and AMG Center for ALS Platform Trial, the MND-SMART trial, and the TRICALS MAGNET trial [68–70].

Bayesian Statistics

Since the inception of the randomized-controlled trial in the 1940s, clinical trial design has largely relied on frequentist statistics [71]. This approach has changed in recent times, with clinical trialists more frequently employing Bayesian statistics. Bayesian statistics express probability based on a "degree of belief" in an event, where this belief is based on "prior knowledge." Bayesian statistics can have beneficial characteristics for adaptive trial designs. For example, the posterior predictive probability feature of the Bayesian approach allows for more frequent monitoring of trial data and subsequent adaptation of the trial methodology, by incorporating the data into the prior knowledge [72].

EDUCATION

Education is a more recent topic with regard to clinical trials in ALS and can be achieved with a two-pronged approach.

From a patient perspective, having access to information about available clinical trials can empower patients and their caregivers to have an active role in their care and encourage them to ask their physician about specific trials. Disseminating information to patients also has a profound impact on recruitment. From our perspective, providing accessible clinical trial information sessions for patient support groups and other patient-focused events can lead to great success in increasing recruitment. Early patient engagement in understanding research is also crucial. Our research team makes every effort to engage with and discuss research with all patients in our ALS clinic, regardless of whether they are currently participating in research, be it a clinical trial of an investigational intervention or an observational study. In this modern age of having access to large amounts of information on the internet and through social media platforms, guidance on interpreting this information, including being wary of unsupported claims, is important for supporting health literacy on ALS among patients and their families. As an example, publicity surrounding new experimental therapies that have yet to be fully validated by current standards can be detrimental to clinical trial recruitment and clinical care [66].

From a clinical perspective, there is a need for broader education on early diagnosis of ALS. As sponsors try to enrich their participant populations and reduce heterogeneity in their trials, there is a current trend in narrowing inclusion criteria to a shorter interval between symptom onset and diagnosis. Community neurologists and family practitioners must be familiar with early signs and symptoms of ALS, as they need to refer potential cases of ALS to a specialist to confirm the diagnosis as soon as possible. Timely diagnosis of patients with ALS will ultimately provide more opportunities to participate in trials in which the window between symptom onset and diagnosis is a criterion for eligibility.

PEOPLE MAKE OR BREAK A TRIAL

It is currently an unprecedented time of enthusiasm for clinical trials in ALS, as more than 100 biotech or pharmaceutical companies have ALS therapies in clinical trials or their drug development pipeline. These include, at the time of this publication, Alexion Pharmaceuticals Inc., Amylyx Pharmaceuticals, Avexis, Biogen, Brainstorm Cell Therapeutics, Cytokinetics Inc., Medicinova Inc., Orion Corporation, Orphazyme, Pfizer (partnership with Sangamo Therapeutics), and Sanofi (partnership with Denali Therapeutics), to name a few. Ultimately, the people involved at every step of the process and their respective capabilities are critical for successfully conducting clinical trials in ALS.

Now more than ever, the pharmaceutical industry and the community of clinicians and scientists need to engage with each other to share expertise on this disease and the lessons learned from past failures. They also need staff who are engaged with the community and are passionate about solving this disease. Trial sponsors, whether from industry or academia, will need to look at the most novel and rapid trial design approaches for well-designed trials to get much-needed treatments to patients. Clinical care and clinical research sites need to work with patients as research partners, not just trial subjects, to address the challenges associated with participant recruitment and retention.

Offering a synergistic approach to both research and clinical care provides a positive experience that can encourage participation in clinical trials. To this day, multidisciplinary care is still the only management option available that extends life to a significant degree in ALS [73, 74]. Therefore, combining clinical trials alongside exceptional patient care provides the most optimal setting to meet recruitment targets and avoid dropouts. Due to their complex nature and a high burden on patients, ALS trials should be conducted only by centers with experience in caring for patients living with ALS, and with access to multidisciplinary care. Having research staff interact directly with patients contributes significantly to successful recruitment and retention. As an example, our clinic at the Montreal Neurological Institute-Hospital saw a staggering increase in recruitment after the research coordinator was fully integrated into the multidisciplinary care team. Furthermore, this integration, and seamless interface between research and clinical care, allows the research staff to continuously monitor prospective patients and react quickly to ensure that potential participants are identified and informed early, which is important for trials with restrictive inclusion criteria. Conversely, this setup also ensures that the care team is kept informed, in real time, of the medical, physical, and social needs of the patients and their caregivers.

Conclusion

Despite a lackluster history, today we are closer than ever to seeing promising therapies become available to patients living with ALS. This dedicated field has extensively studied past failures to ensure that mistakes of the past are not repeated in future trials. Trial design in ALS is becoming more innovative and efficient as our understanding of the disease pathology progresses and novel biomarkers and outcome measures become available. By using all of the available information about ALS, it is hoped that the clinical research community will continue to work together to design better trials to identify the best possible treatments for our patients.

ACKNOWLEDGMENTS

We would like to thank both Dr. Trisha Rao and Dr. Hannah Kaneb for providing editorial support in the writing of this chapter. We would also like to thank the ALS

Team at the Montreal Neurological Institute-Hospital Clinical Research Unit, as well as the Multidisciplinary ALS Clinic, for their insight and perspectives on ALS trial challenges and solutions. Finally, thank you to all of the ALS patients who have participated in clinical trials in the past, without whom the field would not be as advanced as it is today, and to those patients who will participate in clinical trials in the future, all of whom are contributing to a future without ALS.

CONFLICT OF INTEREST

Kristiana Salmon reports no conflict of interest. Angela Genge currently serves on the advisory boards of Avexis, Alexion, AL-S Pharma, Biogen, Brainstorm, Akcea, Cytokinetics, Sanofi, Mitsubishi, and Novartis.

COPYRIGHT AND PERMISSION STATEMENT

To the best of our knowledge, the materials included in this chapter do not violate copyright laws. All original sources have been appropriately acknowledged and/or referenced. Where relevant, appropriate permissions have been obtained from the original copyright holder(s).

REFERENCES

1. Van Damme, P., Robberecht, W., and Van Den Bosch, L. (2017). Modelling amyotrophic lateral sclerosis: progress and possibilities. *Dis Model Mech* 10 (5): 537–549.
2. Miller, R.G., Bouchard, J.P., Duquette, P. et al. (1996). Clinical trials of riluzole in patients with ALS. *Neurology* 47 (4 Suppl 2): 86S–92S.
3. Writing, G. and Edaravone, A.L.S.S.G. (2017). Safety and efficacy of edaravone in well defined patients with amyotrophic lateral sclerosis: a randomised, double-blind, placebo-controlled trial. *Lancet Neurol* 16 (7): 505–512.
4. D'Arcy, H.P. (1999). A change in scientific approach: from alternation to randomised allocation in clinical trials in the 1940s. *BMJ* 319 (7209): 572–573.
5. van den Berg, L.H., Sorenson, E., Gronseth, G. et al. (2019). Revised airlie house consensus guidelines for design and implementation of ALS clinical trials. *Neurology* 92 (14): e1610–e1623.
6. Goyal, N.A., Berry, J.D., Windebank, A. et al. (2020). Addressing heterogeneity in amyotrophic lateral sclerosis CLINICAL TRIALS. *Muscle Nerve* 62: 156–166.
7. Taylor, J.P., Brown, R.H. Jr., and Cleveland, D.W. (2016). Decoding ALS: from genes to mechanism. *Nature* 539 (7628): 197–206.
8. Fournier, C. and Glass, J.D. (2015). Modeling the course of amyotrophic lateral sclerosis. *Nat Biotechnol* 33 (1): 45–47.

9. Cudkowicz, M.E., McKenna-Yasek, D., Sapp, P.E. et al. (1997). Epidemiology of mutations in superoxide dismutase in amyotrophic lateral sclerosis. *Ann Neurol* 41 (2): 210–221.

10. van Eijk, R.P.A., Westeneng, H.J., Nikolakopoulos, S. et al. (2019). Refining eligibility criteria for amyotrophic lateral sclerosis clinical trials. *Neurology* 92 (5): e451–e460.

11. Cedarbaum, J.M., Stambler, N., Malta, E. et al. (1999). The ALSFRS-R: a revised ALS functional rating scale that incorporates assessments of respiratory function. BDNF ALS study group (phase III). *J Neurol Sci* 169 (1-2): 13–21.

12. Proudfoot, M., Jones, A., Talbot, K. et al. (2016). The ALSFRS as an outcome measure in therapeutic trials and its relationship to symptom onset. *Amyotroph Lateral Scler Frontotemporal Degener* 17 (5-6): 414–425.

13. Bedlack, R.S., Vaughan, T., Wicks, P. et al. (2016). How common are ALS plateaus and reversals? *Neurology* 86 (9): 808–812.

14. Czaplinski, A., Yen, A.A., and Appel, S.H. (2006). Forced vital capacity (FVC) as an indicator of survival and disease progression in an ALS clinic population. *J Neurol Neurosurg Psychiatry* 77 (3): 390–392.

15. Pinto, S. and de Carvalho, M. (2019). SVC is a marker of respiratory decline function, similar to FVC, in patients with ALS. *Front Neurol* 10: 109.

16. Fortis, S., Corazalla, E.O., Wang, Q., and Kim, H.J. (2015). The difference between slow and forced vital capacity increases with increasing body mass index: a paradoxical difference in low and normal body mass indices. *Respir Care* 60 (1): 113–118.

17. Lechtzin, N., Cudkowicz, M.E., de Carvalho, M. et al. (2018). Respiratory measures in amyotrophic lateral sclerosis. *Amyotroph Lateral Scler Frontotemporal Degener* 19 (5-6): 321–330.

18. Melo, J., Homma, A., Iturriaga, E. et al. (1999). Pulmonary evaluation and prevalence of non-invasive ventilation in patients with amyotrophic lateral sclerosis: a multi-center survey and proposal of a pulmonary protocol. *J Neurol Sci* 169 (1-2): 114–117.

19. Shefner, J.M., Liu, D., Leitner, M.L. et al. (2016). Quantitative strength testing in ALS clinical trials. *Neurology* 87 (6): 617–624.

20. Gordon, P.H., Corcia, P., Lacomblez, L. et al. (2009). Defining survival as an outcome measure in amyotrophic lateral sclerosis. *Arch Neurol* 66 (6): 758–761.

21. Paganoni, S., Cudkowicz, M., and Berry, J.D. (2014). Outcome measures in amyotrophic lateral sclerosis clinical trials. *Clin Investig (Lond)* 4 (7): 605–618.

22. Cudkowicz, M.E., van den Berg, L.H., Shefner, J.M. et al. (2013). Dexpramipexole versus placebo for patients with amyotrophic lateral sclerosis (EMPOWER): a randomised, double-blind, phase 3 trial. *Lancet Neurol* 12 (11): 1059–1067.

23. Cudkowicz, M.E., Titus, S., Kearney, M. et al. (2014). Safety and efficacy of ceftriaxone for amyotrophic lateral sclerosis: a multi-stage, randomised, double-blind, placebo-controlled trial. *Lancet Neurol* 13 (11): 1083–1091.

24. Group UK-LS, Morrison, K.E., Dhariwal, S. et al. (2013). Lithium in patients with amyotrophic lateral sclerosis (LiCALS): a phase 3 multicentre, randomised, double-blind, placebo-controlled trial. *Lancet Neurol* 12 (4): 339–345.

25. Pascuzzi, R.M., Shefner, J., Chappell, A.S. et al. (2010). A phase II trial of talam-panel in subjects with amyotrophic lateral sclerosis. *Amyotroph Lateral Scler* 11 (3): 266–271.

26. Aggarwal, S. and Cudkowicz, M. (2008). ALS drug development: reflections from the past and a way forward. *Neurotherapeutics* 5 (4): 516–527.

27. Shefner, J.M. (2008). Designing clinical trials in amyotrophic lateral sclerosis. *Phys Med Rehabil Clin N Am* 19 (3): 495–508, ix.

28. Cudkowicz, M.E., Katz, J., Moore, D.H. et al. (2010). Toward more efficient clinical trials for amyotrophic lateral sclerosis. *Amyotroph Lateral Scler* 11 (3): 259–265.

29. Shefner, J.M., Wolff, A.A., Meng, L. et al. (2016). A randomized, placebo-controlled, double-blind phase IIb trial evaluating the safety and efficacy of tirasemtiv in patients with amyotrophic lateral sclerosis. *Amyotroph Lateral Scler Frontotemporal Degener* 17 (5-6): 426–435.

30. Shefner, J.M., Cudkowicz, M.E., Hardiman, O. et al. (2019). A phase III trial of tirasemtiv as a potential treatment for amyotrophic lateral sclerosis. *Amyotroph Lateral Scler Frontotemporal Degener* 0 (0): 1–11.

31. Cykokinetics. (2019). Cytokinetics announces results of FORTITUDE-ALS, a Phase 2 clinical trial of reldesemtiv in patients with ALS, presented at American Academy of Neurology Annual Meeting. Press release (6 May).

32. Nipp, R.D., Hong, K., and Paskett, E.D. (2019). Overcoming barriers to clinical trial enrollment. *Am Soc Clin Oncol Educ Book* 39: 105–114.

33. Treweek, S., Pitkethly, M., Cook, J. et al. (2018). Strategies to improve recruitment to randomised trials. *Cochrane Database Syst Rev* 2: MR000013.

34. de Carvalho, M., Pinto, S., Costa, J. et al. (2010). A randomized, placebo-controlled trial of memantine for functional disability in amyotrophic lateral sclerosis. *Amyotroph Lateral Scler* 11 (5): 456–460.

35. Gordon, P.H., Moore, D.H., Miller, R.G. et al. (2007). Efficacy of minocycline in patients with amyotrophic lateral sclerosis: a phase III randomised trial. *Lancet Neurol* 6 (12): 1045–1053.

36. Miller, R., Bradley, W., Cudkowicz, M. et al. (2007). Phase II/III randomized trial of TCH346 in patients with ALS. *Neurology* 69 (8): 776–784.

37. Schoenfeld, D.A. and Cudkowicz, M. (2008). Design of phase II ALS clinical trials. *Amyotroph Lateral Scler* 9 (1): 16–23.

38. US Food and Drug Administration. (2019). Amyotrophic lateral sclerosis: developing drugs for treatment guidance for industry. Center for Drug Evaluation and Research (CDER).

39. European Medicines Agency. (2015). Guideline on clinical investigation of medicinal products for the treatment of amyotrophic lateral sclerosis (ALS). Committee for Medicinal Product for Human Use.

40. European Medicines Agency. (2019). Withdrawal assessment report: Radicava. Committee for Medicinal Product for Human Use.

41. de Boer, A.S. and Eggan, K. (2015). A perspective on stem cell modeling of amyotrophic lateral sclerosis. *Cell Cycle* 14 (23): 3679–3688.

42. Berry, J.D., Taylor, A.A., Beaulieu, D. et al. (2018). Improved stratification of ALS clinical trials using predicted survival. *Ann Clin Transl Neurol* 5 (4): 474–485.

43. Jahandideh, S., Taylor, A.A., Beaulieu, D. et al. (2018). Longitudinal modeling to predict vital capacity in amyotrophic lateral sclerosis. *Amyotroph Lateral Scler Frontotemporal Degener* 19 (3-4): 294–302.

44. Taylor, A.A., Fournier, C., Polak, M. et al. (2016). Predicting disease progression in amyotrophic lateral sclerosis. *Ann Clin Transl Neurol* 3 (11): 866–875.

45. Miller, R.G., Block, G., Katz, J.S. et al. (2015). Randomized phase 2 trial of NP001-a novel immune regulator: safety and early efficacy in ALS. *Neurol Neuroimmunol Neuroinflamm* 2 (3): e100.

46. Neuraltus Pharmaceuticals. (2018). Reports results from phase 2 NP001 study in amyotrophic lateral sclerosis (ALS). Press release (26 April).

47. Turner, M.R. (2018). Progress and new frontiers in biomarkers for amyotrophic lateral sclerosis. *Biomark Med* 12 (7): 693–696.

48. Xu, Z., Henderson, R.D., David, M., and McCombe, P.A. (2016). Neurofilaments as biomarkers for amyotrophic lateral sclerosis: a systematic review and meta-analysis. *PLoS One* 11 (10): e0164625.

49. Thompson, A.G., Gray, E., Thezenas, M.L. et al. (2018). Cerebrospinal fluid macrophage biomarkers in amyotrophic lateral sclerosis. *Ann Neurol* 83 (2): 258–268.

50. Verber, N.S., Shepheard, S.R., Sassani, M. et al. (2019). Biomarkers in motor neuron disease: a state of the art review. *Front Neurol* 10: 291.

51. Majumder, V., Gregory, J.M., Barria, M.A. et al. (2018). TDP-43 as a potential biomarker for amyotrophic lateral sclerosis: a systematic review and meta-analysis. *BMC Neurol* 18 (1): 90.

52. Neuwirth, C., Braun, N., Claeys, K.G. et al. (2018). Implementing motor unit number index (MUNIX) in a large clinical trial: real world experience from 27 centres. *Clin Neurophysiol* 129 (8): 1756–1762.

53. Rutkove, S.B., Caress, J.B., Cartwright, M.S. et al. (2012). Electrical impedance myography as a biomarker to assess ALS progression. *Amyotroph Lateral Scler* 13 (5): 439–445.

54. Berry, J.D., Miller, R., Moore, D.H. et al. (2013). The combined assessment of function and survival (CAFS): a new endpoint for ALS clinical trials. *Amyotroph Lateral Scler Frontotemporal Degener* 14 (3): 162–168.

55. Rudnicki, S.A., Berry, J.D., Ingersoll, E. et al. (2013). Dexpramipexole effects on functional decline and survival in subjects with amyotrophic lateral sclerosis in a phase II study: subgroup analysis of demographic and clinical characteristics. *Amyotroph Lateral Scler Frontotemporal Degener* 14 (1): 44–51.

56. US Food and Drug Administration. (2019). Adaptive design clinical trials for drugs and biologics guidance for industry. Center for Drug Evaluation and Research (CDER).

57. Bhattacharyya, A. and Rai, S.N. (2019). Adaptive signature design- review of the biomarker guided adaptive phase -III controlled design. *Contemp Clin Trials Commun* 15: 100378.

58. Pallmann, P., Bedding, A.W., Choodari-Oskooei, B. et al. (2018). Adaptive designs in clinical trials: why use them, and how to run and report them. *BMC Med* 16 (1): 29.

59. Mahajan, R. and Gupta, K. (2010). Adaptive design clinical trials: methodology, challenges and prospect. *Indian J Pharmacol* 42 (4): 201–207.

60. Gordon, P.H., Cheung, Y.K., Levin, B. et al. (2008). A novel, efficient, randomized selection trial comparing combinations of drug therapy for ALS. *Amyotroph Lateral Scler* 9 (4): 212–222.

61. Levy, G., Kaufmann, P., Buchsbaum, R. et al. (2006). A two-stage design for a phase II clinical trial of coenzyme Q10 in ALS. *Neurology* 66 (5): 660–663.

62. Cudkowicz, M., Bozik, M.E., Ingersoll, E.W. et al. (2011). The effects of dexpramipexole (KNS-760704) in individuals with amyotrophic lateral sclerosis. *Nat Med* 17 (12): 1652–1656.

63. Abstracts of the 20th International Symposium on Amyotrophic Lateral Sclerosis/ Motor Neuron Diseases (ALS/MND). December 8-10, 2009. Berlin, Germany. Amyotroph Lateral Scler. 2009; 10 Suppl 1 : 7-205.

64. Biogen. (2020). NCT02623699: An efficacy, safety, tolerability, pharmacokinetics and pharmacodynamics study of BIIB067 in adults with inherited amyotrophic lateral sclerosis (ALS) (VALOR [Part C]). https://clinicaltrials.gov/ct2/show/NCT02623699.

65. Merck Sharp & Dohme Corp. (2019). NCT01295827: Study of pembrolizumab (MK-3475) in participants with progressive locally advanced or metastatic carcinoma, melanoma, or non-small cell lung carcinoma (P07990/MK-3475-001/KEYNOTE-001) (KEYNOTE-001). https://clinicaltrials.gov/ct2/show/NCT01295827.

66. Sipp, D. (2011). The unregulated commercialization of stem cell treatments: a global perspective. *Front Med* 5 (4): 348–355.

67. Schultz, A., Saville, B.R., Marsh, J.A., and Snelling, T.L. (2019). An introduction to clinical trial design. *Paediatr Respir Rev* 32: 30–35.

68. Platform Communications: Abstract Book -30th International Symposium on ALS/ MND (Complete printable file). Amyotroph Lateral Scler Frontotemporal Degener. 2019; 20 (sup1): 1-99.

69. University of Edinburgh. (2020). NCT04302870: Motor neurone disease - systematic multi-arm adaptive randomised trial (MND-SMART). https://clinicaltrials.gov/ct2/show/NCT04302870.

70. TRICALS. (2020). MAGNET trial. https://www.tricals.org/trials/magnet/.

71. Lee, J.J. and Chu, C.T. (2012). Bayesian clinical trials in action. *Stat Med* 31 (25): 2955–2972.

72. Yin, G., Lam, C.K., and Shi, H. (2017). Bayesian randomized clinical trials: from fixed to adaptive design. *Contemp Clin Trials* 59: 77–86.

73. Traynor, B.J., Alexander, M., Corr, B. et al. (2003). Effect of a multidisciplinary amyotrophic lateral sclerosis (ALS) clinic on ALS survival: a population based study, 1996–2000. *J Neurol Neurosurg Psychiatry* 74 (9): 1258–1261.

74. Rooney, J., Byrne, S., Heverin, M. et al. (2015). A multidisciplinary clinic approach improves survival in ALS: a comparative study of ALS in Ireland and Northern Ireland. *J Neurol Neurosurg Psychiatry* 86 (5): 496–501.

CHAPTER 10

Future Priorities and Directions in ALS Research and Treatment

Jessica R. Morrice[1], Michael Kuo[2], and Christopher A. Shaw[1–4]

[1] *Experimental Medicine Program, University of British Columbia, Vancouver, British Columbia, Canada*
[2] *Department of Ophthalmology and Visual Sciences, University of British Columbia, Vancouver, British Columbia, Canada*
[3] *Department of Pathology, University of British Columbia, Vancouver, British Columbia, Canada*
[4] *Program in Neuroscience, University of British Columbia, Vancouver, British Columbia, Canada*

INTRODUCTION

After close to 150 years since amyotrophic lateral sclerosis (ALS) was first described by Charcot [1], and nearly 30 years since causative mutations in superoxide dismutase 1 (SOD1) enzyme were discovered [2], ALS remains a disease whose sporadic origins are still largely unknown. While examples exist for the possible toxin-based etiology in geographical isolates such as Guam [3], applying these to the rest of the world's ALS cases has not yielded clear correlates. The past decade has revealed a number of causative mutations (see Chapter 2), risk factors including toxic factors and susceptibility genes (see Chapters 3 and 4), and pathological features both common and unique to etiological subgroups (see Chapters 5–7). All of these provide support for a spectrum nature of ALS and highlight the clinical heterogeneity of this disease (see Chapter 1).

Researchers and clinicians are increasingly beginning to appreciate this heterogeneity in disease presentation and progression, although we may still be in the infancy of understanding the heterogeneity of pathogenic features. In particular, such heterogeneity in presentation, and presumably mechanism, likely impacts efforts to advance the field by discovering one or more reliable biomarker(s) and developing effective therapeutics. The ultimate goal is to make ALS a treatable disease regardless of potentially unique origins of ALS subtypes on the disease spectrum. Currently, patients remain limited in their therapeutic options (see Chapter 9), and indeed this desperation has driven some to seek out alternative, scientifically untested treatments [2].

As poignantly described by Ted Stehr in the Preface, people living with ALS are precariously clinging to life, supported by the efforts of their loved ones and health care providers, and are desperately seeking hope for a better future – if not for themselves, then for future ALS patients. In this context, it remains critical to continue to expand our findings from the laboratory and reflect on the patient population they are intended to represent (see Chapter 8), and perhaps to fully embrace the complex nature of this disease rather than attempting to simplify it by applying overly reductionist approaches.

ETIOLOGICAL HETEROGENEITY OF ALS

Currently, 2–3/100 000 people are diagnosed with ALS, where 50% also present with cognitive impairment and an estimated 10–15% of ALS patients are diagnosed with frontotemporal dementia (ALS-FTD). Disease presentation in others is restricted to lower motor neurons or upper motor neurons, as in progressive muscular atrophy (PMA) and primary lateral sclerosis (PLS), respectively [4, 5]. Some ALS patients initially present with dysfunction in lower limbs, upper limbs, or bulbar-innervated regions or have respiratory symptom onset (see [6] for further review). Further, certain patients have an aggressive disease course, while others live for decades [6], as in the case of Stephen Hawking. Some of these features can be predicted by specific gene mutations [7], but in most cases, the features of disease course appear to be unique to each patient.

The past decade has revealed the majority of genes causing disease in families, or at least those following a pattern of Mendelian inheritance. Mutations in SOD1 are important to highlight as this was the first gene identified in familial ALS (fALS) [2] and the first used to model pathological features *in vitro* and *in vivo*; consequently, it has the best-characterized pathology. Models of this mutation have uncovered pathogenic features such as glutamate excitotoxicity, mitochondrial dysfunction, and proteinopathy. However, it is important to note that mutations in SOD1 have unique pathological features as compared to other gene mutations, such as an absence of TAR DNA-binding protein 43 (TDP-43) pathology, the latter being evident in up to 97% of sporadic ALS (sALS) cases, and no evidence to support RNA toxicity due to the lack of an RNA binding motif [8]. This result suggests that the mechanism, at least in part, underlying mutant SOD1-induced motor neuron degeneration may not be representative of all ALS subtypes. Indeed, symptom onset in the bulbar region is common in ALS patients with a mutation in chromosome 9 open reading frame 72 (*C9orf72*) and very rare in patients with a mutation in SOD1 [6]. Further, the transcriptomic profile of motor neurons in patients with SOD1 mutations and *C9orf72* pathological repeat expansions are distinct [9], suggestive of a unique cellular dysfunction underlying these mutations. This may be true of each specific etiology, and it will be interesting to pursue this concept as pathological features underlying mutations to different genes, environmental stressors, or gene-toxin models continue to be described in various gene and environmental models as such research progresses.

The same can be said for the mechanisms underlying sALS and whether the same features in fALS are also evident in sALS. The mechanism underlying sALS remains less well characterized in comparison to gene mutations, as there are fewer validated models available, although some notable *in vivo* sALS models exist [10–13]. The majority of data available for sALS is based on patient data, which is not available to a similar level of analysis through scientific manipulation as in laboratory models. As such, much of the current literature on sALS is based on *post mortem* samples, providing critical insight into end-stage disease features only. At this time, studies on early and midcourse pathological mechanisms in sALS patients remain unattainable: as patients present with symptoms of motor dysfunction after an estimated 70% of neuronal loss [14], with an additional year to diagnosis [15], many motor neurons have undergone degeneration. Importantly, it is of note that some studies in sALS patients are based on surviving motor neurons in post mortem tissue [16, 17], although it is unclear whether these motor neurons are representative of upstream pathogenesis or harbor qualities that render them more resistant to degeneration.

One feature that seems to be representative of most ALS cases is TDP-43 proteinopathy, and perhaps aggregated fused in sarcoma (FUS), as Tyzack et al. have recently reported [18]. As this feature has proven to be a nearly universal pathological finding, it warrants prioritization in both characterizing the pathobiology and exploiting its diagnostic and therapeutic potential.

ALS RISK FACTORS

As briefly discussed throughout this book, a number of risk factors have been described for sALS. Despite long being suspected of having an important role in sALS, no single environmental factor has demonstrated a clear causal role in disease. It remains to be determined if disease onset is triggered by multiple accumulating factors or a genetic susceptibility to a specific environmental factor or, indeed, if sALS – or at least a subset of cases – is an omnigenic or polygenic disease.

It will be interesting to uncover whether all risk factors follow a similar pathway of motor neuron dysfunction or if upstream mechanisms are unique yet lead to a common downstream pathology in motor neurons. Indeed, a number of features make motor neurons more vulnerable to dysfunction than other cells. Motor neurons have extremely high metabolic requirements, and fast-fatigable and fast-resistant motor neurons appear to be more vulnerable to degeneration compared to slow motor neurons in mutant SOD1 (mSOD1) models [19]. Also, these cells are post-mitotic and therefore unable to lessen the burden of misfolded or pathologically aggregated proteins by division to daughter cells through mitosis. These are among the largest neurons in the body, highlighting how dysfunction in axonal transport may render these cells more vulnerable than other cell types. Further, motor neurons vulnerable to degeneration have unique gene expression and metabolic profiles [20], suggesting a genetic predisposition to stress or dysfunction.

Although environmental factors have been associated with sALS, a clear etiology underlying environmental associations with disease remains unclear. As different pathologic mechanisms are believed to underlie specific gene mutations (i.e. gain of toxic function [21] or loss of function [22]), the same may be true of different environment-associated disease mechanisms. An array of environmental factors, including a variety of toxins/toxicants, are being investigated by different groups to tease out causal roles, including gene-toxin interactions [23–25]. Such gene-toxin studies are in their infancy in ALS, and careful investigation may provide critical insight into the etiology behind a genetic predisposition to toxic agents.

Microbial etiology, specifically a viral basis of disease, remains an active and intriguing area of research. Considering that viruses have been integrating into the human genome for millions of years, it may not be surprising that ~8% of our genome is viral [26]. Indeed, evidence for enteroviruses, retroviruses, and herpesvirus are evident in ALS patients and thus are suspected to be involved in some cases of disease [27]. In fact, enteroviruses have been demonstrated to reproduce ALS-like features *in vivo* [13]. It therefore remains plausible that viral agents induce or participate in ALS susceptibility.

The escalation in depth and volume of genetic studies in ALS demonstrates that the description of the genetic architecture in ALS is expanding [28]. As more genes and genetic factors are being revealed, a greater comprehensive description of the genetic aspects of ALS is being exposed. Further, common biological themes may continue to reveal possible mechanisms underlying pathological hallmarks features such as proteinopathy. It will be of utmost importance to continue these studies in an etiologic-specific context, as it is important to determine whether upstream mechanisms underlying each sALS and fALS case are unique.

One of the most important risk factors of ALS is age. Aside from specific cases involving a mutation in the *ALS2*, SETX, and FUS genes that causes disease in younger individuals [29–31], advanced age is a strong risk factor for ALS. This disease most commonly strikes in an individual's 50–60th year [6]; however, age of onset can also be variable. On average, patients with fALS tend to develop disease an estimated five years earlier than sALS [32], although the ALS variant on Guam also affected younger individuals [32]. Patients with older age of symptom onset are less likely to have upper motor neuron involvement and are more prone to bulbar symptom onset [6]. Also, aging has an inverse relationship with disease course. Patients who present with symptoms at a later age tend to follow a more aggressive disease course as compared to patients with younger disease onset, particularly with onset after age 80 [6]. Aging thus may represent loss of compensatory function to dysfunction or accumulation of cellular stressors or toxins.

As described in Chapter 1, ALS is a clinically heterogeneous disease. This observation may reflect a mechanistically heterogeneous pathology with common end-stage features, a mechanistically homogenous pathology with the involvement of heterogeneous modifying factors, or simply that the medical field has used an umbrella term of *ALS* for multiple different diseases with progressive motor neuron degeneration in common.

CELLULAR DYSFUNCTION IN ALS

Proteinopathy is a hallmark feature in ALS. mSOD1 models first demonstrated that mutations in SOD1 cause the protein to misfold and aggregate. The specific misfolded conformation can be mutation-specific [33, 34]; thus there are groups focused on developing different antibodies targeting each misfolded SOD1 isoform. Likewise, the remaining ALS cases show evident nuclear depletion and pathologic cytoplasmic aggregates of the RNA-binding proteins TDP-43 and also FUS [18, 35]. Many groups focus on the role of proteinopathy in driving disease, which is a feature common not only to all cases of ALS but also to other neurodegenerative diseases, including Alzheimer's disease and Parkinson's disease [36]. There is also evidence that RNA dysregulation and altered metabolism are common features in most cases of ALS [37]. This work may alternatively suggest that proteinopathy is a consequence of RNA pathology, which in turn may be downstream to defects evident in the nuclear pore complex [38]. The relationship between RNA dysregulation and proteinopathy remains to be fully understood in various genetic and environmental models.

ALS is known to be a non-cell-autonomous disease where glial cells, including microglia, play a key role, indicating the importance of the immune system in disease. Although the specific mechanism of the immune system's role in disease is not comprehensively understood, most evidence suggests that the central and peripheral immune systems appear to be implicated in disease progression. Microglia appear to be in a neuroprotective phenotype during early disease and transition to a more neurotoxic state during later stages of neurodegeneration [39] (see Chapter 7). Likewise, cells in the peripheral immune system appear to transition from a neuroprotective to a neurotoxic state during disease progression (see [40] for further review). Evidence from patient studies propose that different peripheral immune cell types are dysregulated, suggesting that distinct immune cell types have differential roles in disease progression. Systemic inflammation of peripheral immune cells such as T cells and neutrophils infiltrate tissues that are pathologically relevant to ALS like the affected regions of the spinal and atrophied muscle tissue [41]. Whether this finding is a cause or consequence of more initiating upstream pathology, such as from the breakdown of the blood-brain barrier, remains an open question in the field [41].

Disappointingly, many immune therapies that have gone to clinical trials have failed. The anti-inflammatory agent minocycline, which blocks microglial function, demonstrated promising therapeutic effects in animal models [42] but failed in clinical trials as it caused an accelerated progression of disease [43]. These results highlight how our understanding of the immune system's role in ALS is still insufficient and adds scrutiny to the applicability of using monogenetic disease models for a heterogeneous disease (see Chapter 8). However, the immune system remains a prioritized therapeutic target for ALS, and different Phase II/III clinical trials targeting inflammation and T regulatory cells in ALS are currently underway [44, 45].

A more recent finding in ALS is the possible involvement of the microbiome (see Chapter 5). Research in this field is in its infancy as compared to other pathologic mechanisms, but initial studies demonstrate that dysbiosis aggravates disease, and studies using genetic animal models demonstrate that restoring the balance of microbial diversity in the gut can alleviate features of disease [46]. Considering that the microbiome can be altered based on environmental factors such as diet, restoring a healthy microbiome in patients is an intriguing method of intervention well worth further pursuit.

Despite much research characterizing pathogenesis in different models, efforts have shifted to be more heavily weighted toward screening therapeutics on different ALS models, perhaps because studies based on mechanistic studies have not proven as successful in therapeutic translation as had been anticipated (see Chapter 9). This reflects the flawed design of clinical trials, issues with patient recruitment and retention in clinical studies, and the lack of fruitful efforts to thoroughly characterize the pathophysiology in ALS. One potential reason for the latter is that the causal factors in disease initiation may be unique to ALS subgroups and lead to common downstream pathogenic features that have been well-described in ALS studies.

ALS AS A "TREATABLE" DISEASE

It may not be surprising that targeting a compensatory mechanism is of little therapeutic benefit to patients. The heterogeneity in disease expression in patients is strongly suggestive of heterogeneity in the underlying pathology, with common cellular responses to stress and dysfunction, although other explanations are possible. A more thorough description of disease mechanisms in different ALS subgroups targeting upstream triggers of dysfunction may lead to a more appropriate clinical trial design, which may then lead to more successful therapeutic outcomes. For this reason, more complete analyses based on describing the timeline of cellular dysfunction are warranted.

Regarding the above, a significant obstacle to the efficacy of disease interventions is the time point of therapeutic application. Currently, the average patient is diagnosed with ALS approximately one year after presenting with signs and symptoms of the disease. A primary reason for this delay is a current lack of reliable biomarkers to diagnose disease; in addition, diagnosis relies on clinical criteria and exclusion criteria of other, more common pathologies such as stroke and post-polio syndrome [47].

Efforts to make ALS a "treatable" disorder are laudable but have not yet been successfully realized. The problems in this endeavor are several-fold and generally widely known. First, therapeutic trials are often based on animal models, such as SOD1 mutations in rodents, which may not be reflective of the heterogeneity of disease expression in humans. Second, as described in Chapter 9, current challenges in clinical design may impede therapeutic approval. A third problem is that considerable damage to motor neurons in the motor cortex and spinal cord has occurred before patients are finally diagnosed with the disease, making a successful application of possible therapeutics of more limited utility. Regarding this last point, the only possible treatment currently available is at late stage of disease. Intervention at this point can at best stop the progressive cascade of pathological events, not reverse it. Clearly, the earlier therapeutic interventions could be applied, the better for the final outcome.

THE IMPORTANCE OF EFFECTIVE BIOMARKERS

All of the above would argue for much earlier detection in humans, ideally prior to a point where significant damage to motor neurons has occurred. Reflecting this paramount need for an effective and reliable biomarker, many groups have pursued different types of cellular and imaging markers for their use in diagnostic and monitoring of disease progression. Saliva [48], proteins [49] and microRNA and extracellular RNA [50] in blood and cerebral spinal fluid (CSF), measures of tongue pathology [51], skin changes [52], and surface electromyography [53] are a short list of recent examples of emerging biomarker studies.

A biomarker can be used for different purposes, and the route of sample collection is important to consider for each purpose. As discussed above, earlier detection of disease is critical for earlier disease intervention. However, since ALS is a rare disease, it would be unrealistic to implement a biomarker collected from CSF as a general disease screen in public health like mammary and prostate exams. A more applicable biomarker to screen for early detection would ideally be based on a more peripheral marker like saliva, blood, or urine, as cited earlier. More invasive and costly biomarkers may have better clinical applications for diagnostics of disease progression.

Biomarkers for ALS would need to be both highly sensitive and reliable. The twin problems of selectivity and sensitivity feature in any discussion of biomarkers for any disease. While some notable efforts have been made toward finding ALS biomarkers [54, 55], it is not clear that any of these are in widespread use at present.

Such problems with the endeavor to find a biomarker will naturally be made more complex by the emerging views on disease heterogeneity, in which biomarkers for one form of ALS may not be the same as for another form, at least at early preclinical stages of the disease. Seeking a universal biomarker for a heterogeneous disease such as ALS may be an idealistic but unrealistic endeavor. A panel of ALS-subtype-specific markers may prove more appropriate for this type of disease spectrum, although pursuing a widespread feature such as TDP-43 pathology may prove well worth investigating.

These are not simple problems to solve, yet doing so will be essential if we ever hope to advance from treating ALS patients post-diagnosis at a stage where the impact of any therapy might be minimal to non-existent. It is for this very reason that a concerted search for biomarkers should become a top priority in ALS research.

FUTURE THERAPEUTIC AVENUES FOR A HETEROGENEOUS DISEASE

The importance of characterizing a clear pathobiology of disease is to target upstream cellular dysfunction or a feature common to both sALS and fALS. This has proven to be a challenging endeavor in ALS; however, clinical trials of a novel therapeutic may be underway. A copper chaperone, (Copper(II)-diacetyl-bis(N(4)-methylthiosemicarbazone) (CuATSM), has been approved for clinical use in positron emission tomography (PET) imaging studies of hypoxia [56]. Recently, CuATSM is being investigated for its therapeutic effect in ALS.

The encouraging therapeutic potential of CuATSM in mSOD1 mouse models garnered considerable momentum, leading clinicians to fast-track human clinical trials on both fALS and sALS [57–59]. While the compound itself generally is not a broadspectrum antioxidant [60], CuATSM restores mSOD1's capacity for reactive oxygen clearance, thereby minimizing oxidative stress [60–66], which is the central theme for it being therapeutic in mSOD1 models. How this translates in sALS remains unclear. However, results from Beckman and colleagues [64] raised the intriguing possibility that the misregulation of copper homeostasis might be a common, ideally early, feature of various neurological diseases.

In support of this, a pilot study was recently conducted in our laboratory to examine whether CuATSM has a therapeutic benefit in a sALS *in vivo* model using exposure to a steryl glucoside toxin [67]. The study by Kuo et al. demonstrated that CuATSM treatment prevented toxin-induced motor deficits and prevented motor neuron degeneration observed in the toxin-treated group [57]. While steryl glucoside toxin-induced motor neuron degeneration in mice displays clinical outcomes and a histological profile consistent with the distinct and progressive features of sALS, the underlying pathological mechanism remains to be clarified. As such, this seems to suggest a potential oxidative stress-induced pathology, or perhaps even a SOD1 dysfunction in the steryl glucoside toxin-induced model of sALS. This view is reflected in a recent study by Paré et al., reporting the presence of misfolded SOD1 pathology in sALS patients [68].

ONGOING CLINICAL TRIALS USING CuATSM

Clinical trials have now completed a multicenter, open-label Phase I trial with oral CuATSM [57]. An extended study was conducted after the proposed timeline in Phase I to further assess CuATSM's safety and therapeutic potential for an additional 24 months [58]. Researchers found that participants showed improved lung and cognitive abilities, while the rate of averaged disease progression slowed [69]. With this data, Phase II clinical trial was approved for late 2019, with a randomized, placebo-controlled design currently recruiting both sALS and fALS patients [59]. The therapeutic potential of CuATSM is indeed promising but again highlights the urgent need for earlier treatment regimes, a need that will ultimately depend on biomarkers for earlier detection of ALS preclinical status, as discussed above.

Excessive reactive oxygen species (ROS) and subsequent oxidative stress is a common pathological feature of many neurodegenerative diseases, including ALS [70, 71]. Oxidative stress has been proposed as a factor that plays a potential role in the pathogenesis of neurodegenerative diseases, and thus indications of increased oxidative stress [72–77] and decreased antioxidant responses [78, 79] are of potential significance as disease biomarkers. Antioxidants have also been examined as potential therapeutics for ALS. Of these, three antioxidants have undergone clinical trials. In large clinical trials, edaravone demonstrated clinical efficacy, while creatine monohydrate and coenzyme Q10 (CoQ10) failed, but not necessarily because they were truly ineffective.

Creatine is an essential nitrogenous organic acid necessary for tissue mass expansion and adenosine triphosphate (ATP) production and recycling [80, 81]. Different groups have speculated that it might have antioxidant properties because its precursor amino acid, arginine, has demonstrated a protective role against oxidative stress [82, 83]. Creatine was subsequently demonstrated to remove superoxide anions, peroxynitrite, hydrogen peroxide, and lipid peroxides *in vitro* [84]. More importantly, in the context of ALS, this molecule was selected for its role in supporting the special energy requirements of different neuronal and glial cell types in the central nervous system (CNS) through proper mitochondrial modulation [85]. Creatine showed neuroprotective effects in the mSOD1^{G93A} mouse model [86], which prompted several clinical trials in the following decade. None of these trials were able to achieve a positive therapeutic effect [87–94].

The therapeutic effects of CoQ10 have been demonstrated in a pre-disease state animal model [95, 96]. CoQ10 is an essential cofactor in the electron transport chain responsible for shuttling electrons between complex II and cytochrome b of complex 3 while potentially boosting mitochondrial function [97, 98]; and it plays a role as an antioxidant in both mitochondria and lipid membranes [99–101], mitigating membrane damage and DNA damage and lipid peroxidation caused by oxidative stress [96, 102]. CoQ10 fed to mSOD1 G93A mice extended mean survival [95], yet the therapeutic translation from mouse models to humans failed in clinical trials [103, 104].

The discrepancy between the positive results seen in pre-disease state models and failures in human clinical trials can perhaps be attributed to the timing of treatment application. The mSOD1 mice were treated with creatine or CoQ10 at age day 50 or 70, respectively [86, 95], which is still within the pre-symptomatic window described to be more likely to produce positive effects than at a later age (100+ days) [105]. Such time points represent the equivalent to of treating ALS patients years before clinical onset. This pre-symptomatic window in animal models is often chosen during drug evaluation for a proof-of-concept purpose [106]. Subsequent evaluation of potential drugs at or post clinical onset in models should be conducted, which would better reflect human patients post diagnosis.

Therapeutic analysis of edaravone, on the other hand, was initiated at the symptom onset of mSOD1 mice and produced positive results including slowed symptom progression and motor neuron degeneration [107]. Edaravone is an intravenous free-radical scavenger that is widely used for treatment of acute cerebral infarction [108]. It has additionally been shown to provide neuroprotective effects against oxidative damages [109, 110]. Building on these findings, the clinical trials [111–114] that followed were successful [115–120], allowing approval for ALS treatment first in Japan in 2015 and then in the US in 2017. This treatment has a marginally positive effect on patient survival and motor function as determined by the ALS Functional Rating Scale Revised (ALSFRS-R) in a subgroup of ALS patients, although considerable adverse effects were observed [121].

A therapeutic approach distinct from those currently available to patients is to apply a personalized medicine approach. The use of induced pluripotent stem cells (iPSCs) for this concept of tailored therapy is gaining traction in the field and current Phase III clinical trials are focused on the therapeutic benefit of stem cells [122]. An exciting future application of iPSCs may be in a personalized medicine approach to model an individual patient's disease profile (see [123] for further review). Organoids may be more appropriate for this use as they allow for modeling cellular interactions [124], which is vital for modeling a non-cell-autonomous disease.

CONCLUSIONS AND THE ROAD FORWARD IN ALS RESEARCH AND TREATMENT

As discussed above, unless and until initial detection of early ALS onset is possible, early disease treatments that are most efficacious in halting disease progression cannot reasonably be expected. For this reason, to make ALS a treatable disease, we are forced to apply therapeutic treatments that were developed in animal models to humans who are at variable, but inevitably late, stages of disease progression.

Perhaps now is the time for the ALS field to step back and consider what is meant when we talk about finding a "cure" for ALS. Do we propose that lost motor neurons can be restored and thus function normally? Instead, if by "cure" we mean that we can find a way to discover biomarkers and early therapeutic applications to make ALS more like polio, then there is more potential for success.

Polio, a virus-induced motor neuron disease, is interesting in this regard. In many cases of polio, the effective response of an individual's immune response to the poliovirus limits the resulting level of motor dysfunction. While there can be latter "post-polio" symptoms, those who do recover from polio have a number of years of life in which the initial deficits do not progress to greater dysfunction [125]. For polio, this is as close to a "cure" as one may expect to achieve. If this same view is taken for ALS and the currently inevitable disease progression could be interrupted, would patients consider this a "cure"?

The current official goal of ALS Canada is to make "ALS a treatable disease." Perhaps this is a more realistic goal, and one that can yet be accomplished once disease heterogeneity and etiology are fully appreciated in disease modeling, therapeutic development, and clinical trial design.

CONFLICT OF INTEREST

The authors declare no potential conflict of interest with respect to research, authorship, and/or publication of this manuscript.

COPYRIGHT AND PERMISSION STATEMENT

To the best of our knowledge, the materials included in this chapter do not violate copyright laws. All original sources have been appropriately acknowledged and/or referenced. Where relevant, appropriate permissions have been obtained from the original copyright holder(s).

REFERENCES

1. Charcot, J.-M. (1874). Amyotrophies spinales deuteropathiques sclérose latérale amyotrophique & Sclérose latérale amyotrophique. *Bureaux du Progrès Médical* 2 (Oeuvres Complétes): 234–266.

2. Rosen, D.R., Siddique, T., Patterson, D. et al. (1993). Mutations in Cu/Zn superoxide dismutase gene are associated with familial amyotrophic lateral sclerosis. *Nature* 362 (6415): 59–62.

3. Reed, D.M. and Brody, J.A. (1975). Amyotrophic lateral sclerosis and parkinsonism-dementia on Guam, 1945–1972. I. Descriptive epidemiology. *American Journal of Epidemiology* 101 (4): 287–301.

4. Saberi, S., Stauffer, J.E., Schulte, D.J., and Ravits, J. (2015). Neuropathology of amyotrophic lateral sclerosis and its variants. *Neurologic clinics* 33 (4): 855–876.

5. Couratier, P., Corcia, P., Lautrette, G. et al. (2017). ALS and frontotemporal dementia belong to a common disease spectrum. *Revue Neurologique* 173 (5): 273–279.

6. Swinnen, B. and Robberecht, W. (2014). The phenotypic variability of amyotrophic lateral sclerosis. *Nature Reviews Neurology* 10 (11): 661–670.

7. Renton, A.E., Chiò, A., and Traynor, B.J. (2014). State of play in amyotrophic lateral sclerosis genetics. *Nature Neuroscience* 17 (1): 17–23.

8. Butti, Z. and Patten, S.A. (2018). RNA dysregulation in amyotrophic lateral sclerosis. *Frontiers in Genetics* 9: 712.

9. Wong, C.O. and Venkatachalam, K. (2019). Motor neurons from ALS patients with mutations in C9ORF72 and SOD1 exhibit distinct transcriptional landscapes. *Human Molecular Genetics* 28 (16): 2799–2810.

10. Tabata, R.C., Wilson, J.M.B., Ly, P. et al. (2008). Chronic exposure to dietary sterol glucosides is neurotoxic to motor neurons and induces an ALS–PDC phenotype. *Neuromolecular Medicine* 10 (1): 24–39.

11. Morsch, M., Radford, R., Lee, A. et al. (2015). in vivo characterization of microglial engulfment of dying neurons in the zebrafish spinal cord. *Frontiers in Cellular Neuroscience* 9: 321.

12. Qian, K., Huang, H., Peterson, A. et al. (2017). Sporadic ALS astrocytes induce neuronal degeneration in vivo. *Stem Cell Reports* 8 (4): 843–855.

13. Xue, Y.C., Ruller, C.M., Fung, G. et al. (2018). Enteroviral infection leads to transactive response DNA-binding Protein 43 pathology in vivo. *The American Journal of Pathology* 188 (12): 2853–2862.

14. Marino, S., Ciurleo, R., Di Lorenzo, G. et al. (2012). Magnetic resonance imaging markers for early diagnosis of Parkinson's disease. *Neural Regeneration Research* 7 (8): 611–619.

15. Salameh, J.S., Brown, R.H. Jr., and Berry, J.D. (2015). Amyotrophic lateral sclerosis: review. *Seminars in Neurology* 35 (4): 469–476.

16. Krach, F., Batra, R., Wheeler, E.C. et al. (2018). Transcriptome-pathology correlation identifies interplay between TDP-43 and the expression of its kinase CK1E in sporadic ALS. *Acta Neuropathologica* 136 (3): 405–423.

17. Dachet, F., Liu, J., Ravits, J., and Song, F. (2019). Predicting disease specific spinal motor neurons and glia in sporadic ALS. *Neurobiology of Disease* 130: 104523.

18. Tyzack, G.E., Luisier, R., Taha, D.M. et al. (2019). Widespread FUS mislocalization is a molecular hallmark of amyotrophic lateral sclerosis. *Brain: A Journal of Neurology* 142 (9): 2572–2580.

19. Pun, S., Santos, A.F., Saxena, S. et al. (2006). Selective vulnerability and pruning of phasic motoneuron axons in motoneuron disease alleviated by CNTF. *Nature Neuroscience* 9 (3): 408–419.

20. Ragagnin, A.M.G., Shadfar, S., Vidal, M. et al. (2019). Motor neuron susceptibility in ALS/FTD. *Frontiers in Neuroscience* 13: 532.

21. Kaur, S.J., McKeown, S.R., and Rashid, S. (2016). Mutant SOD1 mediated pathogenesis of amyotrophic lateral sclerosis. *Gene* 577 (2): 109–118.

22. Weinreich, M., Shepheard, S.R., Verber, N. et al. (2020). Neuropathological characterization of a novel TANK binding kinase (TBK1) gene loss of function mutation associated with amyotrophic lateral sclerosis. *Neuropathology and Applied Neurobiology* 46 (3): 279–291.

23. Powers, S., Kwok, S., Lovejoy, E. et al. (2017). Editor's highlight: embryonic exposure to the environmental neurotoxin BMAA negatively impacts early neuronal development and progression of neurodegeneration in the Sod1-G93R zebrafish model of amyotrophic lateral sclerosis. *Toxicological Sciences: An Official Journal of the Society of Toxicology* 157 (1): 129–140.

24. Wills, A.M., Landers, J.E., Zhang, H. et al. (2008). Paraoxonase 1 (PON1) organophosphate hydrolysis is not reduced in ALS. *Neurology* 70 (12): 929–934.

25. Kamel, F., Umbach, D.M., Lehman, T.A. et al. (2003). Amyotrophic lateral sclerosis, lead, and genetic susceptibility: polymorphisms in the delta-aminolevulinic acid dehydratase and vitamin D receptor genes. *Environmental Health Perspectives* 111 (10): 1335–1339.

26. Li, W., Lee, M.H., Henderson, L. et al. (2015). Human endogenous retrovirus-K contributes to motor neuron disease. *Science Translational Medicine* 7 (307): 307ra153.

27. Celeste, D.B. and Miller, M.S. (2018). Reviewing the evidence for viruses as environmental risk factors for ALS: a new perspective. *Cytokine* 108: 173–178.

28. Ghasemi, M. and Brown, R.H. Jr. (2018). Genetics of amyotrophic lateral sclerosis. *Cold Spring Harbor Perspectives in Medicine* 8 (5).

29. Sheerin, U.M., Schneider, S.A., Carr, L. et al. (2014). ALS2 mutations: juvenile amyotrophic lateral sclerosis and generalized dystonia. *Neurology* 82 (12): 1065–1067.

30. Ma, L., Shi, Y., Chen, Z. et al. (2018). A novel SETX gene mutation associated with juvenile amyotrophic lateral sclerosis. *Brain and Behavior* 8 (9): e01066.

31. Yu, X., Zhao, Z., Shen, H. et al. (2018). Clinical and genetic features of patients with juvenile amyotrophic lateral sclerosis with fused in sarcoma (FUS) mutation. *Medical Science Monitor: International Medical Journal of Experimental and Clinical Research* 24: 8750–8757.

32. Mehta, P.R., Jones, A.R., Opie-Martin, S. et al. (2019). Younger age of onset in familial amyotrophic lateral sclerosis is a result of pathogenic gene variants, rather than ascertainment bias. *Journal of Neurology, Neurosurgery, and Psychiatry* 90 (3): 268–271.

33. Ayers, J.I., Diamond, J., Sari, A. et al. (2016). Distinct conformers of transmissible misfolded SOD1 distinguish human SOD1-FALS from other forms of familial and sporadic ALS. *Acta Neuropathologica* 132 (6): 827–840.

34. Rakhit, R., Robertson, J., Vande Velde, C. et al. (2007). An immunological epitope selective for pathological monomer-misfolded SOD1 in ALS. *Nature Medicine* 13 (6): 754–759.

35. Blair, I.P., Williams, K.L., Warraich, S.T. et al. (2010). FUS mutations in amyotrophic lateral sclerosis: clinical, pathological, neurophysiological and genetic analysis. *Journal of Neurology, Neurosurgery, and Psychiatry* 81 (6): 639–645.

36. Dugger, B.N. and Dickson, D.W. (2017). Pathology of Neurodegenerative diseases. *Cold Spring Harbor Perspectives in Biology* 9 (7): a028035.

37. Xue, Y.C., Ng, C.S., Xiang, P. et al. (2020). Dysregulation of RNA-binding proteins in amyotrophic lateral sclerosis. *Frontiers in Molecular Neuroscience* 13: 78.

38. Chou, C.C., Zhang, Y., Umoh, M.E. et al. (2018). TDP-43 pathology disrupts nuclear pore complexes and nucleocytoplasmic transport in ALS/FTD. *Nature Neuroscience* 21 (2): 228–239.

39. Cartier, N., Lewis, C.A., Zhang, R., and Rossi, F.M. (2014). The role of microglia in human disease: therapeutic tool or target? *Acta Neuropathologica* 128 (3): 363–380.

40. McCombe, P.A., Lee, J.D., Woodruff, T.M., and Henderson, R.D. (2020). The peripheral immune system and amyotrophic lateral sclerosis. *Frontiers in Neurology* 11: 279.

41. Kakaroubas, N., Brennan, S., Keon, M., and Saksena, N.K. (2019). Pathomechanisms of blood-brain barrier disruption in ALS. *Neuroscience Journal* 2019: 2537698.

42. Zhu, S., Stavrovskaya, I.G., Drozda, M. et al. (2002). Minocycline inhibits cytochrome c release and delays progression of amyotrophic lateral sclerosis in mice. *Nature* 417 (6884): 74–78.

43. Gordon, P.H., Moore, D.H., Miller, R.G. et al. (2007). Efficacy of minocycline in patients with amyotrophic lateral sclerosis: a phase III randomised trial. *The Lancet Neurology* 6 (12): 1045–1053.

44. The Methodist Hospital System. (2019). T-regulatory cells in ALS (tregs in ALS). https://clinicaltrials.gov/ct2/show/NCT04055623.

45. MediciNova. (2019). Evaluation of MN-166 (Ibudilast) for 12 months followed by an open-label extension for 6 months in patients with ALS. https://clinicaltrials.gov/ct2/show/NCT04057898.

46. Zhang, Y.G., Wu, S., Yi, J. et al. (2017). Target intestinal microbiota to alleviate disease progression in amyotrophic lateral sclerosis. *Clinical Therapeutics* 39 (2): 322–336.

47. Kiernan, M.C., Vucic, S., Cheah, B.C. et al. (2011). Amyotrophic lateral sclerosis. *Lancet (London, England)* 377 (9769): 942–955.

48. Carlomagno, C., Banfi, P.I., Gualerzi, A. et al. (2020). Human salivary Raman fingerprint as biomarker for the diagnosis of amyotrophic lateral sclerosis. *Scientific Reports* 10 (1): 10175.

49. Oeckl, P., Weydt, P., Thal, D.R. et al. (2020). Proteomics in cerebrospinal fluid and spinal cord suggests UCHL1, MAP 2 and GPNMB as biomarkers and underpins importance of transcriptional pathways in amyotrophic lateral sclerosis. *Acta Neuropathologica* 139 (1): 119–134.

50. Hosaka, T., Yamashita, T., Tamaoka, A., and Kwak, S. (2019). Extracellular RNAs as biomarkers of sporadic amyotrophic lateral sclerosis and other neurodegenerative diseases. *International Journal of Molecular Sciences* 20 (13): 3148.

51. Alix, J.J.P., McDonough, H.E., Sonbas, B. et al. (2020). Multi-dimensional electrical impedance myography of the tongue as a potential biomarker for amyotrophic lateral sclerosis. *Clinical Neurophysiology: Official Journal of the International Federation of Clinical Neurophysiology* 131 (4): 799–808.

52. Yasui, K., Oketa, Y., Higashida, K. et al. (2011). Increased progranulin in the skin of amyotrophic lateral sclerosis: an immunohistochemical study. *Journal of the Neurological Sciences* 309 (1-2): 110–114.

53. Tankisi, H. (2020). Surface electromyography - a diagnostic and monitoring biomarker for amyotrophic lateral sclerosis? *Clinical Neurophysiology: Official Journal of the International Federation of Clinical Neurophysiology* 131 (4): 936–937.

54. Vu, L.T. and Bowser, R. (2017). Fluid-based biomarkers for amyotrophic lateral sclerosis. *Neurotherapeutics: The Journal of the American Society for Experimental Neuro Therapeutics* 14 (1): 119–134.

55. Ryberg, H. and Bowser, R. (2008). Protein biomarkers for amyotrophic lateral sclerosis. *Expert Review of Proteomics* 5 (2): 249–262.

56. Vāvere, A.L. and Lewis, J.S. (2003). Cu-ATSM: a radiopharmaceutical for the PET imaging of hypoxia. *Dalton Transactions (Cambridge, England)* 2007 (43): 4893–4902.

57. Collaborative Medicinal Development Pty Limited. (2016). Phase 1 Dose Escalation and PK Study of Cu(II)ATSM in ALS/MND. Phase 1, Australia, interventional. https://clinicaltrials.gov/ct2/show/NCT02870634.

58. Collaborative Medicinal Development Pty Limited. (2017). ALS Treatment Extension Study. Phase 1, phase 2, Australia, interventional. https://clinicaltrials.gov/ct2/show/NCT03136809.

59. Collaborative Medicinal Development Pty Limited. (2019). CuATSM Compared With Placebo for Treatment of ALS/MND. Phase 2, phase 3, Australia, interventional. https://clinicaltrials.gov/show/NCT04082832.

60. Hung, L.W., Villemagne, V.L., Cheng, L. et al. (2012). The hypoxia imaging agent CuII(atsm) is neuroprotective and improves motor and cognitive functions in multiple animal models of Parkinson's disease. *Journal of Experimental Medicine* 209 (4): 837–854.

61. Soon, C.P., Donnelly, P.S., Turner, B.J. et al. (2011). Diacetylbis(N(4)-methylthiosemi-carbazonato) copper(II) (CuII(atsm)) protects against peroxynitrite-induced nitrosative damage and prolongs survival in amyotrophic lateral sclerosis mouse model. *The Journal of Biological Chemistry* 286 (51): 44035–44044.

62. McAllum, E.J., Lim, N.K., Hickey, J.L. et al. (2013). Therapeutic effects of CuII(atsm) in the SOD1-G37R mouse model of amyotrophic lateral sclerosis. *Amyotrophic Lateral Sclerosis and Frontotemporal Degeneration* 14 (7-8): 586–590.

63. Roberts, B.R., Lim, N.K., McAllum, E.J. et al. (2014). Oral treatment with Cu(II)(atsm) increases mutant SOD1 in vivo but protects motor neurons and improves the phenotype of a transgenic mouse model of amyotrophic lateral sclerosis. *The Journal of Neuroscience: The Official Journal of the Society for Neuroscience* 34 (23): 8021–8031.

64. Williams, J.R., Trias, E., Beilby, P.R. et al. (2016). Copper delivery to the CNS by CuATSM effectively treats motor neuron disease in SOD(G93A) mice co-expressing the Copper-Chaperone-for-SOD. *Neurobiology of Disease* 89: 1–9.

65. Hilton, J.B., Mercer, S.W., Lim, N.K. et al. (2017). Cu(II)(atsm) improves the neurological phenotype and survival of SOD1(G93A) mice and selectively increases enzymatically active SOD1 in the spinal cord. *Scientific Reports* 7: 42292.

66. Vieira, F.G., Hatzipetros, T., Thompson, K. et al. (2017). CuATSM efficacy is independently replicated in a SOD1 mouse model of ALS while unmetallated ATSM therapy fails to reveal benefits. *IBRO Reports* 2: 47–53.

67. Kuo, M.T.H., Beckman, J.S., and Shaw, C.A. (2019). Neuroprotective effect of CuATSM on neurotoxin-induced motor neuron loss in an ALS mouse model. *Neurobiology of Disease* 130: 104495.

68. Paré, B., Lehmann, M., Beaudin, M. et al. (2018). Misfolded SOD1 pathology in sporadic amyotrophic lateral sclerosis. *Scientific Reports* 8 (1): 14223.

69. Rowe, D., Mathers, S., Smith, G. et al. (2018). Theme 9 Clinical trials and trial design. *Amyotrophic Lateral Sclerosis and Frontotemporal Degeneration* 19 (sup1): 264–281.

70. Li, J., Wuliji, O., Li, W. et al. (2013). Oxidative stress and neurodegenerative disorders. *International Journal of Molecular Sciences* 14 (12): 24438–24475.

71. Niedzielska, E., Smaga, I., Gawlik, M. et al. (2016). Oxidative stress in neurodegenerative diseases. *Molecular Neurobiology* 53 (6): 4094–4125.

72. Yavuz, B.B., Yavuz, B., Halil, M. et al. (2008). Serum elevated gamma glutamyltransferase levels may be a marker for oxidative stress in Alzheimer's disease. *International Psychogeriatrics* 20 (4): 815–823.

73. Li, J., Liu, D., Sun, L. et al. (2012). Advanced glycation end products and neurodegenerative diseases: mechanisms and perspective. *Journal of the Neurological Sciences* 317 (1-2): 1–5.

74. Pinchuk, I., Shoval, H., Dotan, Y., and Lichtenberg, D. (2012). Evaluation of antioxidants: scope, limitations and relevance of assays. *Chemistry and Physics of Lipids* 165 (6): 638–647.

75. Ho, E., Karimi Galougahi, K., Liu, C.C. et al. (2013). Biological markers of oxidative stress: applications to cardiovascular research and practice. *Redox Biology* 1: 483–491.

76. Zitka, O., Krizkova, S., Skalickova, S. et al. (2013). Electrochemical study of DNA damaged by oxidation stress. *Combinatorial Chemistry and High Throughput Screening* 16 (2): 130–141.

77. Miller, E., Morel, A., Saso, L., and Saluk, J. (2014). Isoprostanes and neuroprostanes as biomarkers of oxidative stress in neurodegenerative diseases. *Oxidative Medicine and Cellular Longevity* 2014: 572491.

78. Kadiiska, M.B., Basu, S., Brot, N. et al. (2013). Biomarkers of oxidative stress study V: ozone exposure of rats and its effect on lipids, proteins, and DNA in plasma and urine. *Free Radical Biology and Medicine* 61: 408–415.

79. Gomez-Mejiba, S.E., Zhai, Z., Della-Vedova, M.C. et al. (2014). Immuno-spin trapping from biochemistry to medicine: advances, challenges, and pitfalls. Focus on protein-centered radicals. *Biochimica et Biophysica Acta* 1840 (2): 722–729.

80. Brosnan, J.T., da Silva, R.P., and Brosnan, M.E. (2011). The metabolic burden of creatine synthesis. *Amino Acids* 40 (5): 1325–1331.

81. Barcelos, R.P., Stefanello, S.T., Mauriz, J.L. et al. (2016). Creatine and the liver: metabolism and possible interactions. *Mini-Reviews in Medicinal Chemistry* 16 (1): 12–18.

82. Vergnani, L., Hatrik, S., Ricci, F. et al. (2000). Effect of native and oxidized low-density lipoprotein on endothelial nitric oxide and superoxide production: key role of L-arginine availability. *Circulation* 101 (11): 1261–1266.

83. Wu, G. and Meininger, C.J. (2000). Arginine nutrition and cardiovascular function. *Journal of Nutrition* 130 (11): 2626–2629.

84. Lawler, J.M., Barnes, W.S., Wu, G. et al. (2002). Direct antioxidant properties of creatine. *Biochemical and Biophysical Research Communications* 290 (1): 47–52.

85. Hemmer, W. and Wallimann, T. (1993). Functional aspects of creatine kinase in brain. *International Journal of Developmental Neuroscience* 15 (3-5): 249–260.

86. Klivenyi, P., Ferrante, R.J., Matthews, R.T. et al. (1999). Neuroprotective effects of creatine in a transgenic animal model of amyotrophic lateral sclerosis. *Nature Medicine* 5 (3): 347–350.

87. National Center for Research Resources (NCRR). (2000). Clinical trial of creatine in amyotrophic lateral sclerosis (ALS). Phase 2, USA, interventional, updated 24 June 2005. https://clinicaltrials.gov/ct2/show/NCT00005674.

88. National Center for Research Resources (NCRR). (2000). Clinical trial of creatine in amyotrophic lateral sclerosis. Phase 2, USA, interventional, updated 24 June 2005. https://clinicaltrials.gov/ct2/show/NCT00005766.

89. The Avicena Group. (2003). Study of creatine monohydrate in patients with amyotrophic lateral sclerosis. Phase 3, USA, interventional, updated 24 June 2005. https://clinicaltrials.gov/ct2/show/NCT00069186.

90. National Center for Complementary and Integrative Health (NCCIH). (2003). Creatine for the treatment of amyotrophic lateral sclerosis. Phase 2, USA, interventional, updated 4 August 2006. https://clinicaltrials.gov/ct2/show/NCT00070993.

91. Columbia University. (2006). Combination therapy selection trial in amyotrophic lateral sclerosis. Phase 2, USA, interventional, updated 1 February 2011. https://clinicaltrials.gov/ct2/show/NCT00355576.

92. Massachusetts General Hospital. (2011). Safety and efficacy study of creatine and tamoxifen in volunteers with amyotrophic lateral sclerosis (ALS). Phase 2, USA, interventional, updated 4 December 2014. https://clinicaltrials.gov/ct2/show/study/NCT01257581.

93. Groeneveld, G.J., Veldink, J.H., van der Tweel, I. et al. (2003). A randomized sequential trial of creatine in amyotrophic lateral sclerosis. *Annals of Neurology* 53 (4): 437–445.

94. Shefner, J.M., Cudkowicz, M.E., Schoenfeld, D. et al. (2004). A clinical trial of creatine in ALS. *Neurology* 63 (9): 1656–1661.

95. Matthews, R.T., Yang, L., Browne, S. et al. (1998). Coenzyme Q10 administration increases brain mitochondrial concentrations and exerts neuroprotective effects. *Proceedings of the National Academy of Sciences of the United States of America* 95 (15): 8892–8897.

96. Beal, M.F. (2002). Coenzyme Q10 as a possible treatment for neurodegenerative diseases. *Free Radical Research* 36 (4): 455–460.

97. Lenaz, G., Fato, R., Formiggini, G., and Genova, M.L. (2007). The role of Coenzyme Q in mitochondrial electron transport. *Mitochondrion* 7 (Suppl): S8–S33.

98. Crane, F.L. (2001). Biochemical functions of coenzyme Q10. *Journal of the American College of Nutrition* 20 (6): 591–598.

99. Beyer, R.E. (1992). An analysis of the role of coenzyme Q in free radical generation and as an antioxidant. *Biochemistry and Cell Biology* 70 (6): 390–403.

100. Noack, H., Kube, U., and Augustin, W. (1994). Relations between tocopherol depletion and coenzyme Q during lipid peroxidation in rat liver mitochondria. *Free Radical Research* 20 (6): 375–386.

101. Dallner, G. and Sindelar, P.J. (2000). Regulation of ubiquinone metabolism. *Free Radical Biology and Medicine* 29 (3–4): 285–294.

102. Lass, A. and Sohal, R.S. (2000). Effect of coenzyme Q(10) and alpha-tocopherol content of mitochondria on the production of superoxide anion radicals. *FASEB Journal: Official Publication of the Federation of American Societies for Experimental Biology* 14 (1): 87–94.

103. Columbia University. (2005). Clinical trial of high dose CoQ10 in ALS. Phase 2, phase 3, USA, interventional, updated 28 February 2014. https://clinicaltrials.gov/ct2/show/NCT00243932.

104. Kaufmann, P., Thompson, J.L., Levy, G. et al. (2009). Phase II trial of CoQ10 for ALS finds insufficient evidence to justify phase III. *Annals of Neurology* 66 (2): 235–244.

105. Gurney, M.E., Pu, H., Chiu, A.Y. et al. (1994). Motor neuron degeneration in mice that express a human Cu, Zn superoxide dismutase mutation. *Science (New York;, NY)* 264 (5166): 1772–1775.

106. Ludolph, A.C., Bendotti, C., Blaugrund, E. et al. (2007). Guidelines for the preclinical in vivo evaluation of pharmacological active drugs for ALS/MND: report on the 142nd ENMC international workshop. *Amyotrophic Lateral Sclerosis: Official Publication of the World Federation of Neurology Research Group on Motor Neuron Diseases* 8 (4): 217–223.

107. Ito, H., Wate, R., Zhang, J. et al. (2008). Treatment with edaravone, initiated at symptom onset, slows motor decline and decreases SOD1 deposition in ALS mice. *Experimental Neurology* 213 (2): 448–455.

108. Watanabe, T., Yuki, S., Egawa, M., and Nishi, H. (1994). Protective effects of MCI-186 on cerebral ischemia: possible involvement of free radical scavenging and antioxidant actions. *Journal of Pharmacology and Experimental Therapeutics* 268 (3): 1597–1604.

109. Shichinohe, H., Kuroda, S., Yasuda, H. et al. (2004). Neuroprotective effects of the free radical scavenger Edaravone (MCI-186) in mice permanent focal brain ischemia. *Brain Research* 1029 (2): 200–206.

110. Uno, M., Kitazato, K.T., Suzue, A. et al. (2005). Inhibition of brain damage by edaravone, a free radical scavenger, can be monitored by plasma biomarkers that detect oxidative and astrocyte damage in patients with acute cerebral infarction. *Free Radical Biology and Medicine* 39 (8): 1109–1116.

111. Mitsubishi Tanabe Pharma Corporation. (2006). Efficacy and safety study of MCI-186 for treatment of amyotrophic lateral sclerosis (ALS). Phase 3, Japan, interventional, updated 17 May 2017. https://clinicaltrials.gov/ct2/show/NCT00330681.

112. Mitsubishi Tanabe Pharma Corporation. (2007). Expanded controlled study of safety and efficacy of MCI-186 in patients with amyotrophic lateral sclerosis (ALS). Phase 3, Japan, interventional, updated 23 August 2018. https://clinicaltrials.gov/ct2/show/NCT00424463.

113. Mitsubishi Tanabe Pharma Corporation. (2006). Efficacy and safety study of MCI-186 for treatment of amyotrophic lateral sclerosis (ALS) who met severity classification III. Phase 3, Japan, interventional, updated 20 December 2017]. https://clinicaltrials.gov/ct2/show/NCT00415519.

114. Mitsubishi Tanabe Pharma Corporation. (2011). Phase 3 study of MCI-186 for treatment of amyotrophic lateral sclerosis. Phase 3, Japan, interventional, updated 31 December 2018. https://clinicaltrials.gov/ct2/show/NCT01492686.

115. Abe, K., Itoyama, Y., Sobue, G. et al. (2014). Confirmatory double-blind, parallel-group, placebo-controlled study of efficacy and safety of edaravone (MCI-186) in amyotrophic lateral sclerosis patients. *Amyotrophic Lateral Sclerosis and Frontotemporal Degeneration* 15 (7–8): 610–617.

116. Takahashi, F., Takei, K., Tsuda, K., and Palumbo, J. (2017). Post-hoc analysis of MCI186-17, the extension study to MCI186-16, the confirmatory double-blind, parallel-group, placebo-controlled study of edaravone in amyotrophic lateral sclerosis. *Amyotrophic Lateral Sclerosis and Frontotemporal Degeneration* 18 (sup1): 32–39.

117. Takei, K., Takahashi, F., Liu, S. et al. (2017). Post-hoc analysis of randomised, placebo-controlled, double-blind study (MCI186-19) of edaravone (MCI-186) in amyotrophic lateral sclerosis. *Amyotrophic Lateral Sclerosis and Frontotemporal Degeneration* 18 (sup1): 49–54.

118. Writing, G. and Edaravone, A.L.S.S.G. (2017). Safety and efficacy of edaravone in well defined patients with amyotrophic lateral sclerosis: a randomised, double-blind, placebo-controlled trial. *The Lancet Neurology* 16 (7): 505–512.

119. Writing Group On Behalf Of The Edaravone Als 18 Study G (2017). Exploratory double-blind, parallel-group, placebo-controlled study of edaravone (MCI-186) in amyotrophic lateral sclerosis (Japan ALS severity classification: grade 3, requiring assistance for eating, excretion or ambulation). *Amyotrophic Lateral Sclerosis and Frontotemporal Degeneration* 18 (sup1): 40–48.

120. Writing Group On Behalf Of The Edaravone Als 19 Study G (2017). Open-label 24-week extension study of edaravone (MCI-186) in amyotrophic lateral sclerosis. *Amyotrophic Lateral Sclerosis and Frontotemporal Degeneration* 18 (sup1): 55–63.

121. Writing Group; Edaravone (MCI-186) ALS 19 Study Group (2017). Safety and efficacy of edaravone in well defined patients with amyotrophic lateral sclerosis: a randomised, double-blind, placebo-controlled trial. *The Lancet Neurology* 16 (7): 505–512.

122. Brainstorm-Cell Therapeutics. (2017). Safety and efficacy of repeated administrations of NurOwn® in ALS patients. https://clinicaltrials.gov/ct2/show/NCT03280056.

123. Payne, N.L., Sylvain, A., O'Brien, C. et al. (2015). Application of human induced pluripotent stem cells for modeling and treating neurodegenerative diseases. *New Biotechnology* 32 (1): 212–228.

124. Iefremova, V., Manikakis, G., Krefft, O. et al. (2017). An organoid-based model of cortical development identifies non-cell-autonomous defects in Wnt signaling contributing to Miller–Dieker syndrome. *Cell Reports* 19 (1): 50–59.

125. Kidd, D., Williams, A.J., and Howard, R.S. (1996). Poliomyelitis. *Postgraduate Medical Journal* 72 (853): 641–647.

Index

Spectrums of Amyotrophic Lateral Sclerosis: Heterogeneity, Pathogenesis and Therapeutic Directions,
First Edition. Edited by Christopher A. Shaw and Jessica R. Morrice.
© 2021 John Wiley & Sons Ltd. Published 2021 by John Wiley & Sons Ltd.